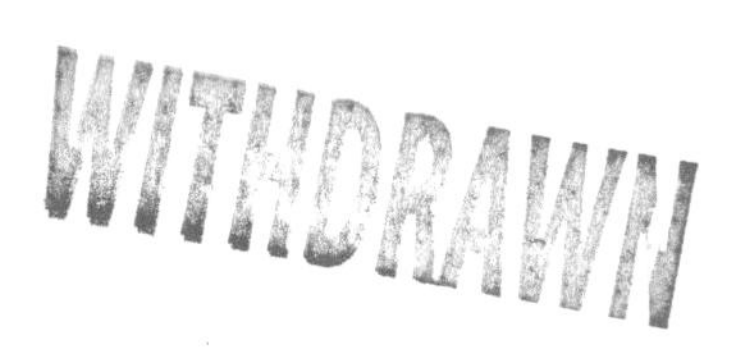

EMERGING INFECTIOUS DISEASES

Trends and Issues

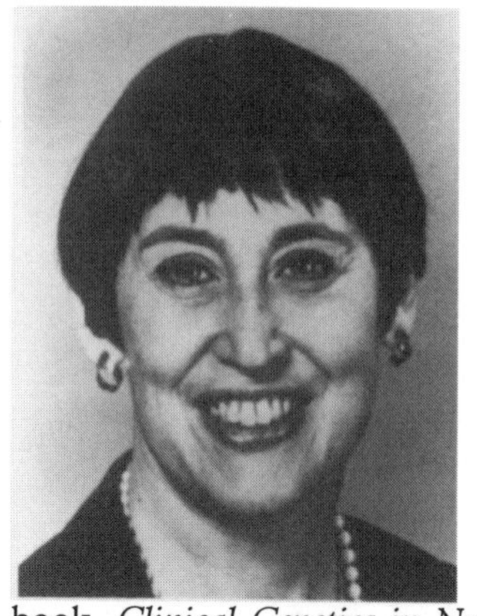

Felissa R. Lashley, (formerly Cohen) RN, PhD, ACRN, FABMG, FACMG, FAAN, is professor and Dean of the School of Nursing, Southern Illinois University Edwardsville. She is also clinical professor of pediatrics at the School of Medicine, Southern Illinois University, Springfield. She is a fellow of the American Academy of Nursing.

Dr. Lashley is certified as a PhD medical geneticist by the American Board of Medical Genetics (the first nurse to be so certified), and a founding fellow of the American College of Medical Genetics.

Dr. Lashley has authored more than 250 publications. The first and second editions of her book, *Clinical Genetics in Nursing Practice*, received Book of the Year Awards from the *American Journal of Nursing*. Two of her other books have received AJN Book of the Year awards: *The Person with AIDS: Nursing Perspectives* (Durham and Cohen, Eds.), and *Women, Children and HIV/AIDS* (Cohen and Durham); *Tuberculosis: A Sourcebook for Nursing Practice* (Cohen and Durham) received a Book of the Year Award from *Nurse Practitioner*. The third edition of *The Person with AIDS: Nursing Perspectives* (Durham and Lashley, editors) was published in 2000. Dr. Lashley was a member of the charter AIDS Research Review Committee, National Institute of Allergy and Infectious Disease, National Institutes of Health (NIH).

Dr. Lashley is an AIDS-certified registered nurse and is immediate past president and a board member of the HIV/AIDS Nursing Certifying Board. She received the 2000 nurse researcher award from the Association of Nurses in Aids Care honoring her research. In 2001, she was given the SAGE award for outstanding mentorship by the Illinois Nurse Leadership Institute. She was a member of the invited interdisciplinary workgroup assembled to advise the National Institute of Nursing Research, NIH, on research opportunities and challenges in emerging infections.

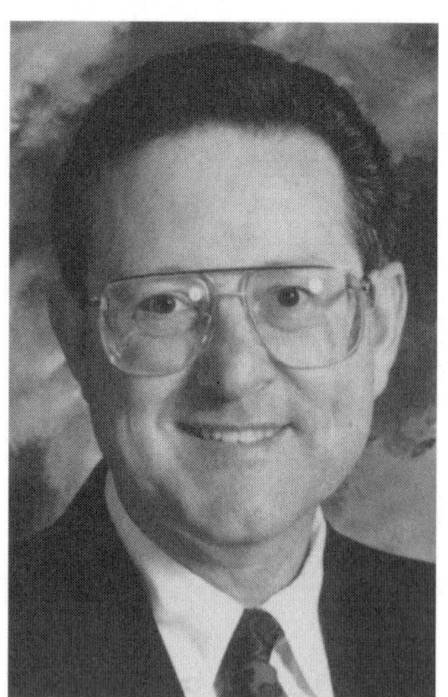

Jerry D. Durham, PhD, RN, FAAN, is Vice Chancellor for Academic Affairs and Professor of Nursing at the University of Missouri—St. Louis. He holds six degrees from four universities, including graduate degrees in medical-surgical (Saint Louis University) and psychiatric mental health nursing (University of Illinois Chicago) and a doctorate in higher education administration (Saint Louis University). He is the coeditor of award-winning books focusing on HIV/AIDS, tuberculosis, and private practice in nursing. He has also served as a reviewer and member of the editorial boards of several nursing journals. Earlier in his career, he worked as a staff nurse, nurse manager, private practitioner, and consultant. He has held faculty and administrative positions in nursing at the University of Illinois Chicago, Illinois Wesleyan University, Indiana University, and the University of Missouri. At the University of Missouri, St. Louis, he previously served as dean of the Barnes College of Nursing.

EMERGING INFECTIOUS DISEASES

Trends and Issues

Felissa R. Lashley, RN, PhD, ACRN, FAAN
Jerry D. Durham, RN, PhD, FAAN, Editors

Springer Publishing Company

Springer Publishing Company, Inc.
536 Broadway
New York, NY 10012-3955

Acquisitions Editor: Ruth Chasek
Production Editor: Pamela Lankas
Cover design by Susan Hauley

02 03 04 05 06/ 5 4 3 2 1

Library of Congress Cataloging-in-Publication Data

Emerging infectious diseases : trends and issues / Felissa R. Lashley, Jerry D. Durham, editors.
p. m.
Includes bibliographical references and index.
ISBN 0-8261-1474-1
1. Communicable diseases. 2. Drug resistance in microorganisms. 3. Epidemiology. I. Lashley, Felissa R., 1941- II. Durham, Jerry D.
RA643.E465 2002
616.9—dc21
2001057684
CIP

Printed in the United States of America by Sheridan Press.

To my wonderful and growing family: Pete, Julie, Benjamin, and Hannah Cohen; Heather Cohen and Chris Ahmann; Neal, Anne, and Jacob Cohen; my mother, Ruth Lashley, and in memory of my father, Jack Lashley. In special memory of my loving deceased friend, Tony Oliver, who gave me a new kind of courage and belief.

—Felissa R. Lashley

To Kathy, whose kindness, love, patience, and support have encouraged me to explore, to dream, and to grow.

—Jerry D. Durham

Contents

Part III Special Considerations

Foreword

As a result of improvements in sanitation and overall living conditions during the early part of the 20th century and the subsequent introduction of many vaccines and antibiotics, infectious-disease mortality declined dramatically in the United States from 1900 through 1980. As a result, considerable complacency developed regarding infectious diseases, which many regarded as either preventable by immunization or treatable by antibiotics. Infectious diseases are the second leading cause of death worldwide and the leading killer of infants and children, however. The World Health Organization (WHO) estimates that approximately 17 million (30%) of the 56 million deaths that occurred worldwide in 1999 were caused by microbial agents. In the United States, infectious diseases are the third leading cause of death and infectious-disease mortality increased during the last 20 years of the century. In addition, over the past 25 years there have been numerous reminders regarding the challenges infectious diseases will continue to pose domestically and globally.

Experiences with emerging and reemerging diseases should have alerted health care workers, microbiologists, researchers, public health officials, policymakers, and the public to the critical importance of ensuring the capacity to detect, respond to, and control these infections. The Institute of Medicine (IOM) published a report entitled *Emerging Infections: Microbial Threats to Health in the United States* in 1992. This report, developed under the leadership of Drs. Joshua Lederberg, Robert Shope, and Stanley Oaks, emphasized the global context of emerging infectious diseases, highlighted the complacency that existed regarding infectious diseases, and identified six important factors in disease emergence and reemergence. These factors included changes in human demographics and behavior; advances in technology and industry; economic development and changes in land use; dramatic increases in the frequency and speed of global travel and commerce; microbial adaptation and change in response to selective pressures; and deterioration in the public health system at the local, state, national, and global levels. The IOM committee made 15 recommendations that stressed the need to improve surveillance and response capacity and identified research and training priorities.

Experience in the United States and around the world since publication of the IOM report reinforces the importance of responding to these recommendations. For example, a number of food-borne outbreaks have been linked to imported foods (e.g., *Cyclospora* gastroenteritis in the United States and Canada associated with raspberries imported from Guatemala). Drug resistance is well recognized as a national and global problem (e.g., the continued emergence and intercountry spread of penicillin resistance in *Streptococcus pneumoniae* and the recent identification of *Staphylococcus aureus* infections caused by strains with partial resistance to vancomycin in Japan, France, and the United States). Human infections caused by an avian strain of influenza in Hong Kong in 1997 provided a reminder of the threat posed by the next influenza pandemic. Outbreaks of Nipah virus infection in Malaysia and Singapore illustrated the challenges posed by zoonotic disease. The emergence of West Nile virus in New York City in 1999 and its subsequent spread through the eastern half of the country emphasized the threats and challenges posed by vector-borne disease.

Each of these outbreaks illustrates the need for health care providers to be aware of emerging diseases in their own and other countries, the critical importance of adequate surveillance and response capacity, the vital role of the modern diagnostic laboratory, and the potential national and global implications of local problems.

The ability to address these emerging and reemerging microbial threats requires adequate surveillance and response capacity, ongoing research programs, effective prevention and control programs, and strengthening of the public health system locally, at the state and national levels, and internationally. The challenges that these diseases will continue to pose require a multidisciplinary approach and a supply of trained health professionals.

The events of September 11, 2001, introduced us to a new era of concern regarding threats to our national security. The subsequent unprecedented bioterrorism attacks involving *Bacillus anthracis* disseminated through the postal system further dramatized the critical importance of preparedness and response capacity at the local, state, and national levels. Health care professionals first recognized the illnesses caused by these outbreaks, reinforcing the importance of heightened vigilance and of familiarity with clinical manifestations of diseases that may result from bioterrorism.

Strengthening partnerships and linkages among the clinical, research, infection control, and public health communities are essential if these challenges are to be confronted. This book should serve as a valuable and timely source of information for members of these communities who need to be involved in preparedness planning and who will strive to monitor, diagnose, treat, and prevent the myriad of potential infectious diseases that patients may experience as we enter the next millennium.

–JAMES M. HUGHES, MD
Assistant Surgeon General
Director, National Center for Infectious Diseases
Centers for Disease Control and Prevention

Preface

Over the past two decades, interest in emerging and reemerging infectious diseases has gained momentum, both within the scientific, public health, and medical communities and in the general public. This interest followed decades of complacency as a result of the antibiotic era, successful vaccination programs, vector control initiatives, and a trust in the ability of medical science to conquer infectious diseases. Indeed, in 1962, Sir MacFarlane Burnet, the famous Nobel-laureate immunologist, wrote in the Preface to his well-known book, *Natural History of Infectious Disease*, that "at times one feels that to write about infectious disease is almost to write of something that has passed into history" (Burnet, 1962, p. 3). Current accelerating interest in emerging infectious diseases among the public, especially in developed nations, is largely a result of concerns about outbreaks that have captured headlines in the world's newspapers including HIV/AIDS, Ebola and other viral hemorrhagic fevers, multidrug-resistant tuberculosis, hantavirus pulmonary syndrome, Lyme disease, West Nile encephalitis in the United States, cryptosporidiosis, *Escherichia coli* O157:H7 infections, cyclosporiasis, transmissible spongiform encephalopathies, and others.

The understanding that science cannot readily triumph over a growing number of infectious diseases has also increased concerns about emerging infections. The 1992 Institute of Medicine report followed by reports from the Centers for Disease Control and Prevention called attention to the increasing emergence of infectious diseases resulting from newly recognized diseases caused by known microorganisms, newly recognized microorganisms causing diseases, diseases and microorganisms found in new geographic areas, microorganisms resistant to antimicrobial agents, microorganisms of animals that have extended their host range to newly infect humans, new reservoirs for microorganisms, microorganisms that have become more virulent, as well as diseases that have markedly increased in incidence. Many reasons exist for the emergence and reemergence of infectious diseases and agents including changes in hosts, microorganisms, and environment resulting from changes in social and cultural behaviors; the relative ease and rapidity of global travel for people and goods; changes in traditional natural boundaries; demand for exotic foods and fast-foods; the effects of civil unrest and wars; deliberate release of biological agents; advances in diagnostic techniques to identify microbes undetectable previously; advances in agricultural practices, deforestation, irrigation, and dam building, which change ecology; weather and climate effects as well as natural disasters; decline in funding of the public health infrastructure in many countries; increasing contact of humans and animals through recreation and living proximity; and advances in medical science changing host immunity, increasing organ transplantation, or increasing use of new devices. Broad efforts to reduce the inappropriate use of antimicrobial therapy in both animals and humans, especially in light of the emergence of microbes that are resistant to treatment (e.g., vancomycin-resistant enterococci), reflect growing concerns.

Also contributing to the growing interest in emerging infectious diseases is a mounting fear that microorganisms hold the potential to serve as an instrument of war among terrorists and rogue nations. In the face of such threats, public health scientists have worked diligently to develop local, regional, and national plans aimed at combating bioterrorism. These plans, which focus on early detection and response to bioterrorism threats, require coordination of the efforts of clinicians, scientists, and law-enforcement personnel. Such efforts are likely to grow appreciably as a result of the September 11, 2001 attacks by terrorists on the World Trade Center and the Pentagon, and the October 2001 occurrence of anthrax cases thought to be either biocrimes or bioterrorism. These instances have jarred public awareness that terrorists are capable of employing weapons of mass destruction, including infectious agents, to achieve their goals. It is no longer unthinkable that terrorists might consider unleashing smallpox, anthrax, botulism, or plague on an unsuspecting population. These realistic concerns about bioterrorism will loom large in the arena of public opinion and public policy in the future.

Both epidemiologists and the general public now understand that, with respect to infectious diseases, we live in a global community in which the health of developed and developing nations is intertwined. In this global community, infectious diseases can spread rapidly around the world, making global surveillance of emerging infections vital to world health. These organisms may migrate from one part of the world to another on wind currents, among migratory fowl, or among travelers. Exotic infectious diseases on distant continents, once seen as posing little threat to the developed world, are now viewed with growing concern among scientists worldwide. Ecological changes and changes wrought by peoples of the world have contributed to the emergence of infectious diseases. These "advances of mankind" include movement of humans and domestic animals into new habitats, deforestation, irrigation, urbanization, and increased air travel. Moreover, public policy and politics, for example, decisions influencing poverty, economic development, population movements, refugees and migrants, and cooperation among governments that can exert enormous influence on the detection, surveillance, and treatment, and prevention of emerging infectious diseases also shape patterns of emerging reemerging infectious diseases. In addition, the decline of public health systems around the world serves to render the world more susceptible to infectious diseases of all kinds.

Over the past two decades, new national and international organizations confront the threat of emerging infectious diseases. Important health organizations with a national or worldview of disease (e.g., the Centers for Disease Control and Prevention and the World Health Organization) have restructured themselves to place greater emphasis on infectious diseases and rapid responses to epidemics, wherever they emerge. Developed nations, recognizing the threat to their economic welfare and social stability, have poured increasing resources into prevention, detection, surveillance, and treatment of emerging infectious diseases and pledged to fight infectious diseases around the world. In the face of mounting criticism, pharmaceutical companies have begun to rethink their pricing policies of drugs that treat infectious diseases in the developing world. Funds to support research aimed at understanding and controlling emerging infectious diseases have increased significantly over the past decade as governments have recognized the importance of this threat.

This book provides readers the knowledge to better understand factors contributing to the emergence and reemergence of infectious diseases and microbial resistance in a wide context. In addition, several chapters focus on specific EIDs of increasing interest to both the scientific community and the general public. These disease-specific chapters examine the epidemiology, microbiology, clinical picture, treatment, and prevention of these diseases. A chapter on bioterrorism explores this topic and potential agents for such use. In the final section, emerging infectious diseases are viewed in broader context, such as their contribution to chronic diseases and cancer, their connection to travel and recreation, the behavioral and cultural influences contributing to the spread of emerging infectious diseases, followed by a look into the future. The future is upon us, and how we prevent and respond to outbreaks of emerging infectious diseases will influence our social, political, and economic status as well as our security for the coming decades.

—FELISSA R. LASHLEY
—JERRY D. DURHAM

REFERENCE

Burnet, F. M. (1962). *Natural history of infectious disease* (3rd. ed.). Cambridge: Cambridge University Press.

Contributors

Victoria L. Anderson, RN, MSN, FNP-C, is nurse practitioner, Laboratory of Host Defenses, National Institute of Allergy and Infectious Diseases, National Institutes of Health, Bethesda, Maryland.

Richard E. Besser, MD, is Acting Chief, Epidemiology Section, Respiratory Diseases Branch, Division of Bacterial and Mycotic Diseases, National Center for Infectious Diseases, Centers for Disease Control and Prevention, Atlanta, Georgia.

Scott Chavers, MPH, is research instructor in the Department of Diagnostic Sciences, School of Dentistry, University of Alabama at Birmingham, Birmingham, Alabama.

James E. Cheek, MD, MPH, is Deputy Director, Division of Community and Environmental Health, Indian Health Service, and Principal Epidemiologist for Infectious Diseases, Epidemiology Program, Indian Health Service, Albuquerque, New Mexico.

Inge B. Corless, RN, PhD, is professor in the graduate program in nursing at the MGH Institute of Health Professions, Boston, Massachusetts.

Victoria Davey, RN, MPH, is Deputy Chief Consultant, Public Health Strategic Health Care Group, Department of Veterans Affairs, Washington, D.C.

Wayne E. Ellis, RN, PhD, CRNA, is assistant professor in the School of Nursing, Southern Illinois University Edwardsville, Edwardsville, Illinois.

Barbara Jeanne Fahey, RN, MPH, is in the Hospital Epidemiology Service, Clinical Center, National Institutes of Health, Bethesda, Maryland.

Hala Fawal, MPH, MBA, is program manager in the Department of Epidemiology and International Health, School of Public Health, University of Alabama at Birmingham, Birmingham, Alabama.

Alicia M. Fry, MD, MPH, is Epidemic Intelligence Officer, Respiratory Diseases Branch, Division of Bacterial and Mycotic Diseases, National Center for Infectious Diseases, Centers for Disease Control and Prevention, Atlanta, Georgia.

Amy V. Groom, MPH, is National Immunization Coordinator, National Epidemiology Program, Indian Health Service, Albuquerque, New Mexico.

Jeanne B. Hewitt, RN, PhD, is associate professor, School of Nursing, University of Wisconsin, Milwaukee, Wisconsin.

Barbara J. Holtzclaw, RN, PhD, FAAN, is professor emeritus, School of Nursing, University of Texas Health Science Center at San Antonio, San Antonio, Texas.

Nancy Khardori, MD, is professor of medicine and Chief, Division of Infectious Diseases, Department of Internal Medicine, Southern Illinois University School of Medicine, and Medical Director, Hospital Infection Control and Epidemiology, Memorial Medical Center, Springfield, Illinois.

Gladys Mabunda, RN, PhD, is assistant professor in the School of Nursing, Southern Illinois University Edwardsville, Edwardsville, Illinois.

Noreen J. Mocsny, RN, MEd, is retired from the Veterans Administration Medical Center, Cincinnati, Ohio where she was a staff nurse in neurology.

Dennis M. Perrotta, PhD, CIC, is State Epidemiologist and Chief, Bureau of Epidemiology, Texas Department of Health, Austin, Texas.

C. J. Peters, MD, was formerly head of the Special Pathogens Branch at the Centers for Disease Control and Prevention and is professor of microbiology and immunology and of pathology at the University of Texas Medical Branch in Galveston, Texas.

Neil W. Schluger, MD, is Chief, Clinical Pulmonary Medicine, and associate professor of medicine and public health, Columbia University College of Physicians and Surgeons, and Columbia University School of Public Health, New York, New York.

Marlene Wellman Schmid, RN, PhD, CIC, is assistant professor, School of Nursing, University of Wisconsin, Milwaukee, Wisconsin.

Laurie J. Singel, RNC, MSN, is instructor, School of Nursing, University of Texas Health Science Center at San Antonio, San Antonio, Texas.

Gerald V. Stokes, PhD, is associate professor, Department of Microbiology and Tropical Medicine, George Washington University School of Medicine and Health Sciences, Washington, D.C.

Roslyn Sykes, RN, PhD, is professor and acting Associate Dean for Special Projects and Partnerships, School of Nursing, Southern Illinois University Edwardsville, Edwardsville, Illinois.

Donna Tartasky, RN, PhD, is a health care consultant in King of Prussia, Pennsylvania.

Sten H. Vermund, MD, PhD, MSc, is professor in the Department of Epidemiology and International Health, University of Alabama at Birmingham, Birmingham, Alabama.

List of Tables and Figures

APPENDICES

Part I

Background

1

An Introduction to Emerging and Reemerging Infectious Diseases

Scott Chavers, Hala Fawal, and Sten H. Vermund

The historic importance of infectious diseases is widely appreciated (Armstrong, Conn, & Pinner, 1999). Surely great strides have been made in the prevention and control of infectious diseases: the eradication of smallpox has inspired the near eradication of poliomyelitis and dracunculiasis (guinea worm); oral rehydration salts have led to the diminution of mortality from infant diarrhea; vaccine-preventable diseases are uncommon in many parts of the world. From these successes, a popular myth emerged among health professionals in industrialized nations, namely, that infectious diseases largely had been conquered and chronic diseases were the principal new frontier for health sciences (Centers for Disease Control and Prevention, 1999). Of course, this was untrue unless one took a highly ethnocentric point of view, ignoring the developing world, and one was naively optimistic that no new pathogens would emerge or reemerge. Yet the last 2 decades of the 20th century provided sobering evidence that microbes are still powerful threats to national and global health and welfare (Armstrong et al., 1999). Tuberculosis and malaria are more prevalent than ever, and infection with the human immunodeficiency virus (HIV) has actually been labeled a national security threat for the United States, so insidious, disruptive, and pervasive is its impact on health indices and the economy in developing nations.

Why are we seeing such a wide assortment of emerging and reemerging infectious diseases? This book seeks to illuminate an answer to this key question. Among the factors that contribute to emerging and reemerging infectious diseases are

- demographic factors including population growth, migration, housing density, and distribution of population within a region;
- social and behavioral changes such as the increased use of child care, liberalized sexual behavior, outdoor recreational pursuits, alcohol and drug use, patterns and styles of the transportation of goods, and widespread business and leisure travel;
- advances in health care technology including modern chemotherapies, styles and institutions of health care delivery, iatrogenic immunosuppression, health care-associated use of antibiotics and antiseptics with consequent selective pressure and development of drug resistance, and invasive catheter techniques that introduce foreign objects either through natural orifices or parenteral routes;
- changes in the treatment and handling of foodstuffs, including mass production of nearly all food products, water processing, and use of adjunct agricultural practices such as antibiotics in animal feed;
- climatologic changes and environmental alterations such as those associated with the El Niño ocean current centered off the coast of Peru, global warming, natural disasters such as volcanic eruptions, deforestation, and land development (including dams, farming, irrigation, mining) with attendant expansion of vector–reservoir–human contacts;
- microbial evolution including natural variation, mutation, and cross-species zoonotic transmission;
- war and/or natural disasters with the consequent breakdown of public health measures—including disease control activities—with or without economic collapse; and
- deliberate release of microorganisms as a component of war or terrorism as with the 2001 outbreak of anthrax in the United States.

Many of these factors will be addressed here, alerting the reader to the relationships between social or behavioral phenomena and the risk of emerging pathogens (Lederberg, Shope, & Oaks, 1992).

Factors that contribute immediately to the emergence of a given agent are often conceptualized as an ecological triangle, framing the emergence of an infectious disease via interactions of (a) the causal agent, (b) the human host, and (c) the social and biological environment, often mediated through an animal reservoir and/or an insect vector. The agents involved in emerging infectious diseases are as diverse as the agents in nature: viruses, bacteria, fungi, protozoa, helminths, and even prions (which are communicable proteins that do not meet conventional definitions of a microorganism but are nonetheless infectious from person to person or from animal to person). Host characteristics include biological and genetic predictors of susceptibility and infectiousness, often mediated by the complex behavioral, social, economic, political, religious, and technological features of a host environment. Environmental influences increase or diminish the degree to which an infectious agent and vulnerable humans come into contact, or the likelihood that humans will become infected with the given agent. For example, higher temperature and humidity are obvious influences on insect vectors of disease and also are associated with wearing loose, light clothing that facilitates insect biting. Environmental pollution that changes vector breeding patterns, natural disasters, water use patterns, human waste and garbage sanitation, and social conditions that influence behavior all are critical contributors to disease incidence. The all-important political response that can temper or exacerbate disease is a variable often overlooked except in extreme times of war or famine (Garfield, Frieden, & Vermund, 1987). It is a misconception that a natural balance between the infectious agent, the host, and the environment results in stability, keeping emerging diseases in check. Rather, recurrent epidemics and plagues, along with high endemic rates of many infectious diseases, are dynamic and evolving contributors to human history even in modern times.

We live in a world of change. As humans, we can alter how we behave with each other and how we interact with the environment. Two dominant themes underscore the risk of emerging pathogens: technological advances and population pressures (see Table 1.1). How we interact socially, sexually, politically, and economically can often be linked to migrant labor and urbanization, which are in turn related to the influences of technology and population growth. Yet diseases

TABLE 1.1 Factors Contributing to Emerging and Reemerging Infectious Diseases

Contributing Factor	Specific Examples of the Contributing Factor	Selected Diseases Related to the Contributing Factor
Demographic factors	Population growth, migration, housing density, population distribution, aging	Dengue, tuberculosis (TB), influenza, HIV, malaria, tropical parasitic diseases such as filariasis and leishmaniasis
Social and behavioral changes	Increased use of child care, liberalized sexual behavior, outdoor recreational pursuits, alcohol and drug use, transportation and distribution of goods, changes in travel frequency	HIV and other sexually transmitted diseases (STDs), hepatitis A-B-C, pelvic inflammatory disease, measles, diphtheria, pertussis, Lyme disease
Advances in health care technology	Modern chemotherapies, styles and institutions of health care delivery, iatrogenic immuno-suppression, health care-associated antibiosis and antisepsis, invasive catheter techniques	Multidrug-resistant tuberculosis, methicillin-resistant *Staphylococcus aureus* (MRSA), vancomycin-resistant enterococci (VRE), opportunistic infections in immunosuppressed persons
Changes in treatment and handling of water/ foodstuffs	Mass production of nearly all food products, water processing, use of adjunct agricultural practices such as antibiotic supplementation of feed	Cryptosporidiosis, guinea worm, schistosomiasis, diarrheal diseases, hookworm, listeriosis, hemolytic uremic syndrome, cyclosporiasis, salmonellosis, Creutzfeldt-Jakob disease, VRE, leptospirosis
Climatologic changes and environmental alterations	El Niño, global warming, natural disasters, deforestation, land use/ development	Tick-borne diseases, highland malaria, hantavirus pulmonary syndrome, plague
Microbial evolution	Natural variation, mutation, cross-species zoonotic transmission	Influenza, HIV, leptospirosis, plague, trichinellosis, African sleeping sickness, antibiotic-resistant bacteria
War and/or natural disasters	Breakdown of public health measures	Vaccine preventable diseases, cholera, STDs, TB
Deliberate release of pathogens	Bioterrorism, biowarfare	Anthrax, smallpox, plague, tularemia botulism, salmonellosis

can also emerge from nature without these mediating influences. A prevalent mammalian hantavirus emerges in humans when a drought drives deer mice into proximity with human dwellings. Ebola virus emerges mysteriously and disappears just as inexplicably. HIV enters human populations through traditional means of hunting and bush-meat preparation, yet becomes pandemic through modern travel, use of dirty medical injection needles, and sexual promiscuity (Vermund, Tabereaux, & Kaslow, 1999). While our environment is manipulated in order to facilitate a higher quality of life, the very act of manipulation can carry new infectious risks. Construction of dams may create new vector and intermediate host environments conducive for malaria, onchocerciasis (river blindness), schistosomiasis, or filariasis. Great advances in technology may diminish many historic infectious risks, yet these same advances create new, sometimes unforeseen problems at the time of implementation. Both drug and insecticide resistance are examples. Infectious diseases are also emerging due to our ability to detect them; some were always present, but hitherto unrecognized because of technical limitations and/or due to low numbers of afflicted persons in previous years. Cryptosporidiosis, cyclosporiasis, Legionnaires' disease, hantavirus, and Lyme disease all emerged without specific diagnostic techniques optimized to detect them. It is notable how quickly diagnostic approaches were developed for these particular emerging pathogens. Yet how many other organisms that might cause diabetes, multiple sclerosis, Alzheimer's disease, certain cancers, cardiovascular disease, or autoimmune diseases remain undiagnosed, owing perhaps to our technological limitations (see chapter 21)?

As many popular books now highlight, changes in the dynamics of human activity within the context of nature, mediated by new technologies, may help explain the emergence and reemergence of infectious diseases. Emerging infectious diseases can be considered in several categories:

1. truly new diseases that emerge in humans from zoonotic environmental sources;
2. newly recognized diseases that may have been prevalent or may have been uncommon, but only now are appreciated;
3. reemerging diseases that represent well-known infections that are now increasing in frequency, often after decades or centuries of declining rates, due to failures in disease control strategies, the emergence of co-infections (like HIV) that facilitate spread-

ing, expansion into geographic areas or populations such as immunosuppressed persons (see chapter 23), and/or as a result of increasing resistance to antimicrobial therapy; and

4. unexplained syndromes whose definitive diagnosis awaits new technical or scientific insights.

These factors do not exist in a vacuum; social, behavioral, and biological origins of the change in the agent-host-environment-vector relationship contribute to the emergence of infectious diseases (see Table 1.1).

DEMOGRAPHIC FACTORS

Population pressures in a world with over 6 billion inhabitants contribute dramatically to infectious diseases. It is estimated that the world's population now grows by 70 million persons each year. In the year 2005, one half of the human race will live in an urban setting and by 2030, 65% of the human race will live in cities (Dantley, 1977; Gelbard, Haub, & Kent, 1999; Lederberg et al., 1992). Population demographics are altered by population growth, migration, and differential mortality. Redistribution of rural populations to urban environments, especially in the developing world, increases crowding and person-to-person contact. In addition, personal behavior is no longer subject to the scrutiny of a tightly knit community with an intact cultural identity.

Overcrowding, poverty, poor hygiene and sanitation, and unsafe water typically accompany urbanization, due to the emergence of shantytowns and other unplanned living quarters. Close quarters may increase tuberculosis and other diseases that exploit increased host susceptibility, especially among the very young, the elderly, or persons who are immunocompromised (Lederberg et al., 1992). The redistribution of migrating populations exposes susceptible individuals to infectious diseases that may be more endemic in their new environment. "Microbial traffic" accompanies the migration of its human host. The influx of new individuals may overwhelm public health infrastructures and disrupt natural reservoirs, by deforestation and other environmental disruptions such as the building of roads and dams, irrigation schemes, agricultural development, and the establishment of housing settlements in order to accommodate the influx of immigrants or refugees from more rural settings (CISET, 1995; Cohen & Larson,

1996; Krause, 1998; Lederberg et al., 1992; Morse, 1993; World Health Organization, 1999).

Urbanization and environmental disruption allow arthropod vector-borne viral infectious diseases to thrive in areas where they have not previously been a risk to humans. An especially important emerging agent is the dengue virus (see chapter 7). Dengue is most often transmitted by the *Aedes aegypti* mosquito, although other species can also transmit virus (e.g., *Ae. albopictus, Ae. polynesiensis*) (Gubler, 1998; Gubler & Clark, 1995). The public health impact of dengue is being increasingly noted in the Americas, corresponding to the deterioration of mosquito control programs that were extensively promulgated in the 1950s and 1960s (Gubler & Clark, 1995; Istúriz, Gubler, & Brea del Castillo, 2000). There are an estimated 50–100 million cases of dengue fever, and 250,000–500,000 cases of dengue hemorrhagic disease worldwide (World Health Organization, 2000). Furthermore, there are large geographic areas of concern such as the southeastern United States, where ecological conditions and endemic mosquito vectors favor future dengue transmission.

The impact of demographic changes can be seen in other infectious diseases. Tuberculosis is a disease of crowding and limited resources (Castro, 1998). Influenza thrives when population density rises and when humans live in proximity to pigs or fowl (Snacken, 1999; Snacken, Kendal, Haaheim, & Wood, 1999). Housing density correlates with risk for a number of other respiratory and vaccine-preventable diseases. Demographic shifts result when an increase in mean life expectancy occurs in a population, resulting in more immunosuppression related to chronic disease or old age, an increasing age of hospitalized patients, and consequent hospital-acquired infections. Economic development may result in migration-related disease or in expanding vector breeding. For example, irrigation programs may result in expanded vector breeding for tropical parasitic and viral diseases that now infect hundreds of millions of people worldwide. Migration can result in persons moving from a zone of high endemicity, introducing infections to other hospitable zones.

SOCIAL CHANGE AND HUMAN BEHAVIOR

Industrialized societies have experienced profound changes in the ways they conduct day-to-day business. Child care is often within a social setting, rather than a family setting, with more social mixing than before. In rural societies, hunting and food gathering, and in industrialized nations, certain occupations or recreation, often result in contact with natural disease vectors (such as ticks or mosquitoes) or infected animals (such as rodents or birds). Plague disproportionately affects Native Americans in the United States due to risk derived from hunting, and preparing small feral animals for food, such as squirrels, that are plague reservoirs. Increased illicit drug and alcohol abuse may result in expansion of previously exotic needle-related diseases or in familiar infections of the "street" lifestyle such as tuberculosis. Transportation of goods and people can itself become a vehicle for spread of infection, as noted with truck drivers and HIV. Immigration, business or leisure travel, and humanitarian missions can all result in appearance of previously distant organisms in local environments.

Changes in modern reproductive technology have led to changes in personal health behaviors, and reproductive choices have helped reduce unwanted pregnancies. Greater personal freedom and social standing for women has accompanied lower pregnancy-related mortality. Current research is assessing what part, if any, these technologies may have played in the spread of infectious diseases. Oral contraceptive pill use may augment the risk of chlamydial and gonococcal cervicitis. These may be associated with increased cervical ectopy that may, in turn, be associated with increased risk of sexually transmitted infections including HIV. Vaginal douching has been linked with increased risk of pelvic inflammatory disease, presumably from disruption of the normal vaginal ecology ideally dominated by hydrogen peroxide-producing lactobacilli. If the oral contraceptive pill and the intrauterine device are used as sole methods of birth control, rather than combined with condom use, then risk of sexually transmitted infections may be increased due to the absence of a barrier to sexually acquired microbes.

The HIV pandemic captures many elements of social and behavioral contributions to infectious disease spread. HIV is more common where men are away from their families for long periods of time. It spreads rapidly when sexual partners or needle-sharing partners are exchanged more freely. Travelers spread HIV worldwide. Ineffective political responses are the norm, facilitating further spread. Poverty and crowding are relevant, but sociocultural norms governing sexual behavior and prevention of sexually transmitted infections are even more important in predicting HIV spread (Vermund, Kristensen, & Bhatta, 2000).

One of the greatest technological advances in the 20th century has been the increase in the speed and volume of international travel. As travel technology has changed, our ability to journey to previously inaccessible areas has increased. In past millennia, the invention of the wheel and domestication of animals for carrying riders and supplies allowed trade caravans and armies to travel into new lands, contacting previously isolated populations. With the advent of sailing vessels came the ability to journey to new continents previously unreachable except by remote land bridges. The invention of the steam engine made it possible to reach destinations much faster and increased the number of individuals who could travel at one time. In the age of flight, we can now circumnavigate the globe in three flight segments taking less than 2 days, compared to over a year in the clipper ship era of prior centuries. In the 1990s, more than 500 million travelers crossed international borders yearly by aircraft alone. Predictions have been made that this number will grow by 10% per annum. In the mid-1990s, between 500,000 and 1,500,000 legal immigrants were admitted to the United States each year, accompanied by many thousand illegal immigrants (Cetron, Keystone, Shlim, & Steffen, 1998). Along with this increase in travel and migration is an efficient pathway for the rapid spread of infectious diseases around the globe. Just as smallpox, measles, and tuberculosis devastated susceptible indigenous populations in the Americas after Columbus, modern travel carries the potential to introduce microbes and their vectors into previously unexposed populations (see chapter 22). Returning soldiers from World War I contributed to the rapidity and magnitude of the Spanish flu pandemic of 1918 and 1919. Without intermediate animal hosts, diseases such as HIV, tuberculosis, chlamydia, influenza, measles, diphtheria, pertussis, and hepatitis A, B, and C have spread throughout the globe entirely through human contact. Each year, over 1,000 cases of malaria are diagnosed in the U.S. from returning travelers or from immigrants. Autochthonous cases from local vector-borne transmission are reported every few years in such locations as Long Island, New York and southern California (Centers for Disease Control and Prevention, 2000) (see chapter 15). Vigilance is needed to avoid the vector breeding conditions that might sustain expanded disease transmission.

MODERN MEDICAL TECHNOLOGIES

Advances in health care technology have clashed with aging populations, especially in those industrialized societies that can afford a higher level of technological care. Cancer, rheumatologic disease, and infectious diseases can be treated, but the therapies themselves may induce immunosuppression and risk from other infectious agents. Inpatient care typically involves catheters, indwelling lines, and other physical facilitators of infectious inoculation. Hospitals and other health care settings often harbor multiresistant organisms that emerge due to the use—often inappropriate—of antibiotics. Intensive care settings may be foci for the most virulent of organisms. Health care-associated exposures to organisms that have been subjected to selective antibiotic pressure and development of resistant bacteria are common sources of serious complications around the world (Tenover & Hughes, 1996).

The dynamics of a hospital setting are more complex than one might imagine. Persons with serious infections may expose visitors and especially hospital staff. Visitors and hospital staff may, in turn, expose patients to infections from outside the hospital. This is particularly hazardous among patients whose immunologic and other host defenses have been impaired by modern medical treatments. Medical treatments that decrease the capacities of the immune system are numerous, including bone marrow or solid organ transplants, chemotherapy, chronic corticosteroid therapy, renal dialysis, and indwelling medical devices. The use of such medical devices and the invasive procedures that incorporate them facilitate the transmission of hospital infections. Devices help circumvent the normal integumentary and mucosal defenses against microbial invasion by allowing normal bacteria as well as hospital pathogens direct entrance into the body.

Health-care-acquired infections afflict millions of persons annually worldwide. Ironically, the sickest patients, those in intensive care units, are at the highest risk of hospital-acquired infections. The Institute of Medicine reports that preventable adverse patient events are responsible for 44,000–98,000 deaths annually at a cost of U.S. $17–$29 billion in the United States alone (Kohn, Corrigan, & Donaldson, 1999). Even such staggering statistics do not prompt full infection control procedure adherence such as handwashing among medical personnel between their contacts with patients (see chapter 25).

The antibiotic era dates from the late 1930s. Since that time, bacteria have emerged that are resistant to all known antibiotics. The multiple drug-resistant *Mycobacterium tuberculosis* that has been associated with the HIV epidemic has generated tuberculosis strains that have proven fatal despite rapid diagnosis and the highest sophistication in therapy (see chapter 16). We stay barely one step ahead of resistant microorganisms in our biomedical research, at increasingly higher costs for drug discovery and antibiotic purchases.

FOODBORNE AND WATERBORNE DISEASES

Urbanization necessitates food production, storage, transport, and distribution. Food production, especially of meats, often involves antibiotic treatment of animal feed designed to improve animal growth or productivity. Such therapies have been associated directly with human disease from antibiotic-resistant bacteria (Holmberg, Osterholm, Senger, & Cohen, 1984; Krause, 1998; Witte, 2000; Witte, Tschape, Klare, & Werner, 2000). Improper storage or transport can introduce or help multiply microorganisms (Keene, 1999). Distribution can introduce agents from food handlers, at proximal or distal arms of the food handling process. Waterborne diseases are more common in tropical and resource-poor nations. Yet deteriorating infrastructures in older industrialized cities can result in surprising outbreaks, as with the lethal Milwaukee, Wisconsin cryptosporidiosis epidemic in 1993, possibly the largest point source waterborne outbreak in recorded history (see chapter 5). Water can result in disease transmission by harboring the organism, by being in short supply such that water washing for human hygiene is not feasible, by being the source of insect vector breeding, or by being the source of organisms that harbor intermediate hosts of infectious agents, as with the invertebrate cyclops for guinea worm or the snail for schistosomiasis (White, Bradley, & White, 1972). Poor sanitation alone can result in disease transmission from diarrheal diseases or hookworm. Hence, food, sanitation, and water, staples of human existence, are all vehicles for infectious agents.

In the early 20th century, changes in food-processing technology greatly reduced the incidence of foodborne diseases in industrialized countries, including sanitation improvements, refrigeration, improved food storage, and governmental regulations and monitoring. The role of the "muckraking" journalists like Upton Sinclair was substantial in raising public awareness of dangers within the food industry. At the same time, these new technologies were integrated with changes in agricultural practices that sowed the seeds for new hazards. Farmers moved away from growing multiple crops for local needs and began growing single cash crops for sale and regional or even international export. The cultivation of fruits and vegetables and animal husbandry moved from small private farms to large industrialized farms where massive amounts of vegetables and animals are subjected to the same environmental agents. These modern methods have increased the efficiency and reduced the cost of food products by centralizing the processing of food products, but this centralization increases the chances of accidental contamination of large volumes of food products all at once. When combined with the global economy of many food manufacturers, the contamination of food at any stage in delivery may result in contaminated food products being distributed across the world (Keene, 1999).

Foodborne illnesses are responsible for an estimated 6–80 million illnesses and 500–9,000 deaths in the United States each year. The huge range in these estimates indicates our ignorance as to the actual burden of such illness, which may be responsible for $5 billion in economic losses yearly in the U.S. In more than half the investigations of foodborne illnesses in the United States, the pathogen is not identified; in fact, most cases of foodborne illnesses are never specifically diagnosed or reported. Although foodborne illnesses often cause diarrhea, *Listeria monocytogenes* can cause abortion in pregnancy or meningitis/sepsis in individuals with reduced immune system responses. *Escherichia coli* strain O157:H7 (see chapter 9) is a leading cause of hemolytic uremic syndrome and kidney failure, typically from eating undercooked, contaminated meat products. Preferences for any raw or lightly cooked foods can also place people at increased risk for foodborne illness. Consumption of raw foods of animal origin, including raw shellfish, unpasteurized milk, and ground beef, or unpasteurized fruit beverages is particularly hazardous.

As consumers have increased their consumption of fresh produce the number of recognized outbreaks associated with produce has increased. Seasonally, greater than 75% of fresh fruits and vegetables are imported and consumed within days of harvest. The surfaces of fruits and vegetables may become contaminated by soil or feces/manure from humans or animals. Cyclosporiasis has been associated with the consumption of raspberries and lettuce imported to the United States (see chapter 6). Use of unclean water supplies can lead to the contamination of produce because water is used to irrigate and wash produce and to make ice used to keep produce cool during trucking. Pathogens identified in fruit and vegetable-associated illnesses in North America in the 1990s included viruses, bacteria, fungi, and parasites such as hepatitis A, *Salmonella* spp, *E. coli* O157:H7, *Shigella flexneri*, and *Cyclospora cayetanensis*.

Food and waterborne outbreaks have the potential to afflict thousands of persons from a single contamination (Cook, Dobbs, Hlady, Wells, Barrett, Puhr, et al., 1998). In 1985, a salmonellosis associated with contaminated milk from a large dairy resulted in approximately 250,000 illnesses (Keene, 1999; van den Bogaard & Stobberingh, 2000). In 1994, a nationwide outbreak of *Salmonella enteritis* occurred when ice cream premix was hauled in tanker trucks that had not been thoroughly sanitized after transporting raw liquid egg leading to an estimated 224,000 cases of salmonellosis. Epidemiologic techniques traced an outbreak of *Salmonella enteritidis* to a single egg-producing farm that housed greater than 400,000 egg-laying hens in five henhouses. Two large multistate outbreaks of enterohemorrhagic E. coli disease have resulted from the consumption of undercooked beef hamburgers served by large fast-food chains. Epidemic investigations have shown that the restaurants' cooking practices were insufficient to kill the bacteria, an observation that has now transformed the fast-food industry's technical approaches and safety precautions.

The use of antibiotics to enhance growth and prevent illnesses in domesticated animals has been implicated in the development of antibiotic resistance and the emergence of new, drug-resistant strains of bacterial disease in humans. Supplementing animal feed with antimicrobial agents to enhance growth has been common practice for more than 30 years and is estimated to constitute more than half the total antimicrobial use worldwide. Accumulating evidence now indicates that the use of the glycopeptide avoparcin as a growth promoter has created in food animals a major reservoir of *Enterococcus faecium* resistant to the standard drug treatment with vancomycin (van den Bogaard & Stobberingh, 2000; Witte, Tschabe, Klare, & Werner, 2000) (see chapter 19).

Animal feed production practices have also been implicated in the development of new pathogens such as prions (Tan, Williams, Khan, Champion, & Nielsen, 1999). Over 170,000 cases of bovine spongiform encephalopathy were confirmed in more than 34,000 herds in Britain through 1999, and extension of the epidemic of "mad cow" disease to Europe's mainland occurred in 2000. Supplementation of the diets of calves and dairy cattle with meat and bone meal produced by commercial rendering plants may have been the source of the disease, probably because of contamination with infected neural tissue; cows fed diets containing material from scrapie-infected sheep may have initiated the outbreak. After the disease had been transmitted to cows, it was spread further by the addition of material from infected cows to cattle feed. The onset of the epidemic followed changes in the rendering process started in the 1970s, including the use of continuous heating instead of batch heating and the inclusion of more tallow in the bone meal; both changes were likely to increase the likelihood of infection. The variant human disease, Creutzfeldt-Jakob, is an incurable and devastating neurological condition now on the rise in Europe (Brown, Will, Bradley, Asher, & Detwiler, 2001) (see chapter 17).

Agricultural development can lead to infection independent of the food supply per se. Hantavirus causes more than 100,000 infections a year in China. The virus is an infection of a field mouse, *Apodemus agarius*, that flourishes in rice fields. People usually contract the disease during the rice harvest through contact with infected rodents. Leptospirosis can be acquired the same way and has even been reported among participants in an international sporting event in Indonesia that involved swimming across a river.

CLIMATE AND ECOLOGICAL CHANGES

Climatologic changes typically happen so slowly that they evade intervention by politicians who are reelected based on 2–4 year achievements and whose scope of vision may not extend much beyond the limited, short-term economic interests of their homelands. Global warming, a consequence of high energy utilization in resource-ample countries combined with deforestation and environmental degradation in resource-poor nations, is contributing to higher disease rates from such conditions as malaria and arboviruses whose insect vectors are nurtured in such a warming climate (Haines, McMichael, Kovats, & Saunders, 1998; McMichael, Patz, & Kovats, 1998). Environmental alterations such as land development can expand water for insect or snail breeding with dams or irrigation. While farming can be nurtured in environmentally benign ways, slash and burn technologies are often practiced, bringing humans into direct contact with remote jungle organisms. Natural phenomena like the El Niño ocean current off the Peruvian coast, volcanic eruptions, and earthquakes often result in disease-related alterations of the environment and the human condition. Expansion of vector–reservoir–human contacts are the most critical elements of the climatologic threat to human health.

Climate has affected the timing and intensity of
throughout history. Yet modern technologies, pa
volume burning of fossil fuels like gas, oil, and coal
ble for changes of historic proportions in the
average global temperature has increased by 0.6°
revolution; 9 of the 11 hottest years of the 20th century occu
1985. Scientists from the Intergovernmental Panel on Climate Change forecast a 1° C to 3.5° C increase in average global temperature by 2100. Such temperature increases expand the niche for insect vectors that depend on higher temperature and humidity for their breeding and sustenance. Sweden has experienced a northern expansion in the distribution of tick vectors probably due to increasing temperatures in the north. During the 1980s and 1990s there has been a resurgence of highland malaria in Latin America, central and east Africa, and Asia, corresponding to warming and to increases in insect populations. Global warming is implicated in these disease shifts. A widespread and accelerating retreat of tropical summit glaciers, the growth of plants at higher altitudes, a diminution of the freezing zone by 150 meters, and the acceleration of global warming since 1970 all bode ill for further climate change that will facilitate disease expansion.

MICROBIAL EVOLUTION

Inherent in the microbial world is the natural variation and mutation of organisms. Influenza mutates within its porcine or avian primary hosts and quickly spreads to humans with new pandemic viral types each and every year. Cross-species zoonotic transmission can happen precipitously with cataclysmic consequences, as with HIV in the 20th century (Gao, Bailes, Robertson, Chen, Rodenburg, Michael, et al., 1999). Alternatively, it can occur periodically and routinely as with influenza and with many zoonoses (e.g., leptospirosis, plague, and trichinellosis) that afflict persons in endemic locales. Some organisms such as trypanosomes, the parasitic cause of African sleeping sickness, continually reinvent their surface antigen profiles in order to evade the host immune responses. In 2000, poliomyelitis reemerged in both the Dominican Republic and Haiti after vaccine coverage rates dropped. This occurred nearly a decade after the Americas were declared polio-free, a dramatic event that presaged hoped-for global eradication in the early 21st century. The Hispaniola outbreak may

...e resulted from circulating mutant vaccine-strain poliovirus in a ...onimmune population; there is no substitute for vigilance and persistence in eradication efforts.

Pandemic influenza and other zoonotic diseases have agricultural origins so intimate with human society as to defy intervention. In China, farmers raise pigs and ducks together. Because population density is high and land is scarce, it is common for fowl, pigs, and humans to live in close proximity. Waterfowl are a major reservoir of influenza viruses; pigs can serve as recombinant mixing vessels for new mammalian influenza strains. Integrated pig–duck agriculture puts these two species in contact with each other and with man, enabling efficient reproduction of recombinant mutant viruses and transfer to humankind.

The inherent variability and adaptability of microorganisms guarantee that they will never be eliminated as sources of human disease. Our public health strategy must be one of control and containment. Furthermore, we must not be lulled into the false promises of elimination of infectious diseases as important contributors to human disease; the inherent variability of these organisms alone guarantees future emerging and reemerging infectious diseases.

WAR AND NATURAL DISASTERS

Humankind has learned much about the control of infectious diseases. Soap, water, personal hygiene, clean drinking and cooking water, safe fecal disposal, uncrowded housing, basic medical care, and rodent control (see Appendix C, Table C.6) can all prevent infection and disease. Such basic sanitation is taken for granted in many parts of the world. Yet in areas of chronic poverty and war, or in conditions of natural disaster, all these may fail with tragic results. The breakdown of public health measures, including disease control activities, can occur even in relatively prosperous countries in conditions of war or disaster. In poorer nations, war, civil strife, or natural disaster is often accompanied with economic collapse, famine, and homelessness; the decline in public health control measures is exacerbated by the general economic decline. Few conditions are more conducive to infectious disease spread or emergence of novel pathogens than wars or disasters. Makeshift refugee camps that are associated with attendant miseries consequent to privation and violence, rape, sexually transmitted diseases, burn injuries, vaccine-preventable diseases, and water/sanitation/rodent-related diseases are all too common.

Even in conditions of improving government services to control infectious diseases, war can undermine control strategies when health care workers, representing the government, are targeted by rebel forces. The breakdown in public health control measures was responsible for malaria expansions in Nicaraguan war zones after the U.S.-sponsored "contra" rebels began attacking government health workers and clinics (Garfield et al., 1987). This is especially tragic in settings where progress is being made in public health, but is interrupted or reversed by the civil unrest. Countries with war- or strife-related public health crises in 2000 and 2001 included Afghanistan, Bosnia and Herzegovina, Central African Republic, Chechnya, Congo Democratic Republic, Gaza, Haiti, Indonesia, Iran, Iraq, Kosovo, Kyrgyz Repulic, Liberia, Macedonia, Pakistan, Sierra Leone, Solomon Islands, Somalia, Sudan, Tajikistan, and Yemen.

DELIBERATE RELEASE OF ORGANISMS

As we enter the 21st century, a long-anticipated deliberate use of infectious agents as biological weapons has been seen in the United States with the intentional spread of anthrax via the postal system (Centers for Disease Control and Prevention, 2001). The use of biological agents as weapons is a significant threat to the general public's physical, social, and psychological well-being. The 1984 inoculation of salad bars with *Salmonella typhimurium* in an area of Oregon (described in chapter 24) was seen as more of an oddity than a true threat to the public health (Török, Tauxe, Wise, Livengood, Sokolow, Mauvais, et al., 1997). Both outbreaks resulted in considerable mental health, economic, and societal burdens—salmonellosis on a local scale, anthrax on an international scale. The most recent episode and additional fears have galvanized the United States and world communities to address these concerns with initiatives as diverse as vaccinia vaccine production for smallpox to education of health care workers for disease recognition. The reality of biological weapons has resulted in a renewed emphasis on the importance of our prevention infrastructure; coping with biological agents depends on the integrity of the public health system (World Health Organization, 2001).

SUMMARY

Technologies can expand infectious diseases. Technologies can also help control infectious diseases. Some interventions are daunting in their complexity, such as how to slow global warming by reducing energy consumption; however, many nations with high fossil fuel energy consumption are unmotivated to change their comparatively luxurious lifestyles. Other interventions, feasible in a shorter time frame, include increased coverage with vaccinations, oral rehydration fluids, and HIV prevention strategies. Some interventions are of intermediate complexity, such as the provision of clean water and sanitation, the reform of food processing, improved antibiotic practices in hospital settings, and expanded primary healthcare with essential drugs. Health professionals, engineers, politicians, and others must work together to find solutions (Cohen & Larson, 1996). This book seeks to articulate both the problems we face and the solutions we must exploit to address the challenge of emerging and reemerging diseases.

REFERENCES

Armstrong, G. L., Conn, L. A., & Pinner, R. W. (1999). Trends in infectious disease mortality in the United States during the 20th century. *Journal of the American Medical Association, 281*, 61–66.

Brown, P., Will, R. G., Bradley, R., Asher, D. M., & Detwiler, L. (2001). Bovine spongiform encephalopathy and variant Creutzfeldt-Jakob disease: Background, evolution, and current concerns. *Emerging Infectious Diseases, 7*, 6–16.

Castro, K. G. (1998). Global tuberculosis challenges. *Emerging Infectious Diseases, 4*, 408–409.

Centers for Disease Control and Prevention. (1999). Achievements in public health, 1900–1999: Control of infectious diseases. *Morbidity and Mortality Weekly Report, 48*, 621–629.

Centers for Disease Control and Prevention. (2000). Probable locally acquired mosquito-transmitted *Plasmodium vivax* infection—Suffolk County, New York, 1999. *Morbidity and Mortality Weekly Report, 49*, 495–498.

Centers for Disease Control and Prevention. (2001). Update: Investigation of bioterrorism-related anthrax—November 16, 2001. *Morbidity and Mortality Weekly Report, 50*, 1008–1010.

Cetron, M., Keystone, J., Shlim, D., & Steffen, R. (1998). Travelers' health. *Emerging Infectious Diseases, 4*, 405–407.

Cohen, F., & Larson, E. (1996). Emerging infectious diseases: Nursing responses. *Nursing Outlook, 44*, 164–168.

Committee on International Science, Engineering and Technology. (1995). *Report of the National Science and Technology Council Committee on International Science, Engineering and Technology Working Group on emerging and re-emerging infectious diseases.* Washington, DC: National Science and Technology Council.

Cook, K. A., Dobbs, T. E., Hlady, W. G., Wells, J. G., Barrett, T. J., Puhr, N. D., et al. (1998). Outbreak of *Salmonella* serotype Hartford infections associated with unpasteurized orange juice. *Journal of the American Medical Association, 280,* 1504–1509.

Dantley, R. A. (1997). *Urban problems: Perspectives and solutions.* Chicago: Rand McNally.

Gao, F., Bailes, E., Robertson, D. L., Chen, Y., Rodenburg, C. M., Michael, S. F., et al. (1999). Origin of HIV-1 in the chimpanzee *Pan troglodytes troglodytes. Nature, 397*(6718), 385–386.

Garfield, R. M., Frieden, T., & Vermund, S. H. (1987). Health related outcomes of war in Nicaragua. *American Journal of Public Health, 77,* 615–618.

Gelbard, A., Haub, C., & Kent, M. M. (1999). World population and beyond six billion. *Population Reference Bureau, Inc.* [On-line], *54*(1). Available: www.prb.org/pubs/population_bulletin/bu54-1/54_1_intro.htm

Gubler, D. J. (1998). Resurgent vector-borne diseases as a global health problem. *Emerging Infectious Diseases, 4,* 442–450.

Gubler, D., & Clark, G. G. (1995). Dengue/dengue hemorrhagic fever: The emergence of a global health problem. *Emerging Infectious Diseases, 1,* 55–57.

Haines, A., McMichael, A. J., Kovats, S., & Saunders, M. (1998). Majority view of climate scientists is that global warming is indeed happening. *British Medical Journal, 316,* 1530.

Holmberg, S. D., Osterholm, M. T., Senger, K. A., & Cohen, M. L. (1984). Drug-resistant *Salmonella* from animals fed antimicrobials. *New England Journal of Medicine, 311,* 617–622.

Istúriz, R. W., Gubler, D. J., & Brea del Castillo, J. B. (2000). Dengue and dengue hemorrhagic fever in Latin America and the Caribbean. *Infectious Disease Clinics of North America, 14,* 121–140.

Keene, W. E. (1999). Lessons from investigations of foodborne disease outbreaks. *Journal of the American Medical Association, 281,* 1845–1847.

Kohn, L., Corrigan, J., & Donaldson, M. (1999). *To err is human: Building a safer health system.* Washington, DC: Institute of Medicine, National Academy Press.

Krause, R. M. (1998). Emerging infections. In R. M. Krause (Ed.), *Emerging infections* (pp. 6–7). San Diego: Academic Press.

Lederberg, J., Shope, R. E., & Oaks, Jr., S. C. (1992). *Emerging infections: Microbial threats to health in the United States.* Washington, DC: Institute of Medicine, National Academy Press.

McMichael, A. J., Patz, J., & Kovats, R. S. (1998). Impacts of global environmental change on future health and health care in tropical countries. *British Medical Bulletin, 54,* 475–488.

Morse, S. S. (1993). Examining the origins of emerging virus. In S. S. Morse (Ed.), *Emerging viruses* (pp. 10–28). New York: Oxford University Press.

Snacken, R. (1999). Control of influenza. Public health policies. *Vaccine, 17(Suppl. 3)*, S61–S63.

Snacken, R., Kendal, A. P., Haaheim, L. R., & Wood, J. M. (1999). The next influenza pandemic: Lessons from Hong Kong. *Emerging Infectious Diseases*, *5*, 195–203.

Tan, L., Williams, M. A., Khan, M. K., Champion, H. C., & Nielsen, N. H. (1999). Risk of transmission of bovine spongiform encephalopathy to humans in the United States: Report of the Council on Scientific Affairs. American Medical Association. *Journal of the American Medical Association*, *281*, 2330–2339.

Tenover, F. C., & Hughes, J. M. (1996). The challenges of emerging infectious diseases. Development and spread of multiply-resistant bacterial pathogens. *Journal of the American Medical Association*, *275*, 300–304.

Török, T. J., Tauxe, R. V., Wise, R. P., Livengood, J. R., Sokolow, R., Mauvais, S., et al. (1997). A large community outbreak of salmonellosis caused by intentional contamination of restaurant salad bars. *Journal of the American Medical Association*, *278*, 389–398.

van den Bogaard, A. E., & Stobberingh, E. E. (2000). Epidemiology of resistance to antibiotics. Links between animals and humans. *International Journal of Antimicrobial Agents*, *14*, 327–335.

Vermund, S. H., Kristensen, S., & Bhatta, M. P. (2000). HIV as an STD. In K. H. Mayer & H. F. Pizer (Eds.), *The emergence of AIDS: The impact on immunology, microbiology and public health* (pp. 121–128). Washington, DC: American Public Health Association.

Vermund, S. H., Tabereaux, P. B., & Kaslow, R. A. (1999). Epidemiology of HIV infection. In T. Merigan, D. Bolognesi, & J. Bartlett (Eds.), *Textbook of AIDS medicine* (2nd ed., pp. 101–109). Baltimore: Williams & Wilkins.

White, G. F., Bradley, D. J., & White, A. U. (1972). *Drawers of water: Domestic water use in East Africa*. Chicago: University of Chicago Press.

Witte, W. (2000). Ecological impact of antibiotic use in animals on different complex microflora: Environment. *International Journal of Antimicrobial Agents*, *14*, 321–325.

Witte, W., Tschape, H., Klare, I., & Werner, G. (2000). Antibiotics in animal feed. *Acta Veterinaria Scandinavica Supplement*, *93*, 37–44.

World Health Organization. (1999). *Removing obstacles to healthy development*. Geneva: WHO.

World Health Organization. (2000). Dengue/dengue haemorrhagic fever. Situation in 2000. *Weekly Epidemiological Record*, *75*(24), 193–196.

World Health Organization. (2001). Public health response to biological and chemical weapons. WHO guidance. Projected second edition of *Health aspects of chemical and biological weapons: Report of a WHO group of consultants*, Geneva: WHO (1970). Prepublication issue for restricted distribution.

2

Microbial Resistance to Antibiotics

Gerald V. Stokes

The alarming headlines have become all too common: "*Staphylococcus aureus* with reduced susceptibility to vancomycin . . . (invades) . . . Illinois, 1999" (Centers for Disease Control and Prevention, 2000)—another "superbug" that traditional antibiotics cannot cure has been isolated from unsuspecting patients. A total of four individuals died in this particular instance, but the implications are more far-reaching. During the previous year no other cases had been reported in that region of the country. In the coming years, however, this newly feared superbug strain—resistant to all available antibiotics—may emerge. Health care providers throughout the United States have watched similar scenarios play out in other parts of the world, as bacteria have gained resistance to conventional antibiotics faster than new therapies can be introduced onto the market. But why is the news of vancomycin resistance so dreaded (see also chapter 19)? The answer is simple and best illustrated with the following whimsical example:

> Imagine yourself fighting off a hoard of mean-spirited space aliens, bent on total destruction of the world and all human life-forms. Now imagine the earthlings having a secret weapon, used only for protection against space-alien invasions. Just as the bloodthirsty aliens approach, you, with your back to the wall, confidently reach in your pocket, remove your secret weapon, aim the device at the approaching beasts, and fire. But instead of dying, the critters blink in amazement and continue undisturbed, baring

their fangs, as you stand there totally defenseless. Score: Aliens 1, Humans 0. *Staphylococcus aureus* has survived our secret weapon called vancomycin and now nothing can protect us from the consequences.

Bacteria with acquired antibiotic-resistance properties pose a significant threat to human health and well-being. Vancomycin has truly been our last line of defense (i.e., our "secret weapon") against the "alien" pathogenic strains of *S. aureus* and *Enterococcus* spp. Other highly valued antibiotics have protected us against other pathogens, which, over the course of time, have also developed resistance. In the absence of effective vaccination or containment strategies, the use of effective antibiotics has been our most reliable and effective means of combating the spread of microbial pathogens within susceptible populations. Our casual overconfidence in, and overprescription of, these "magic bullets" have contributed to limitations in their effectiveness.

How did this situation evolve? What practices accelerated the evolution of antibiotic resistance in pathogens? What can we do to buy time and hopefully devise new effective treatments to halt the spread of resistant strains? In discussing these questions, emphasis will be placed on antibiotic resistance in bacteria that cause infections and disease in natural (community-acquired) or hospital (nosocomial) situations.

ANTIBIOTIC RESISTANCE IS AN INEVITABLE EVOLUTION

Antibiotics are naturally occurring compounds that either kill (bactericidal) or restrict (bacteriostatic) the growth of bacteria and other microbials. The active compounds, once identified, isolated, tested, and modified, have served effectively for use against human and animal infections. Other applications have evolved, however, that undermine the effectiveness of these compounds. The prototype antibiotic is penicillin and its many variants. Penicillin is a product produced by the mold *Penicillium chrysogenum*. Glycopeptides, like vancomycin, are produced by bacterial microbes such as *Streptomyces toyocaensis* or *Amycolatopis orientalis*. There are various naturally occurring sources of antibiotics. Multiple gene loci are involved in the synthesis of each antibiotic. Marshall, Lessard, Park, and Wright (1998) suggest genes isolated from the latter organisms may, in fact, have been the naturally occurring source from which other microbes (e.g., *Enterococcus* spp) acquired resistance. Chemical modifications of the naturally occurring compounds have been developed to produce new compounds that display beneficial attributes that enhanced their usefulness (i.e., greater stability, broader spectrum, less toxicity, and greater solubility). Penicillin has been extensively altered to yield compounds that have extended the usefulness of the beta lactam ring-based antibiotics. Many of the modifications were achieved by the additions of new radicals to the basic ring structures. Examples of extended-spectrum penicillins include ampicillin, amoxicillin, carbenicillin, peperacillin, and mezlocillin. Dicloxacillin, cloxacillin, methicillin, nafcillin, and oxacillin are examples of penicillinase-resistant penicillins. Useful antibiotics are selectively toxic against certain bacterial species or groups while displaying little or no significant adverse effects on host cells, tissues, and organ systems. Other compounds have similar effects on other microbials such as yeasts, molds, fungi, parasites, and viruses. The goal of chemical modifications of these naturally occurring compounds is to make them more stable, more effective, but less toxic for use in the treatment of infections or applications in agriculture. Knowledge of the molecular structure and advanced organic chemistry has made this task feasible. New analogues are synthesized and then tested for their relative effectiveness and chemical properties. The pharmacology of antibiotics varies with each new modification; however, in general, the antimicrobial effect is targeted to a unique function or structure found on bacterial (prokaryotic) cells that distinguishes them from host (eukaryotic) cells. This targeting is by design and represents the desired properties of an effective antibiotic, that is, one that selectively impedes the microbes without causing undue harm to host (animal) tissues and organs. There are many compounds that display antibacterial properties but that are unduly toxic or unstable and, therefore, ineffective as useful therapeutic agents for the general public.

The search for new and alternative sources of antibiotics has been redirected toward plant extracts. Solvent extracts of many traditional plants and herbs display antibacterial activities of varying spectra. Mahasneh and El-Oqlah (1999) demonstrated antibacterial properties of common herbal medicines used daily in middle eastern countries. Commonly used dietary supplements such as garlic (Yoshida, Iwata, Katsuzaki, Naganawa, Ishikawa, Fukuda, et al., 1998) and St. John's wort (Schempp, Pelz, Wittmer, Schopf, & Simon, 1999) show antibacterial properties against a broad range of gram-positive and gram-negative microbes. Whether the active agents from different herbs merit general applications as antibiotics would require extensive basic and clinical research.

SELECTIVE ADVANTAGES OF RESISTANCE

Genes, which encode antibiotic resistance in bacteria, may reside on the bacterial chromosome or on self-replicating extrachromosomal genetic material, namely, plasmids or transposons (Briggs & Fratamico, 1999). The most important bacterial pathogens appear to possess relatively few genetic markers of significance because, by definition, we limit ourselves to those that affect specific individual or multiple drugs. The frequency of mutational changes within the chromosome of bacteria occurs within the range of 10^{-7} to 10^{-9}. Many of the changes have little or no significant effect on antibiotic resistance. A change that confers antibiotic resistance may provide additional survival to the bacteria—enabling it to grow in a previously restricted environment in the absence of other bacteria that would compete for limited nutrients. The sheer randomness of the mutational processes almost guarantees that eventually every conceivable environmental condition will become favorable to the survival of the mutated bacteria. Resistance to the presence of antibiotics is not different from other nonmedical conditions in which bacteria have mastered extremely hostile environments (e.g., deep-sea volcanic vents, hot spring geysers, salt lakes, and arctic glaciers). An example of the randomness in natural mutations is illustrated by the fact that antibiotic-resistant bacteria have been recovered from soil and humans on the Solomon Islands even prior to the introduction of antibiotics to the island population (Gardner, Smith, & Beer, 1968). A new genetic trait, once established, may spread simply by transfer from one generation of microbe to the next, or literally jump from one organism to the next on a plasmid or transposon. Conjugation, genetic transfer via an interlinking sex pilus between donor and recipient, is the primary means of information exchange. Conjugation is the directed transfer of genetic material between two bacteria, via a minute tube structure. One bacterium performs the transfer and is called the donor; the other bacterium receives the donor's genetic information. The source of genetic material transferred between the bacteria can be of chromosomal, plasmid, or other mobile element origin (Carattoli, Villa, Pezzella, Bordi, &

Visca, 2001). The process occurs most often within bacteria of the same species, however cross-species conjugation is highly probable. This mechanism poses the greater threat since wherever microbes from various species interact, as in the case of animal and human microbes, opportunities for zoonotic (animal to human) transfer to occur are present. Genetic material encoded on transposons may be exchanged between gram-positive and gram-negative bacteria as well as between those of similar Gram staining attributes. It has been proposed that part of the human complement of about 30,000 genes were acquired from bacteria (Claverie, 2001).

ANTIBIOTICS ACT ON UNIQUE BACTERIA SITES

Unique features of bacteria such as the cell wall (peptidoglycan) properties, 30s and 50s ribosomal subunit structure, cell-membrane permeability, and metabolic intermediates are the targets of effective antibiotics. There are about 10 selected sites or points in the physiology of bacteria at which antibiotics impinge. Table 2.1 lists several antibiotics and the general target sites in bacteria on which they function. For some long-standing and effective antibiotics the modes of action remain unclear, as in the case of isoniazid and pentamidine (used in the treatment of *Mycobacterium* spp infections). The in vitro mechanics of inhibition may differ from the in vivo mechanisms. Estimates of the relative effectiveness of antibiotics, however, are difficult without sacrificing laboratory animals. The combination of public concerns and financial costs have diminished the use of animals in infectious disease research and development. Most current tests essentially attempt to determine the concentrations of antibiotic necessary to inhibit or impede bacterial growth. That value is then extrapolated into attainable biological levels observed in animal studies under conditions of bacterial challenge.

MEASURING RESISTANCE

Treatment for bacterial infections is most effective if the level of sensitivity to the specific antibiotic is known. In addition, physiological levels of antibiotic concentration in the desired body compartment must reach inhibitory levels in order to be effective against the bacteria.

TABLE 2.1 Antibiotics and Action Sites

Antibiotic	Action Site
Penicillins Cephalosporins Vancomycin Bacitracin	Peptidoglycan synthesis
Streptomycin Tetracyclines Erythromycin Chloramphenicol	Ribosomal subunits
Quinolones Nalidixic Acid	DNA synthesis
Rifampin	mRNA
Polymyxins Amphotericin B	Cell membrane
Isoniazid Pentamidine	Mycolic acid synthesis
Methotrexate Sulfonamides	Folate synthesis

Clinicians, in most cases, treat patients empirically, based on the prevailing recommended regimen for a particular type of infection (e.g., penicillin for lung or genital tract infections) without isolating and identifying the causative bacteria, that is growing up a pure culture, and conducting antibiotic susceptibility studies (tests), before prescribing the drug. (Note the similarity with the first half of Koch's Postulates; Koch, 1881). In most instances the educated guess of the practitioner is accurate in prescribing the most likely effective drug. This approach is not always accurate, however, as the professional experiences of practitioners vary or the infectious agent may have acquired new resistance.

Many reasonable arguments have been presented to justify this empirical approach to prescribing antibiotics. The intent is to circumvent

- time wasted in not treating the patient as rapidly as possible (especially in life-threatening situations),

- time wasted in not reducing the infectious period and thus increasing the chance of spreading the infection,
- cost (expense) associated with keeping patients in the hospital during the investigation period,
- requirement of a skilled technician or special lab equipment and reagents to perform the tests, and
- demands from the patient for immediate therapy (under a veiled threat of possible malpractice litigation).

Ideally the antibiotic susceptibility tests on the suspect microbes should be performed using at least two approved evaluation tests consisting of a rough screening test (e.g., disk diffusion or Kirby Bauer) and a more sensitive quantitative test (e.g., Microscan Walkaway Rapid test). The purpose of the more sensitive test is to determine the smallest amount (concentration) of antibiotic needed to kill or inhibit the bacteria. These values, called the minimal inhibitory concentration (MIC) and minimal bacteriocidal concentration (MBC), respectively, are extremely important in evaluating the drug resistance level of particular isolates. For example, *Staphylococcus aureus*, determined to have an MIC greater than 4 μ/ml vancomycin, is considered to show "reduced susceptibility" (to vancomycin) and therefore could present a major risk to the patient and general population. It is also important to note that laboratorians use different test methods to determine the MIC and MBC levels of different antibiotics. There are many commercial diagnostic devices on the market designed to make these determinations; however, these are not all equally accurate in delivering consistent results (Tenover, Swenson, O'Hara, & Stocker, 1995). Examples of commercial diagnostic devices used to determine the MIC/MBC levels of bacteria are the Microscan Walkway Rapid device (Dade International) and Vitek systems (BioMérieux USA). The prevalence of antibiotic resistance bacteria with an elevated MIC is monitored closely by groups such as the Active Bacterial Core Surveillance (ABCs)/Emerging Infections Program (EIP) Network; Centers for Disease Control and Prevention (CDC) Hospital Infection Program (Centers for Disease Control and Prevention, 1998b); and National Nosocomial Infection Surveillance system. Public health departments in many countries also monitor the frequency of antibiotic-resistant microbes and share this valuable data with other national and international agencies. Worldwide surveillance networks serve a vital role in combating the emergence of antibiotic-resistant organisms. Data compiled by the various networks are used to identify and analyze emerging trends (both anticipated and unexpected), thereby enabling researchers, health care providers, and public health planners to prepare countermeasures.

ANTIBIOTIC PROCESSES

Resistance to antibiotics is mediated by the expression of special sets of genes inherited or acquired by microbes. The overall outcome of this expression may result in varying degrees of resistance against the action of specific or classes of antibiotics. Sometimes resistance can involve multiple (different) drugs since groups of antibiotics may share common structural architecture. A large study monitored the prevalence of drug resistance in *Streptococcus pneumoniae.* More than 50% of those tested showed reduced susceptibility to penicillin G. From that group 80% were also resistant to macrolides (Roussel-Delvllez, Weber, Maugein, Thierry, Laurans, & Fosse, 1999). In general, bacteria display antibiotic resistance through the expression of genes that yield an increase in enzymes that

- degrade or inactivate antibiotics (e.g., the inactivation of penicillin by bacterial penicillinase),
- alter translational (ribosome) machinery, or
- affect bacterial cell targets so that they no longer respond to the action of chemicals that interfere with ribosome function (e.g., mutated resistance to the action of erythromycin) or structural changes in the cell membrane, resulting in altered permeability, thereby impeding the entry (transport) of certain antibiotics (e.g., certain types of tetracycline resistance).

The location of the genetic changes may take place on the bacterial chromosome or on extrachromosomal genetic information (e.g., plasmid, resistance factors, or transposons). Additional factors (e.g., presence or absence of DNA repair enzyme machinery) may affect the rate of genetic change, along with exposure to mutagens, to alter the growth rate of the organism and impose selective pressures that enhance the survival of mutants. In addition, the overall physiology of the bacteria may affect their ability to acquire new (foreign) genetic information that may convey resistance factors. Processes of conjugation and transduction vary within different bacterial species. Resistance factors (R-factors), self-replicating extrachromosomal material that is easily spread between bacteria of the same species, may also spread to bacteria of different genera. The spread of vancomycin resistance from the *Enterococcus* spp to *Staphylococcus* spp is an example of this possibility. Table 2.2 shows several of the most important examples of resistance acquired by bacteria that have had profound affects on human health care delivery. The increased appearance and expansion of antibiotic-resistant strains of bacteria within a population over a given period of time can be interpreted as the emergence of the organism. A variety of factors, including virulence of the organism, number of susceptible hosts, and overall immunological profile of the population, affect the level of emergence and transmission to new populations. Changes in antibiotic sensitivities occur in nearly all microbes; however, the patterns may vary in different parts of the world depending on the prevailing selective pressures.

CONDITIONS/LOCATIONS OF EMERGENCE OF ANTIBIOTIC RESISTANCE

The ease at which a disease becomes established and spreads within a population is dependent on many factors. Antibiotic-resistant bacteria are subject to many of these same variables. Mutations and genetic interactions that affect antibiotic resistance occur at a predictable frequency. Selective pressures determine whether the new organism will survive and spread. The emergence of an *avirulent* strain of bacteria

TABLE 2.2 Recently Acquired Antibiotic Resistance

Resistance	Organism	Consequence
Vancomycin resistance	*Staphylococcus aureus*	High mortality in exposed patients
Vancomycin resistance	Enterococci	High mortality in exposed patients
Multiple drug resistance	*Mycobacterium tuberculosis*	Rapid (epidemic) spread within untreated populations

would be of relatively little public health consequence, whereas a *virulent* strain of the same organism, by definition, would pose possible major health threats. Healthy people carrying avirulent organisms are not likely to seek medical attention; however, sick or ill individuals may seek treatment and therefore bring the new pathogen to the attention of the medical/health care staff. For this reason concerns about antibiotic-resistant organisms center on those organisms that possess additional virulence factors associated with disease (e.g., toxins, invasive properties, cell- or tissue-destroying factors). Factors that contribute to the selection of such pathogens are numerous and often due to a combination of influences. Several of these factors are discussed briefly below.

Crowding

Dense crowding or grouping of people enables easier spread of disease, especially air-borne infections. Military camps, college classrooms, public mass transportation (e.g., rail) systems, and airplanes are locations where people are grouped closely together for extended periods of time. Airborne bacteria, secreted through coughing, sneezing, or simply talking can pollute the air or coat surfaces (fomites) for later uptake by an unsuspecting person. The sharing of foods, kissing, sexual activity, and contamination of water sources provide other opportunities for disease-causing agents to spread. This is a major source of disease transmission in day care centers among preschool children. Hospitals attract sick people, many of whom carry virulent organisms that possess antibiotic resistance. Hospital-acquired (nosocomial) infections are the primary means by which several pathogens are spread. Several studies have shown that the probability of becoming infected with a new ailment increases with the length of time spent in the hospital. Fellow patients, health care staff, and medical devices and procedures may contribute to the spread of nosocomial infections. The simple task of hand washing has been shown very effective in reducing transmission of disease agents.

Nonadherence to Antibiotic Therapy

Nonadherence to antibiotic therapy has been closely associated with the emergence of resistant organisms. Patients who do not complete a prescribed antibiotic treatment period for bacterial infections may develop more resistant organisms that are then spread to other persons or the health care staff. Adherence is especially important in those therapies that require long-term treatment (e.g., tuberculosis which may require months of therapy). Observers are sometimes used to watch each patient (directly observed therapy [DOT]) take the prescribed medication in order to confirm adherence.

Over-Prescribing Antibiotics

A visit to a health care provider, especially in the case of children, too often results in the prescribing of antibiotics. During the winter months when colds and flu are prevalent this practice is common even though antibiotics do not affect the causative agents (viruses). The over-prescription of antibiotics for nonbacterial illnesses likely contributes to the selection of antibiotic-resistant strains (Kam, Luey, Fung, Yiu, Harden, & Cheung, 1995). Clinicians should explain to the parents the inappropriateness of antibiotics for certain illnesses and that nearly all viral illnesses are untreatable. Other measures for reducing the use of unnecessary antibiotics may be found in Cohen and Tartasky (1997). Newly introduced antiviral flu treatments (e.g., Relenza and Tamiflu) reduce the symptoms of discomfort and illness but do not totally eliminate the effects. Pediatricians have prescribed cephalosporin in the treatment of ear infections (otitis media). Studies have shown that in this group of children multidrug-resistant pneumococci were recovered that were resistant to cefotaxime and ceftriaxone (Kam et al., 1995). Clinicians must remain vigilant regarding their use of antibiotics and the possible long-term consequences they pose.

Many hospitals in the U.S. use as part of their standard operating protocols (in certain areas such as hematology and orthopedic units) the administration of vancomycin in cases of major surgery and in the treatment of hospital-acquired (nosocomial) infections. This intervention is believed to be a major factor in the emergence of glycopeptide-resistant enterococci (GRE).

Antibiotics in Food

Growers of certain food animals, especially livestock, poultry and aquaculture, add antibiotics to animal feed or the growing environment. It is believed the antibiotics alter the normal flora of the gut, causing a decreased competition for acquiring metabolites by bacteria and resulting in increased availability for animal cell growth. Both harmful and beneficial bacteria are affected by the practice (Jensen, 1998). The practice was initially used to ward off bacterial pathogens, but now is used primarily to enhance the growth rate of animals. A significant proportion (approximately half the worldwide production) of all antibiotics manufactured goes into animals' feed and therefore has become a major economic factor in their production, sale, and use. Antibiotics may also be sprayed on crops, such as fruit trees, in order to protect against surface bacteria (Levy, 1998). Bacteria possessing tetracycline resistance have been recovered from fruit trees in orchards that were not previously treated, therefore raising questions about the mechanism by which resistance occurs naturally (Schnabel & Jones, 1999). Many of the agricultural antibiotics are analogues of those used in the treatment of human disease and infections. The glycopeptide avoparcin, fed to animals, is nearly identical to vancomycin. Resistance to avoparcin also confers resistance to vancomycin. Since many bacteria are common to both human and animals (e.g., *Enterococcus faecium* and *E. faecalis*), any genetic change induced due to this antibiotic being added to animal feed may result in the transmission of the new resistant strain to humans. One form of vancomycin resistance in *E. faecium* (called the VanA gene cluster) is located on a transposon designated Tn*1546* (Butaye, Devriese, & Haesebrouck, 1999; Wegener, Aarestrup, Jensen, Hammerum, & Bager, 1999). Resistance factors encoded by transposons can easily transfer between different enterococci and even between different bacterial species (e.g., *S. aureus*). Transmission between bacterial species presents the greatest concern to researchers and health care providers. There has been a marked increase in the number of GRE recovered from hospital patients in the U.S. Preliminary evidence suggests that this finding represents possible infections of humans from food or animal origin. The implications of antibiotic-resistant strains recovered from meat products poses a major concern due to changing patterns of food preparation and consumption. The consumption of rare meats, especially poultry, presents a threat due to the increased prevalence of *Salmonella* spp and *Campylobacter* spp recovered from these meats.

In countries where the practice of feeding the antimicrobial growth promoter avoparcin to animals (e.g., pigs and chickens) is a common practice there is a high frequency of recovering vancomycin-resistant enterococci (see chapter 19) (Äärestrup, 1995; Bager, Madsen, Christensen, & Äärestrup, 1997). The U.S. and Sweden do not sanction the use of avoparcin in animal feed and therefore have low rate of resistant strain recovery from livestock and poultry. In the United Kingdom and Denmark, where the practice is common, the recovery rate is high. All evidence supports the theory that animals and humans share many identical bacteria, and that humans often acquire the animal pathogens through the consumption of improperly cooked or processed foods. Normal flora (and their accompanying plasmids) found in the intestinal tract of cattle and swine are readily passed into the human population as a consequence of routine farm practices or through intermediates such as farm rodents, animal bedding, and waste materials (Marshall, Pertowski, & Levy, 1990). Contamination of farm surfaces and colonization of farm workers may extend over periods of months allowing opportunities for secondary bacterial spread beyond the initial location.

Public Access to Antibiotics Is Not Restricted Worldwide

In some countries access to antibiotics over the counter is commonplace. Individuals can easily purchase drugs, share them with others, and even send them abroad. The quality of the antibiotics may be inconsistent between manufacturers. A 1-week treatment period using an inferior quality preparation may not completely eliminate the disease agent but simply enable the selective process for resistance to take place.

The Internet has become an essential means of gathering health care information. This unregulated medium also enables users to share information and create chatrooms or bulletin boards for obtaining antibiotics from nontraditional sources. Use of the Internet to seek out sellers and distributors of antibiotics, from any point on the globe, is now possible. Inadequate or improper regulation of these unregulated drugs, and information on their use, may increase the probability of antibiotic-resistant organisms and their eventual spread to the general population. It is important to rely on reputable, verifiable sources for medical information. The U.S. Food and Drug Administration posts a website advising the public on the hazards and concerns of obtaining drugs over the Internet (United States Food and Drug Administration, 1999).

GEOGRAPHIC DISTRIBUTION OF ANTIBIOTIC RESISTANCE

The genetic changes in bacteria that affect antibiotic resistance can occur anywhere on the globe. Hospitals, farms, fields, campuses, classrooms, military barracks, or any place where people are closely grouped are locations where the change could occur. Locations where people work or live in close proximity to livestock are areas where zoonotic transmissions are more likely to occur. Chicken and swine are animals frequently linked with the transmission of bacteria and viruses to humans. Locations where the indigenous people consume the local wildlife (e.g., the practice of eating monkey, venison, rodents, or rabbit in some parts of the world) have been linked to transmission of disease organisms to humans.

Once change has occurred, spread within the human population is relatively easy. Opportunities are numerous given the nature of humans. Two new factors affect the spread of disease agents—global travel (world access within a day) (see chapter 22) and international trade markets. Once the new resistant organism emerges and spreads within the immediate (human or animal) population it can potentially infect an individual who could carry the organism (during the prodromal or incubation period) to any location on the earth. It is for this reason that elaborate, worldwide surveillance networks have been established to continually monitor the patterns of newly emerging antibiotic-resistant organisms. Such networks include National Nosocomial Infection Surveillance system and Active Bacterial Core Surveillance (ABCs)/Emerging Infections Program (EIP) Network.

World trade agreements have reduced the barriers that restrict the flow of foods and other products between countries. Major concerns occur when highly perishable products are traded without adequate time for thorough screening for pathogens. Fresh fruits and vegetables that may receive preliminary washing before shipment or misting during transit may potentially spread microbes. Fresh meats pose similar threats. Food handlers, dock workers, or product workers who may harbor a resistant pathogen may inadvertently contaminate products at numerous points during the long transportation chain. In theory a child in St. Louis, Missouri can receive the pathogen of a field worker in Guatemala without ever meeting the individual. A business traveler in Hong Kong, dining on sushi and bean sprouts, could transmit resistant bacteria to his friends and family in the U.S., as a carrier, without even experiencing the illness (e.g., *Escherichia coli* O157:H7).

FACTORS INFLUENCING EMERGENCE

The emergence of antibiotic-resistant organisms is a continuous process. Conditions that give a selective advantage to an organism will affect whether it survives and expands within groups and receptive populations. Instances where the presence of antibiotics is high and constant (e.g., certain animal feed programs and hospital units) will only increase the likelihood of emergence. Different host populations are better able to cope with the resistant organisms. Healthy younger individuals are better prepared to survive an exposure compared to older individuals or those with illnesses or immune deficiencies.

Several proposals have been offered as a means of limiting the induction and spread of antibiotic-resistant organisms. These include some of the proposed practices outlined in Table 2.3. Others may be found in Cohen and Tartasky (1997). Overreliance on antibiotics as a prophylactic agent diminishes the special properties of these compounds. Care should be placed on using alternate mechanisms of infection prevention while reserving the use of antibiotics for curative purposes. Some of the alternate approaches to disease and infection control include the following:

1. *Greater use of vaccines.* Bacterial vaccines can prevent infection, thus reducing the need to administer antibiotics. Vaccines used in the prevention of pneumococcal pneumonia, *Haemophilus influenzae*, bacterial meningitis, and Lyme disease reduce the need for antibiotics.

TABLE 2.3 Measures to Reduce Antibiotic Resistance*

Approach	Desired Outcome
Restrict the use of antibiotics, especially in animal feed	Reduce indiscriminate use
Retire the use of select antibiotics	Reserve antibiotic classes for select situations
Alternate the use of certain antibiotics	Reduce selection/emergence of resistance
Require sensitivity testing before prescribing	More efficient use of available antibiotic options

*For additional suggestions see Cohen and Tartasky (1997).

Vaccination also helps to limit the spread of disease within the population (see chapter 1) through the protective benefits of "herd immunity."

2. *Extensive clinical laboratory testing.* Rapid techniques of identifying the causative pathogen and determining antibiotic sensitivity will maximize the effectiveness of antibiotics.

Various professional groups have also been established, such as the Alliance for the Prudent Use of Antibiotics (Grave, Lillehaug, Lunestad, & Horsberg, 1999), which is a nonprofit, international organization solely dedicated to preserving the effectiveness of antibiotics through logical systematic use.

Quarantine is usually not a viable option for disease and infection control. The practice of quarantining individuals has changed significantly due to changing times. The CDC Division on Quarantine has authority to isolate individuals entering the country who appear infected with certain highly infectious bacteria or viruses. These regulations are not directed toward drug-resistant organisms but rather specific diseases (e.g., cholera, smallpox, infectious tuberculosis) (Centers for Disease Control and Prevention, 1996). The practice is effective, however, in holding animals with possible pathogens.

SLOW PACE OF NEW DRUG DEVELOPMENT AND MARKETING

The time required to discover, develop, test, and obtain final approval for a new drug can take over 20 years and cost millions of dollars. Most of the regulations, imposed primarily by the Food and Drug Administration, are designed to protect the citizenry from the consequences of exposure to unsafe and ineffective medical products. A lengthy series of preliminary reports on the basic biology and animal toxicity studies are required prior to the initial tests on humans. The entire process has been a model that many other countries emulate. The process is not foolproof, however, and occasionally harmful drugs reach the general public (e.g., thalidomide, Fen-Phen).

The absence of new antibiotic development is attributed to several factors as discussed below. The time and cost associated with the development of new antibiotics is clearly extensive such that only a few worldwide companies are active in the business of drug discovery.

One factor that motivates them is the parallel cost associated with the annual cost of treating antibiotic-resistant infections. It is estimated that in the U.S. alone over $30 billion is spent in the treatment of antibiotic-resistant infections (Institute of Medicine, 1999). Most are associated with nosocomial infections, immune deficient patients, transplant recipients, dialysis patients, and those affected by respiratory tract infections. The overall costs on a worldwide scale magnify the U.S. expenditures severalfold. Aside from the humanitarian reasons, companies are attracted by the potential monetary rewards from developing and marketing an effective treatment to infections.

New drug development may take as many as 15–20 years. Initial insight into the possible applications of a compound begin at the level of basic scientific studies. Additional studies may attempt to test efficacy using small animals (mice or rats) since the use of primates is very expensive and highly regulated. Restrictions on the use of laboratory animals have increased, resulting in strict regulations on their humane treatments and limits on the types of experimental designs. No animal fully mimics the response of humans to investigational (experimental) drugs. Similarly the types of experiments are highly regulated, especially those involving infectious disease agents. The public still remembers the infamous studies involving syphilis-infected minorities who were denied antibiotic treatment during the 1940s. The experiments, known as the Tuskegee Syphilis Study, included over 600 Black men in a long-term study. Victims of syphilis were denied antibiotic treatment with the drug penicillin. At that point in time the causative agent of syphilis, *Treponema pallidum*, had not acquired antibiotic resistance. Disease progression was monitored in untreated patients over the course of several years. Several died from their infections. Many suffered disease-associated complications. Eventually a national condemnation of the project resulted in its termination and subsequent denunciation (Centers for Disease Control and Prevention, 1999).

Today investigational studies using human subjects are subjected to close scrutiny during the three phases of development. These are essentially grouped as follows: (a) Phase I—Evaluation of clinical pharmacology, usually conducted in volunteers; (b) Phase II—Determination of dose and initial evaluation of efficacy, conducted in a small number of patients; and (c) Phase III—Large comparative study (compound versus placebo and/or established treatment) in patients to establish clinical benefit and safety—includes "blinded" experiments. If the results of these trials prove promising, then the investigators may initiate a series of petitions for final FDA approval of the drug for general use. At any point in the process any reported major side effects or unexpected negative observations could delay, halt, or terminate the entire process. Liability insurance is not underwritten by the government and few companies risk new ventures in product development.

SUMMARY

Infections from organisms resistant to antimicrobial therapy continue to increase, especially in hospitals. The emergence of a new resistant strain in one part of the globe poses a threat to people on the other side of Earth as a plane ride can carry an incubating disease nearly anywhere within the symptomless incubation time. The quality of life and cost of health care are adversely affected with the emergence of each new drug-resistant organism. Only through a combination of scientific research initiatives, education, and prudent hospital management decisions can we maintain the delicate balance of preparedness for inevitable mutational emergence.

REFERENCES

Aärestrup, F. M. (1995). Occurrence of glycopeptide resistance among *Enterococcus faecium* isolates from ecological and conventional poultry farms. *Microbial Drug Resistance, 1,* 255–257.

Bager, F., Madsen, M., Christensen, J., & Aarestrup, F. M. (1997). Avoparcin used as a growth promoter is associated with the occurrence of vancomycin-resistant *Enterococcus faecium* on Danish poultry and pig farms. *Preventive Veterinary Medicine, 31,* 95–112.

Briggs, C. E., & Fratamico, P. M. (1999). Molecular characterization of an antibiotic resistance gene cluster of *Salmonella typhimurium* DT104. *Antimicrobial Agents and Chemotherapy, 43,* 846–849.

Butaye, P., Devriese, L. A., & Haesebrouck, F. (1999). Phenotypic distinction in *Enterococcus faecium* and *Enterococcus faecalis* strains between susceptibility and resistance to growth-enhancing antibiotics. *Antimicrobial Agents and Chemotherapy, 43,* 2569–2570.

Carattoli, A., Villa, L., Pezzella, C., Bordi, E., & Visca, P. (2001). Expanding drug resistance through integron acquisition by IncFI plasmids of *Salmonella enterica* typhimurium. *Emerging Infectious Diseases, 7,* 444–447.

Centers for Disease Control and Prevention. (1996). *Public health screening at U.S. ports of entry: A guide for U.S. immigration, customs and agriculture inspection.* U.S. Public Health Service, CDC-NCID, Division of Quarantine [On-line]. Available: http://www.cdc.gov/ncidod/dq/pdf/hguide.pdf

Centers for Disease Control and Prevention. (1998). *Hospital infections program* [On-line]. Available: www.cdc.gov/ncidod/hip/default.htm

Centers for Disease Control and Prevention. (1999). *The Tuskegee Study: A hard lesson learned* [On-line]. Available: http://www.cdc.gov/nchstp/od/tuskegee/time.htm

Centers for Disease Control and Prevention. (2000). *Staphylococcus aureus* with reduced susceptibility to vancomycin—Illinois, 1999. *Morbidity and Mortality Weekly Report, 48,* 1165.

Claverie, J. M. (2001). What if there are only 30,000 human genes? *Science, 291,* 1255.

Cohen, F. L., & Tartasky, D. (1997). Microbial resistance to drug therapy: A review. *American Journal of Infection Control, 25,* 51–64.

Gardner, P., Smith, D. H., Beer, H., & Moellering, R.C., Jr. (1969). Recovery of resistance (R) factors from a drug-free community. *Lancet, 2,* 774–776.

Grave, K., Lillehaug, A., Lunestad, B. T., & Horsberg, T. E. (1999). Prudent use of antibacterial drugs in Norwegian aquaculture? Surveillance by the use of prescription data. *Acta Veterinaria Scandinavica, 40,* 185–195.

Institute of Medicine. (1999, May). *Institute of Medicine homepage* [On-line]. Available: http://www4.nas.edu/iom/iomhome.nsf/pages/recently+released+reports

Jensen, B. (1998). The impact of feed additives on the microbial ecology of young pigs. *Journal of Animal and Feed Sciences, 7,* 45–64.

Kam, K. M., Luey, K. Y., Fung, S. M., Yiu, P. P., Harden, T. J., & Cheung, M. M. (1995). Emergence of multiple-antibiotic-resistant *Streptococcus pneumoniae* in Hong Kong. *Antimicrobial Agents and Chemotherapy, 39,* 2667–2670.

Koch, R. (1881). Zur untersuchung von pathogenen organismen (Method for the study of pathogenic organisms). *Mittheillungen aus dem Kaiserlichen Gesundheitsamte, 1,* 1–48.

Levy, S. B. (1998). The challenge of antibiotic resistance. *Scientific American, 278*(3), 46–53.

Mahasneh, A. M., & El-Oqlah, A. A. (1999). Antimicrobial activity of extracts of herbal plants used in the traditional medicine of Jordan. *Journal of Ethnopharmacology, 64,* 271–276.

Marshall, C. G., Lessard, I., Park, I., & Wright, G. D. (1998). Glycopeptide antibiotic resistance genes in glycopeptide-producing organisms. *Antimicrobial Agents and Chemotherapy, 42,* 2215–2220.

Marshall, B., Pertowski, D., & Levy, S. B. (1990). Inter- and intraspecies spread of *Escherichia coli* in a farm environment in the absence of antibiotic usage. *Proceedings of the National Academy of Science, USA, 87,* 6609–6613.

Roussel-Delvllez, M., Weber, M., Maugein, J., Thierry, J., Laurans, G., & Fosse, T. (1999). *Résistance du pneumocoque aux antibiotiques en 1997: Résultats de 18 observatoires régionaux. Bulletin Epidémiologique Annuel 1998 report.* Paris, France: National Institute for Public Health Surveillance.

Schempp, C. M., Pelz, K., Wittmer, A., Schopf, E., & Simon, J. C. (1999). Antibacterial activity of hyperforin from St. John's wort, against multiresistant *Staphylococcus aureus* and gram-positive bacteria. *Lancet, 353*, 2129.

Schnabel, E. L., & Jones, A. L. (1999). Distribution of tetracycline resistance genes and transposons among phylloplane bacteria in Michigan apple orchards. *Applied and Environmental Microbiology, 65*, 4898–4907.

Tenover, F. C., Swenson, J. M., O'Hara, C. M., & Stocker, S. A. (1995). Ability of commercial and reference antimicrobial susceptibility testing methods to detect vancomycin resistance in enterococci. *Journal of Clinical Microbiology, 33*, 1524–1527.

United States Food and Drug Administration. (1999). *Buying medical products online* [On-line]. Available: http://www.fda.gov/oc/buyonline/default.htm

Wegener, H. C., Aarestrup, F. M., Jensen, L. B., Hammerum, A. M., & Bager, F. (1999). Use of antimicrobial growth promoters in food animals and *Enterococcus faecium* resistance to therapeutic antimicrobial drugs in Europe. *Emerging Infectious Diseases, 5*, 329–335.

Yoshida, H., Iwata, N., Katsuzaki, H., Naganawa, R., Ishikawa, K., Fukuda, H., et al. (1998). Antimicrobial activity of a compound isolated from an oil-macerated garlic extract. *Bioscience, Biotechnology & Biochemistry, 62*, 1014–1017.

3

Categories and Highlights of Significant Current Emerging Infectious Diseases

Felissa R. Lashley

Like other infectious diseases, emerging infectious diseases (EIDs) may be thought of in various ways: by the category of the organism, by the route of transmission, by the most prevalent method of spread, or by geographic distribution. EIDs will be discussed below in terms of the classification of the infectious agent (bacterial, viral, parasitic, fungal, and prion), and conceptually by their chief mode of dissemination to humans—limited here to those that are food- and/or waterborne, zoonotic or vector-borne, and those that are potentially transmissible by blood transfusion or transplant. Some of the latter categories overlap. For example, malaria is a vector-borne disease that is also transmissible by blood transfusion. After this general discussion, chapters follow highlighting specific EIDs that are of special interest or importance. Numerous tables providing information about a large number of emerging infectious diseases are found in Appendices A and B. As in other chapters, the definition of EIDs includes newly identified diseases caused by a previously known organism; newly identified diseases caused by a previously unknown organism; the recognition of a new organism; a familiar organism whose geographic range has extended, whose host has changed, whose incidence has increased, or one that has changed to become more virulent or antibiotic resistant.

EMERGING INFECTIONS BY MICROORGANISM CLASSIFICATION

Emerging Bacterial Diseases

Bacteria were the first disease-causing microbes to yield to modern pharmacologic interventions. Morbidity from "old" bacterial illnesses such as tuberculosis (TB) and cholera, however, continues to be a problem. Some of these have been identified as emerging or reemerging due to emergence of antimicrobial-resistant forms such as multidrug-resistant-TB (MDR-TB); vancomycin-resistant enterococci (VRE) infections caused by *E. faecalis* or *E. faecium* resulting in significant problems from nosocomial infections; or resistant forms of *Streptococcus pneumoniae*; the major bacterial cause of meningitis, pneumonia, and otitis media (see chapters 16, 18, and 19). Other microorganisms are defined as resurgent due to changes in their geographic distribution or increased incidence of infection often following the decline of the public health system. An example of the latter is the resurgence of diphtheria (caused by *Cornyebacterium diphtheriae*) and pertussis (whooping cough; caused by *Bordetella pertussis*), both vaccine-preventable diseases, in former states of the Soviet Union. Pertussis is also being increasingly seen in adults in the United States. Resistance of bacteria to antibiotics, is becoming of increasing concern. A well-known disease, tuberculosis, has developed multidrug resistance, and is thus defined as reemerging (see chapter 16), and although rare to date, nosocomial outbreaks of fluoroquinolone-resistant *Salmonella* are expected to become more frequent (Olsen, DeBess, McGivern, Marano, Eby, Mauvais, et al., 2001). *Staphylococcus aureus*, a frequent cause of infection in nosocomial settings and the immunosuppressed is becoming resistant to various antibiotics, especially methicillin, and may be known as methicillin-resistant *Staphylococcus aureus* (MRSA) (Paradisi, Corti, & Messeri, 2001). *S. aureus* also may be resistant to vancomycin (Verhoef, 2001). Another mechanism for emergence in bacteria are mutations resulting in new strains of an organism that may be more virulent or seek different hosts. Outbreaks of a new strain of *Escherichia coli*, a familiar bacteria, known as O157:H7, fit this pattern, causing diarrhea and hemolytic uremic syndrome (see chapter 9). Likewise, although cholera is an ancient disease, new virulent strains such as the El Tor strain of *Vibrio cholerae* have emerged and there is an endemic focus of infection in the U.S. as well as increased cases due to imported foods or travelers (see chapter 4). *Clostridium novyi* was associated with illness in injection-drug users in Great Britain in 2000 (Centers for Disease Control and Prevention, 2000d). New bacterial diseases such as Lyme disease, ehrlichiosis, and various rickettsial fevers have been identified (see chapter 14). Emerging bacterial diseases are summarized in Appendix A, Table A.1. Some of these diseases will be briefly discussed below or in individual chapters.

Toxic shock syndrome (TSS), a febrile illness associated with shock, multiorgan dysfunction, and high death rates, was first described in association with staphylococci in 1978 (Todd, Fishaut, Kapral, & Welch, 1978), but came to national attention in 1979–1980 when a new and initially puzzling entity was affecting young healthy women. The connection with menstruation, tampon use (especially the tampon absorbency), and TSS from *Staphylococcus aureus* led to some misperceptions that TSS only occurred in association with these variables. Although TSS did initially appear to occur disproportionately in menstruating women, there is an increasing proportion of nonmenstrual cases, many reported subsequent to surgical procedures (Hajjeh, Reingold, Weil, Shutt, Schuchat, & Perkins, 1999; Reingold, 1998). Some strains of *Staphylococcus aureus* have become methicillin-resistant leading to additional concerns (Paradisi et al., 2001). Methicillin-resistant *Staphylococcus aureus* have also been responsible for community-acquired foodborne gastroenteritis (Jones, Kellum, Porter, Bell, & Schaffner, 2002).

In the mid-1980s a resurgence of severe, invasive group A streptococcal (GAS) infections was seen, leading to toxic shock syndrome and necrotizing fasciitis. GAS infections had been known previously but had appeared to be declining prior to this resurgence, which was attributed to an increased virulence of the organism. It is also known that host susceptibility plays a vital role in predisposition of persons to GAS. Any illness caused by *Streptococcus pyogenes* can result in streptococcal toxic shock syndrome, which is an acute febrile illness often with tissue infection that can progress to shock, multiorgan failure, and death. The death rate is high—30% to 60% (Stevens, 2000). GAS infection resulting in necrotizing fasciitis with or without toxic shock syndrome has emerged, becoming known in the popular press as "flesh-eating" bacteria. Mortality is high with this condition and survivors often need major debridement and/or amputation of limbs. About half of the cases are associated with TSS. Aggressive therapy is needed in treatment (File & Tan, 2000; Stevens, 2001).

Bartonella (formerly called *Rochalimaea*) *quintana* was recognized as the cause of trench fever during World War I, and another species, *B. bacilliformis* was recognized as the cause of Oroya fever and Carrión's disease earlier (Maguiña & Gotuzzo, 2000). Knowledge about the *Bartonella* genus has increased rapidly, and it is now known to include 16 species, some of which resulted from the renaming described above, and some from phylogenetic studies resulting in reclassification of *Grahamella* species to *Bartonella* in 1995 (Breitschwerdt & Kordick, 2000). At least five species are known to cause disease in humans—*B. bacilliformis, B. henselae, B. quintana, B. elizabethae*, and, most recently, *B. clarridgeae* (Maguiña & Gotuzzo, 2000). *B. grahamii* has been found in a patient with neuroretinitis (Kerkhoff, Bergmans, Van der Zee, & Rothova, 1999). The major diseases caused are trench fever, cat scratch fever, bacillary angiomatosis, bacillary peliosis, endocarditis, and bacteremia. *Bartonella* are aerobic, fastidious, gram-negative bacteria, some of which have flagella such as *B. bacilliformis* and *B. clarridgeae.* Some *Bartonella* may be transmitted by a vector such as the body louse, transmitting *B. quintana* and resulting in trench fever (Breitschwerdt & Kordick, 2000; Schmidt, 1998).

B. henselae has been identified as the major cause of cat scratch disease. Cat scratch disease may be the most common *Bartonella* infection. The cat flea may be involved in transmission. Typically, in 95%–99% of cases there is a history of a cat bite, scratch, or lick, and one risk factor is having a cat in the home, especially one under one year of age. Typically, children between 2 and 14 years of age are affected (Koehler, 1998; Schmidt, 1998; Walker, 2001). The disease is usually self-limiting in the immunocompetent in whom it usually occurs, with one or more papules, vesicles, or pustules occurring 3–10 days after the bite or scratch. Lymphadenopathy then develops, commonly axillary, cervical, or inguinal. These can take several months to resolve. Sometimes low-grade fever and malaise may be seen. Antibiotic therapy does not usually alter the course of infection. Complicated or atypical cat scratch disease can include neurologic, ophthalmologic, and systemic manifestations, and is more likely in persons who are immunosuppressed (Conrad, 2001; Koehler, 1998; Maguiña & Gotuzzo, 2000; Walker, 2001).

In 1983, Stoler, Bonfiglio, Steigbigel, and Pereira described atypical skin lesions that became known as bacillary angiomatosis (BA) in persons with AIDS. BA is a vascular, proliferative lesion that occurs most frequently subcutaneously as nodules, or more superficially as papules, warts, or hyperketatotic plaques that are typically reddish purple with a diameter of about one centimeter. Histologically, lobular proliferation of blood vessels is seen, and the lesions may bleed easily. Lesions may occur in other sites such as the gastrointestinal tract, the larynx, and bones (Maguiña & Gotuzzo, 2000). Bacillary peliosis (BP) is a vasculoproliferative lesion resulting in the development of cystic blood-filled spaces that occurs most frequently in the liver parenchyma, spleen, and sometimes lymph nodes, nearly always in persons with AIDS. BA and BP respond to appropriate antibiotic therapy such as erythromycin or doxycycline (Koehler, 1998; Pretorius & Kelly, 2000). BA and BP can result from both *B. quintana* and *B. henselae*. Bacteremia and endocarditis may occur in both the immunocompetent and the immunocompromised often from *B. quintana*, *B. elizabethae*, and *B. henselae* (Koehler, 1998; Pretorius & Kelly, 2000).

Emerging Viral Diseases

The greatest number of emerging infectious diseases are viral. Many of these are hemorrhagic fevers whose agents have been recognized relatively recently, and tend to be seen in certain geographic distributions in North America (such as hantavirus pulmonary syndrome), Asia (such as hemorrhagic fever with renal syndrome), Africa (such as Ebola fever) and South America (such as Bolivian hemorrhagic fever), often with high mortality rates (see chapter 8). The most notorious new viral EID was HIV infection/AIDS which has had a considerable clinical, social, and political impact (see chapter 12). Another recently emerged virus causes West Nile fever (see chapter 20) and Nipah virus infection can result in encephalitis. Less exotic, but nevertheless a very important viral disease, is influenza or the flu, in which new strains have evolved; and newly identified viruses that can cause hepatitis, such as hepatitis C, and other liver diseases (see chapter 11). Specific emerging viral infections are discussed in individual chapters and in Appendix A, Table A.4. Two are considered briefly below.

Influenza itself is not a true emerging infectious disease; however, the virus strains causing influenza mutate frequently resulting in lack of resistance in human populations; influenza has caused pandemics leading to the deaths of millions. Some flu strains have crossed species. For example, in 1997, in Hong Kong, a child died of viral pneumonia and multiorgan failure after an outbreak of H5N1 avian influenza occurred in fowl such as ducks and chickens. It became the first time that an avian influenza virus was isolated from a human with respiratory infection, and led to fears of a new pandemic (Shortridge, Gao, Guan, Ito, Kawaoka, Markwell, et al., 2000). By the end of 1997, there were 18 identified human cases (Horimoto & Kawaoka, 2001). Identification of the source of the virus in the live poultry markets led to bans on import of poultry and the slaughter of approximately 1.2 million chickens and 0.3 million other poultry that included nearly 1,000 retail poultry markets as well as wholesale markets and small farms (Shortridge et al., 2000). Other strains of influenza virus such as H9N2 were isolated from poultry. This strain has also been isolated from pigs and other animals and persons with influenza-like illness and it is also a candidate for causing a pandemic (Shortridge et al., 2000). Because fowl are a reservoir for the influenza virus, the practice of raising pigs and ducks together as they do in China, where crowding is also a factor, allows viruses to recombine, with pigs as a vessel, enabling the virus to cross the species barrier to humans. Altered viral genes can result not only in cross-species transfer but also in altered virulence (Hatta, Gao, Halfmann, & Kawaoka, 2001). This is also an example of how cultural practices and social conditions influence infectious disease spread. An excellent review of the history of influenza is found in a book by Gina Kolata (2001).

A recent example of the recognition of a previously undetected viral disease occurred in Australia as follows. An outbreak of an acute, lethal respiratory disease in Hendra, a suburb of Brisbane, occurred in a group of thoroughbred horses in September, 1994. A trainer and a stablehand became ill and the trainer died of respiratory disease (Selvey, Wells, McCormack, Ansford, Murray, Rogers, et al., 1995). The next reported incident involved a sugarcane farmer in Mackay, near Hendra, who had assisted at autopsies of horses that had died of an acute illness in August, 1994. He was subsequently diagnosed with a viral infection in 1995 that was then called equine morbillivirus (the earlier name for Hendra virus). The farmer died later of meningoencephalitis, which was believed to have been in a latent phase for a year before reactivating to result in his fatal illness. A search for a reservoir of the infection resulted in the isolation of the virus from fruit bats, known also as flying foxes, that were shown to be identical to the virus from the lung of one of the horses who had died. Presumably in both cases the humans were infected by contact with the horses who had been infected by the fruit bats (Mackenzie, 1999; Murray, Eaton, Hooper, Wang, Williamson, & Young, 1998).

Emerging Fungal Diseases

In comparison with the other categories of microbes, fewer known emerging fungal diseases affect humans. Invasive fungi emerge when environmental conditions are permissive or when hosts are susceptible (Walsh, 1998). In many cases, they appear as opportunistic infections threatening patients who are immunosuppressed because of such conditions as HIV infection, malignancy, organ transplantation, or even aging. In immunocompromised persons, the opportunistic infection seen may depend on the infection endemic in the geographic area or on where the patient has travelled. *Penicillium marneffei*, for example, is most commonly seen in southeast Asia where it is a relatively frequent opportunistic infection in persons with HIV infection (Sirisanthana, 2001). Other endemic fungi such as *Coccidioides immitis* in the southwestern United States cause respiratory disease and are increasing in incidence in both the immunologically compromised and in those who have relocated to endemic areas, many of whom are elderly and have some degree of immunosuppression. In addition to *P. marneffei*, *Candida albicans* and non-albicans species, *Aspergillus* spp, *Cryptococcus neoformans*, *Trochosporon* spp, *Sporothrix schenckii*, *Histoplasma capsulatum*, *Malassezia*, and *Fusarium* spp, have been described as emerging, using a definition of emerging as organisms that have increased in frequency, particularly because of their appearance as opportunists in the immunosuppressed (Lashley, 2000; Robinson, 1999; Walsh, 1998). These are summarized in Appendix A, Table A.2.

Emerging Parasitic Diseases

Many of the emerging parasitic diseases were thought of as affecting relatively few people in developed countries. This view began to change when an increased prevalence of what were thought of as rare or exotic infections began to be seen more commonly in connection with the immunosuppression of HIV disease. This view also had to be quickly reevaluated when the outbreak of cryptosporidiosis resulting from the contamination of municipal water supply that affected over 400,000 persons occurred in Milwaukee, Wisconsin in 1993. Many of the parasitic diseases are already known but parasites that have emerged relatively recently are *Cyclospora cayetanensis* (see chapter 6), *Cryptosporidium parvum* (see chapter 5), *Babesia microti* (see chapter 14), and microsporidia. Most are protozoal parasites but increased helminth infections are also being seen. Many are food- or waterborne (see Appendix B, Table B.1) (MacLean, 1998). A familiar parasite, *Trichinella*, usually acquired through ingestion of undercooked pork is now emerging as a result of infected horsemeat in countries in Europe where eating horsemeat is popular. Acquiring the parasite may also result from eating bear meat and other exotic meats as the demand for variety and the unusual expands (Pozio, 2000; Slifko, Smith, & Rose, 2000). Likewise, *Taenia solium*, the pork tapeworm, has been recognized recently to cause neurocysticercosis or infection of the central nervous system. Recognition of neurocysticercosis as a major cause of neurologic disease including epilepsy resulted from improved diagnostic examinations such as computed axial tomography and magnetic resonance imaging scanning; from large numbers of immigrants to the U.S. from developing countries who were diagnosed with neurocysticercosis (for example, in Los Angeles, the diagnosis increased fourfold between 1977 and 1981); and improved serological assays for diagnosis allowing for accurate prevalence estimates. In the U.S. most cases are in immigrants or in persons born in this country who have traveled to rural areas in endemic countries (White, 2000). Locally acquired cases are known in the U.S. In one well known instance, orthodox Jews in one New York community, who would not have themselves been in contact with pork, acquired neurocysticercosis through eating food prepared by immigrant domestic workers who carried *Taenia* (Schantz, Moore, Muñoz, Hartman, Schaefer, Aron, et al., 1992).

While malaria is no longer considered endemic in the United States, it once was, and its range and resistance patterns are extending (Phillips, 2001). While cases of malaria have been diagnosed subsequent to travel, outbreaks of mosquito-borne transmission in New York, New Jersey, California, Texas, and other areas (for a total of 24 episodes in the U.S. since 1985) have been described. These are usually due to *Plasmodium vivax* but some are also due to the more severe *Plasmodium falciparum*. Conditions are met in the U.S. for the potential transmission of malaria including people who have malarial parasites in their blood, and the presence of the appropriate vector—the *Anopheles* mosquito (see chapter 15) (Centers for Disease Control and Prevention, 2000c; Zucker, 1996).

Microsporidia or microsporida are the non-taxonomic terms used to describe protozoal parasites belonging to the phylum *Microspora*. There are nearly 150 genera (Franzen & Müller, 2001). The microsporidia are obligate intracellular parasites that lack mitochondria and can form spores (Mêtênier & Vivarès, 2001). The first human case of microsporidiosis was reported in 1959 in a 9-year-old child with neurological symptoms (Matsubayashi, Koike, Mikata, Takei, & Hagiwara, 1959). In 1973, two new species, *Vittaforma* (formerly *Nosema*) *corneum*, and *Nosema connori* were identified. In 1985, their increasing importance in persons with HIV infection began to be recognized. At present the following genera are known to cause human infection: *Vittaforma*, *Nosema*, *Pleistophora*, *Encephalitozoon*, *Enterocytozoon*, *Trachypleistophora*, *Brachiola*, and lastly *Microsporidium*, into which all species with undetermined status are classified (Franzen & Müller, 2001; Mota, Rauch, & Edberg, 2000; Nichols, 2000). While immunocompromised persons are most susceptible to microsporidiosis, those who are immunocompetent may also develop infection. Microsporidiosis usually results in self-limited diarrhea, but ocular microsporidiosis resulting in keratitis, corneal ulceration, and even blindness can occur. Disseminated microsporidiosis can affect the nervous system (Franzen & Müller, 2001; Mota et al., 2000). In persons with HIV infection, microsporidia such as *Enterocytozoon bieneusi* causing chronic diarrhea and biliary effects, and *Encephalitozoon intestinalis*, causing diarrhea as well as small bowel perforation and dissemination to the respiratory tract, kidney, and eyes, have become problematic. Keratoconjunctivitis from various microsporidia occurs in HIV-infected persons. The source of microsporidial infections is often not known. Person-to-person transmission through the fecal-oral and urinary-oral routes, and direct inoculation to conjunctiva is known, and food- and waterborne transmission have been suggested but not demonstrated (Didier, 1998; Mota et al., 2000). Other emerging parasitic diseases are summarized in Appendix A, Table A.3.

Emerging Prion Diseases

In the past, there have been debates over the nature of prions, a type of protein particle that is devoid of nucleic acids. Prion proteins that are altered usually through conformational changes such as misfolding cause three categories of disease in humans: sporadic, infectious/iatrogenic, and genetic (Alter, 2000; Prusiner, 2001). Although prion diseases have a long incubation period this period is shorter for vCJD. Altered prions cause fatal spongiform encephalopathies. A certain prion protein polymorphism appears to be a determinant of genetic susceptibility to acquired infections and sporadic prion diseases (see chapter 17). The prion diseases that have attracted the most attention are Creutzfeldt-Jakob disease, especially that acquired through iatrogenic means such as growth hormone injections and corneal transplants; variant Creutzfeldt-Jakob disease (vCJD), a human form of bovine transmissible spongiform encephalopathy (BSE), commonly referred to as "mad cow" disease; and kuru, acquired through formerly practiced ritualistic cannibalism in the Fore tribe in Papua New Guinea. While iatrogenic prion diseases represent a small percentage of all prion disease in humans, there may be a considerable potential for transmission generally through blood transfusions; and corneal, dura mater, and other transplants or other iatrogenic means (Centers for Disease Control and Prevention, 1997). Concern has also arisen over the potential transmission of prion diseases through inadequately sterilized instruments or devices. The current BSE epidemic in the United Kingdom emerged in the 1980s, and has been reported in other countries as well. Linkage to vCJD was first noted in a 1996 report (Will, Ironside, Zeidler, Cousens, Estibeiro, Alperovitch, et al., 1996). Continued concern about transmission from infected meats or meat products such as gelatin or even through products such as bone meal has led to various bans of imported products and conferences on approaches for protection (Brown, Will, Bradley, Asher, & Detwiler, 2001). Effects and reactions are political, social, and economic, at times bordering on hysteria. Prion diseases are considered in depth in chapter 17.

SELECTED TRANSMISSION MODES OF EIDS

Vector-Borne Diseases and Zoonoses

Some emerging infectious diseases are transmitted to humans from their usual animal hosts and are known as zoonoses. For a review, see Weiss (2001). Hansen, Woodall, Brown, Jaax, McNamara, and

Ruiz (2001) identify the following as the most important factors associated with emerging zoonotic diseases: the transportation of humans and animals to new areas, increased contact between humans and animals, changes in husbandry practices and in the environment, more immunocompromised persons in the population at large, increased recognition of certain diseases as zoonotic in origin as well as the discovery of new organisms that were not previously recognized. They may appear as human infections in an episodic way, such as happens with Lassa fever (see chapter 8), or may more permanently jump the species barrier often through a mutation in the organism such as is believed to have occurred in the case of HIV infection. It is believed that HIV-1 originated as the simian immunodeficiency virus from the *Pan troglodytes troglodytes* (Gao, Bailes, Robertson, Chen, Rodenburg, Michael, Cummins, et al., 1999), and HIV-2 from the sooty mangebey (Hahn, Shaw, De Cock, & Sharp, 2000) (see chapter 12). Some zoonoses are relatively benign, others cause limited disease, and still others result in more serious and extensive outbreaks. An example of a current geographically localized zoonotic disease with the potential to spread is *Echinococcus multilocularis* infection in Alaska and nearby Canada. It causes alveolar hydatid disease of the lung with an untreated mortality of near 80%. Foxes, small rodents, and domestic dogs are known hosts. Illegal exporting of foxes to the southeastern U.S. may result in a spread of this zoonosis outside of Alaska and the area around the Canadian/U.S. border making it an emerging disease due to extension of geographic boundaries (Butler, Parkinson, Funk, Beller, Hayes, & Hughes, 1999).

Vectors usually are arthropods, especially insects, that are capable of transmitting microorganisms to vertebrate hosts. Arthropods are vectors for viral, bacterial, and parasitic agents. Arthropod-borne viral diseases called arboviruses are more common than bacterial or parasitic diseases spread in this way. More than 40% of viruses that infect mammals move from host to host by arthropod vectors (van den Heuvel, Hogenhout, & van der Wilk, 1999). There are about 100 known arboviruses that are pathogenic for humans—some of which are emerging or reemerging and others that do not fit this classification. Among bacteria, the group known as rickettsiae are often arthropod-associated. Rickettsial diseases include many of the "spotted fevers" as well as ehrlichiosis (Rauolt & Olson, 1999). Examples of emerging vector-borne diseases are listed in Appendix B, Table B.3. Selected important vector-borne EIDs are further discussed in relation to recreational activities and travel in chapters 14 and 22.

Primary vectors are the major species that are involved in transmission of a specific disease, while secondary vectors include species that are involved in transmission of a specific disease only under certain conditions (Goddard, 1999). Thus, not every mosquito can transmit *Plasmodium vivax*, one of the parasites causing malaria, rather *P. vivax* is mainly transmitted by the *Anopheles* mosquito, species of which are distributed throughout the U.S. Arthropods may transmit microorganisms mechanically (e.g., when flies feed on excrement and then walk on food), or biologically (e.g., when the organism multiplies or develops in the arthropod as in the multiplication of *Plasmodium* in mosquitoes transmitting malaria) (Goddard, 1999). Mosquitoes are the major vector of infectious diseases in humans followed by ticks (Parola & Raoult, 2001). Arthropods known to transmit microorganisms leading to disease are listed with a disease example:

- Mosquitoes (*Culex pipiens*, West Nile virus, and West Nile fever)
- Lice (the body louse, *Rickettsia prowazekii*, and epidemic typhus)
- Ticks (the deer tick, *B. burgdorferi*, and Lyme disease)
- Mites (mouse mite, *R. akari*, and rickettsialpox)
- Midges (biting midges, Oropouche virus, and Oropouche fever)
- Fleas (the oriental rat flea, *Yersinia pestis*, and plague)
- Flies (tsetse fly, *Trypanosoma brucei gambiense*, and sleeping sickness or human African trypanosomiasis, Gambian type) (Deubel, Gubler, Layton, & Malkinson, 2001; Goddard, 1999; Rauolt & Olson, 1999; Strickland, 2000)

Of interest in understanding, managing, and ultimately preventing and controlling the vector-borne EIDs is knowledge about (a) the contributions of ecologic, meteorologic, and climactic conditions in influencing environmental, vector, and reservoir variables; (b) the biology of the vector and the host reservoir; and (c) the human characteristics that contribute to emergence. Vector-borne diseases are particularly affected by environmental factors, including climate and weather conditions. For example, the emergence of the Sin Nombre virus resulting in hantavirus pulmonary syndrome initially in the southwestern United States was said to occur following specific weather conditions, leading to an increased prevalence in piñon nuts that fed deer mice carrying the hantavirus, as well as promoting the growth of vegetation providing shelter for them (Engelthaler, Mosley, Cheek, Levy, Komatsu, Ettestad, et al., 1999).

Foodborne and Waterborne Diseases

Overlap exists to some extent between foodborne and waterborne infectious diseases. Those organisms that are ingested and then cause illness (usually gastrointestinal) are usually transmissible through either food or water or both. In addition, food may be contaminated by water sources during activities such as planting, growing, harvesting, processing, preparation, and handling. The fecal-oral and person-to-person modes are the major routes of transmission of foodborne and waterborne EIDs. Causes of emerging foodborne illness include viruses, bacteria, parasites, altered prions, toxins that may or may not be of microbial origin, and other nonmicrobial substances. In a detailed analysis, foodborne illnesses from all causes including nonidentified pathogens was found to account for about 74 million illnesses, 323,914 hospitalizations, and 5,194 deaths per year in the United States, whereas foodborne diseases caused by known microbes are believed to cause about 14 million illnesses, 60,000 hospitalizations, and 1,800 deaths in the United States each year (Mead, Slutsker, Dietz, McCaig, Bresee, Shapiro, et al., 1999). Many of the responsible pathogens such as *Toxoplasma*, *Staphylococcus*, *Streptococcus*, and hepatitis A are not considered typical emerging infectious agents, whereas *Campylobacter jejuni*, *E. coli* O157:H7, *Listeria monocytogenes*, *Cyclospora cayetanensis*, and certain subtypes of *Salmonella* meet that criterion, and are of concern. Viruses are a frequent cause of gastroenteritis from food. The Norwalk-like virus, calciviruses that are a strain of a group of small, round structured viruses were recognized in 1972 in connection with a gastroenteritis outbreak in Norwalk, Ohio that had occurred in 1968 (Atmar & Estes, 2001; Centers for Disease Control and Prevention, 2000b). Rotavirus diarrhea, occurring primarily in children, was first identified in 1973 in Australia (Strickland, 2000). *Cryptosporidium*, usually thought of as a waterborne infection, can also be transmitted directly from food, and was transmitted to 88 people in Washington D.C. through raw produce prepared by an infected foodhandler (Quiroz, Bern, MacArthur, Xiao, Fletcher, Arrowood, et al., 2000).

Several factors are thought to be responsible for the increase in the number and type of foodborne diseases. These include

- demographic changes resulting in growing numbers of the population with immune compromise such as chronic illness, HIV infection, aging, or post-transplant;

- breakdown in surveillance;
- demand for organic foods;
- demand for exotic foods;
- demand for out-of-season produce leading to importation from some developing countries where agricultural practices result in compromised food safety;
- increased consumption of internationally distributed foods—a cholera outbreak in Maryland resulted from ingestion of coconut milk imported from southeast Asia, and an incident of staphylococcal food poisoning in the United States was associated with eating mushrooms canned in China;
- cultural food practices and habits such as eating undercooked pork leading to trichinosis in Laotians in the United States; eating raw or lightly cooked foods of animal origin such as shellfish, fish (as sushi or sashimi), or ground beef (as in steak tartare or served very rare);
- decrease in knowledge of food safety practices in the home such as washing hands thoroughly after handling raw poultry;
- reliance on convenience foods with a higher consumption of food not prepared in the home (this includes food eaten in eat-in restaurants and obtained from take-out facilities such as fast food restaurants and supermarkets; it also includes partial preparation of foods such as melons sliced in the produce section of supermarkets allowing the contamination of the inner surface by microbes on the outer surface);
- greater prevalence of food served in a salad bar or buffet type setting allowing contamination or varying temperature controls;
- economic development changes (e.g., shifting from a cold season oyster harvest to year round harvests in the Gulf of Mexico has been associated with the emergence of *Vibrio vulnificans* in oysters (Slutsker, Altekruse, & Swerdlow, 1998).

Contamination of foods can occur at multiple points from planting, growing, harvesting, and initial processing through transporting, distributing, later processing, preparing, and serving. Contamination can arise from contaminated irrigation water; use of manure or human fertilizer; poor sanitary practices in the fields, in handling areas and during preparation and serving; contaminated wash water; use of unclean vehicles for transportation and/or distribution; and cross-contamination. In a graphic illustration, observers have described Guatemalan raspberries in open containers waiting for shipment being contaminated by bird droppings until they were coated in white. Outbreaks arise from newly recognized pathogens and also from known pathogens contaminating foods not previously known to support their growth such as lettuce, sprouts, and apple cider (*E. coli* O157:H7). Because of changes in food distribution, outbreaks may now be widespread and harder to recognize. For example, an outbreak of *Salmonella* subtype Enteritidis infection was noticed because of an increase of gastroenteritis in southern Minnesota. An ice cream premix that was pasteurized at a plant on-site had to be transported to another plant to be made into a nationally distributed brand of ice cream. The tanker trucks had previously been used to haul raw eggs. Post-pasteurization contamination of the premix resulted in about 250,000 illnesses from eating the ice cream prepared from the premix that became contaminated during transport (Hennessey, Hedberg, Slutsker, White, Besser-Wiek, Moen, et al., 1996).

The consumption of fish, often raw or undercooked, has increased due to several factors—improvements in transport of fish, greater accessibility, awareness of health benefits, cultural influences, and increased per capita income. Sushi bars serving raw fish have multiplied. A new disease, metorchiasis, is caused by the North American liver fluke, *Metorchis conjunctus*, a helminth that is considered to have emerged in 1993. In Montreal, Canada, 27 persons became ill after eating sashimi (raw fish) infected with this organism at a picnic. The long-term oncogenic potential of this infection is unknown (MacLean, 1998). Another popular way of eating fish raw, as ceviche, prepared with lemon or lime juice to "cook" it, has resulted in foodborne infection. Gnathostomosis is another parasitic disease contracted from undercooked fish (Rojas-Molina, Pedraza-Sanchez, Torres-Bibiano, Meza-Martinez, & Escobar-Gutierrez, 1999).

Foodborne illnesses have a public health impact beyond the discomfort of acute gastroenteritis. Many can cause disability and chronic sequelae particularly in those who are immunologically compromised to some degree such as the elderly, children, transplant recipients, and persons with HIV infection. An example is Guillain-Barrê syndrome secondary to *Campylobacter* infection. Foodborne illness is often underreported, particularly when milder or nonspecific in nature (Mead et al., 1999; Yuki, 2001). Some foodborne pathogens are also spread through water or from person to person, and some of these pathogens are probably not yet identified.

Among well-publicized outbreaks of food-related emerging infections have been those of *E. coli* O157:H7 outbreaks through contaminated ground beef, unpasteurized apple cider, and alfalfa sprouts (see chapter 9); *Cyclospora* contamination of Guatemalan raspberries, mesclun lettuce, and fresh basil leaves (see chapter 6); variant CJD and contaminated beef (see chapter 17); *Listeria monocytogenes* and hot dogs, soft cheeses, and deli meats; and strains of *Salmonella enterica* serotype Newport contaminating alfalfa sprouts (Centers for Disease Control and Prevention, 2001a).

Campylobacter jejuni is currently the most frequently diagnosed bacterial foodborne infection in the United States with an approximate 2.1 million to 2.4 million cases occurring each year. A gram-negative rod-shaped bacteria, it was first identified as a diarrheal pathogen in 1973. The average incubation period is 3 days with a range of 1–7 days. Symptoms of *Campylobacter* enteritis typically include abdominal pain that is usually more severe than in shigellosis or salmonellosis, and severe watery diarrhea often with fever and generalized aching as well as nausea, but vomiting is not usual. Serious sequelae of *Campylobacter* infection can include Guillain-Barrê syndrome, and Reiter syndrome, a reactive arthopathy affecting multiple joints. *Campylobacter* has a varied animal reservoir including fowl, dogs, cats, rodents, cattle, hogs, sheep, and reptiles. *Campylobacter* frequently contaminates raw meat and broiler poultry. Raw milk or untreated water may also be sources. Infection often results from foods such as bread or salad that become contaminated from raw meats or poultry during preparation. The organism does not multiply once in food (Altekruse, Stern, Fields, & Swerdlow, 1999; Mandell, Bennett, & Dolin, 2000).

Listeria monocytogenes is a gram-positive bacteria capable of causing various illness in both humans and animals. In the past, it has been mostly associated with disease in those who are immunocompromised. Epidemic illnesses have been largely linked to refrigerated ready-to-eat foods such as coleslaw, hot dogs, deli foods, milk, soft low acid cheeses such as brie and feta, patê, and, recently, to contaminated corn in a salad (Aureli, Fiorucci, Caroli, Marchiaro, Novara, Leone, et al., 2000; Centers for Disease Control and Prevention, 2001a). *L. monocytogenes* can proliferate in biofilms and low temperatures so it can infect food processing plants (Schlech, 2000). The usual clinical picture includes diarrhea, fever, cramps, fatigue, headache, and myalgia. Central nervous system infections, especially meningitis and sepsis can occur. It is the fifth leading cause of bacterial meningitis in all age groups in both immunocompetent and immunocompromised persons. It causes about 2,500 serious illnesses and 500 deaths in the United States per year (Centers for Disease Control and Prevention, 2000a). Seven to twenty days after infection, maternal sepsis can result in abortion, stillbirth, or premature delivery (Schlech, 2000). Vertical transmission from mother to fetus can occur with the potential result of meningitis in newborns.

Salmonella serotype Enteritidis and serotype Typhimurium DT104 are nontyphoidal *Salmonella* that have been long known but which have increased in prevalence in recent years. In the 1970s, *Salmonella* Enteritidis accounted for about 5% of salmonellosis in the U.S. but this increased to about 25% in 1997. Its reservoirs include the periovarian tissue of hens' eggs where the bacteria may then infect the yolk membrane of an egg as it forms, as well as broiler chickens. Mice may be an intermediate host that pass the organism from one chicken flock to another. Better farm hygiene and the use of liquid eggs that can be pasteurized, especially with high-risk populations (e.g., nursing home residents), and egg refrigeration precautions should reduce infection in the United States (Tauxe, 1999). *Salmonella* Typhimurium DT104 has a reservoir in dairy cows where it causes illness. Most outbreaks in the U.S. have resulted from the ingestion of Mexican soft cheese made from raw milk or from raw milk consumption. Both organisms may result in gastroenteritis. *Salmonella* Typhimurium DT104 may cause bacteremia and life-threatening illness more frequently, and infection with multidrug-resistant strains may occur in patients who have or are taking antibiotics. This infection should be considered when a person develops diarrhea on antibiotic therapy (Tauxe, 1999). Other serotypes producing large outbreaks in 1999 were associated with produce vehicles such as unpasteurized orange juice, mangos, and raw sprouts (Centers for Disease Control and Prevention, 2000b).

Waterborne emerging infections may result from ingestion of contaminated drinking water or from contact with contaminated recreational water. Such infections may originate in the community in which the person resides, or may occur in the course of recreational pursuits either in developed areas, during travel to foreign locales or in wilderness areas (see chapter 22 for a discussion of EIDs in relation to travel and recreation). Conditions such as flooding may provide temporary favorable conditions for outbreaks of emerging infectious diseases through a variety of mechanisms including runoff from contaminated fields. The most frequent illnesses resulting from waterborne infections are gastrointestinal illness, dermatitis, and meningoencephalitis, the latter resulting from infection by free-living amoeba such as *Naegleria* when fresh water is forced up the nose of a swimmer or diver during the summer when conditions are favorable for such infection (Barwick, Levy, Craun, Beach, & Calderon, 2000). Contaminated water may contaminate food such as in grocery store spray systems, or result from direct exposure to organisms in these sprays such as *Legionella.* Waterborne infections can also occur from showering. In a recent outbreak of legionellosis in a children's hospital, showering was implicated as the means of exposure to contaminated potable water (Campins, Ferrer, Callis, Pelaz, Cortes, Pinart, et al., 2000). Hospital water supplies and water used for therapeutic purposes can unwittingly become the source for emerging infections such as *Legionella,* and atypical mycobacteria (Emmerson, 2001).

Drinking water systems may be community or noncommunity systems. The latter may be transient or nontransient. Millions of people per year use noncommunity water systems while traveling or working, usually without being aware of this. For example, transient noncommunity systems include highway rest stations, restaurants, and parks with their own water systems. Treatment, standards, and regulations vary according to the type of system (Barwick et al., 2000). Contamination of drinking water may occur through surface or groundwater source contamination, breaks in integrity of well and/or distribution systems, and breaks in disinfection or water treatment. CDC definitions of recreational waters include swimming pools, whirlpools, hot tubs, spas, water parks, and fresh and marine surface waters such as lakes, beaches, and springs (Barwick et al., 2000). *Legionella* infections can be acquired through exposure to sprays from whirlpools, hot tubs, spas and the like, and have even been associated with visiting an aquarium (World Health Organization, 2000). Decorative fountains may also be the source of waterborne disease outbreaks.

During 1997–1998, the most recent data available, 13 states reported 17 outbreaks of waterborne infection associated with drinking water, causing illness in about 2,038 persons. Ten of these outbreaks were of known infectious etiology—6 caused by parasites and 4 by bacteria. In five outbreaks the cause was not identified. Parasitic infections included four caused by *Giardia* (not considered an emerging infectious agent), and two by *Cryptosporidium.* In one of the cryptosporidiosis outbreaks in Texas, about 1,400 persons became ill after a lightening storm caused a spill of raw sewage that resulted in contamination of municipal utility district wells, illustrating how weather conditions can play a role in the emergence of infectious diseases. Earlier, *Cryptosporidium* was responsible for the largest known outbreak of emerging infectious disease contamination of drinking water in the United States, when about 403,000 persons became ill in Milwaukee, Wisconsin in 1993 (MacKenzie, Hoxie, Proctor, Gradus, Blair, Peterson, et al., 1994) (see chapter 5). Bacterial outbreaks were attributed to *E. coli* O157:H7, and *Shigella sonnei*. In one of the *E. coli* O157:H7 outbreaks, 157 persons were affected in Wyoming when an untreated community water system supplied by a spring and two wells was apparently contaminated by wildlife fecal material from the spring (Barwick et al., 2000).

In examining recreational waterborne outbreaks during the same period, 18 states reported 32 outbreaks associated with treated (17) and fresh (15) water, causing illness in about 2,128 persons. Of these, 29 outbreaks were associated with infectious etiology, some causing gastroenteritis (the majority) followed by dermatitis or neurologic disease. Gastroenteritis was most frequently caused by parasites (all *Cryptosporidium*), followed by bacteria (*E. coli* O157:H7 and *Shigella sonnei*), and then by Norwalk-like viruses, and *Leptospira* (see chapter 22). Dermatitis outbreaks were caused by *P. aeroginosa*, and a *Schistosoma* species. Four deaths were caused by primary amebic meningoencephalitis due to infection with *Naegleria* (Barwick et al., 2000). In one outbreak in a water park in Georgia, 26 persons were infected by *E. coli* O157:H7; 7 developed hemolytic uremic syndrome and one died. *E. coli* O157:H7 is discussed in chapter 9. It was believed that the source of the outbreak was a fecal accident in a children's pool in the water park (Gilbert & Blake, 1998). Prevention of food and waterborne infections is discussed in Appendix C, Tables C.1, C.2, and C.3.

Transfusion and Transplant Transmitted Emerging and Reemerging Infections

With the knowledge that HIV infection could be acquired via transfusion of blood or blood products came extensive political pressure to ensure the absolute safety of the transfusion of blood and blood products, especially in the United States. The ability to transmit infection by transfusion depends on a variety of elements including the pathogenicity of the agent, its prevalence in the blood donor population, the ability to persist in a host, and if so in which cell type, and the aspect of recipient immunity. Changes in approaches to blood donation and screening have resulted in minimal risk for transfusion-transmitted diseases in the United States but not in zero risk. Elsewhere the picture is different. More than two thirds of countries do not have policies in place that would ensure safe blood donations, and many of these countries have a heavy burden of emerging infectious agents (Klein, 2000). At times, pockets of specific risk occur that need to be immediately addressed such as the 1997 deferral of blood donations of members of the National Guard who had been exposed to ticks during a training exercise. Several later developed ehrlichiosis or Rocky Mountain spotted fever (Klein, 2000; McQuiston, Childs, Chamberland, & Tabor, for the Working Group on Transfusion Transmission of Tick-borne Diseases, 2000). Other examples of specific deferrals in response to potential emerging/reemerging infectious-disease risk include the decision in the United States to restrict donations as described in chapter 17 for those at risk for acquisition of the agent (altered prions) responsible for bovine spongiform encephalopathy and variant Creutzfeldt-Jakob disease, including deferral for relatives of persons with Creutzfeldt-Jakob disease (see chapter 17), and deferral of Desert Storm veterans because of exposure to *Leishmania donovani*, the parasitic agent of leishmaniasis (Klein, 2000). In light of the wider-than-realized spread of vCJD, most notably in Britain and western Europe, more stringent blood donation restrictions have been put in place (see chapter 17) to exclude persons who may have become infected with vCJD, but who are not symptomatic. Donors of other tissues might also be considered for exclusion (Roos, 2001).

The HIV epidemic focused attention on transfusion and transplant safety issues in regard to emerging infections. Even in the last 20 years, a variety of viral agents with the potential to be transmitted via blood transfusion have emerged. In addition to HIV, they include HTLV-I; HTLV-II; hepatitis C; Kaposi's sarcoma-associated virus or human herpesvirus 8; the hepatitis G or GB virus-C; herpesvirus-6; and the putative hepatitis-linked TT virus (Allain, 1998; 2000). The potential for other nonemerging agents to be transmitted in this way also occurs. These agents include cytomegalovirus, *Toxoplasma* and others, some of which pose particular risk to subsets of recipients such as those who are immunosuppressed (Moor, Dubbelman, VanSteveninck, & Brand, 1999). Concern about the transmission of tick-borne infectious agents via blood transfusion was evidenced by a conference held in January 1999 sponsored by CDC, the Food and Drug Administration, the National Institutes of Health, and the Department of Defense to review current information, identify possible risks, identify research strategies related to diagnostic test development, and assess whether or not policy changes in blood collection to address this potential risk are needed (McQuiston et al., 2000). The agents of focus were *Borrelia burgdorferi* causing Lyme disease, *Ehrlichia chaffeensis* causing human monocytic ehrlichiosis, an agent resembling *Ehrlichia equi/E. phagocytophila* causing human granulocytic ehrlichiosis, *Babesia microti* causing babesiosis, and *Rickettsia rickettsii* causing Rocky Mountain spotted fever which does not fit the usual definitions of an EID (McQuiston et al., 2000). Various other parasitic agents have also been known to be transmitted through transfusion, such as *Trypanosoma cruzi*, the agent of Chagas' disease and *Plasmodium vivax* and *P. falciparum*, agents of malaria. While these pose a minimal degree of risk in the United States and other developed countries overall, they pose a greater risk in areas with a high density of persons who have immigrated from countries where these agents are prevalent. They may also pose a risk to travelers needing a blood transfusion in countries where screening of the blood supply does not occur, and where there are high concentrations of persons who have been infected (some chronically) with infectious agents such as those that cause malaria, HIV infection, hepatitis, dengue, trypanosomiasis, and others. For example, in Latin America, there are 16–18 million persons with Chagas' disease (Strickland, 2000). In the U.S. persons who acquired the disease in childhood and who have immigrated to this country may be chronically infected, even if currently asymptomatic. Thus, the frequency of the organism in human blood varies across the population, being higher in areas of high concentration of immigrants from endemic countries. In the United States and Canada, as of 1999, there were 6 cases of *T. cruzi* transmission through transfusion reported (Dodd, 2000). In the United States from 1963–1999, 93 cases of transfusion-transmitted malaria were reported (Mungai, Tegtmeier, Chamberland, & Parise, 2001).

Currently, the major transfusion-transmitted emerging infections posing risk in the United States are all strains of human immunodeficiency virus (HIV), human T-lymphotropic virus I (HTLV-I), hepatitis B (HBV), and hepatitis C (HCV). (See chapters 11, 12, and 21 for more information.) The majority of these are transmitted by the infected person during the period between infection and the appearance of organisms or antibodies in the blood. The estimated risk for transmission of these through blood transfusions are: HIV (1 in 450,000 to 1 in 677,000 units), HTLV-I (1 in 641,000), HCV (1 in 103,000), and HBV (1 in 63,000) (Glynn, Kleinman, Schreiber, Busch, Wright, Smith, et al., 2000; Ling, Robbins, Brown, Dunmire, Thoe, Wong, et al., 2000). Appendix B, Table B.3 provides information on transfusion-transmitted emerging/reemerging infectious diseases.

The current system used in the United States to ensure blood safety includes sensitive screening tests; education and stringent screening, selection, and deferral procedures for donors; postdonation product quarantine; a safety surveillance system; and donor tracing and notification when needed (Klein, 2000). Newer methods of testing donated blood such as by nucleic acid testing increase blood safety (Chamberland, Alter, Busch, Nemo, & Ricketts, 2001).

Xenotransplantation, the use of tissues and organs for animal to human transplantation, poses a potential risk of the transfer of zoonoses from the animal donor not only to the human recipient but also to persons who come into professional or personal contact with him/her. Of particular concern are viruses, especially those that can cross species barriers. The porcine endogenous retroviruses have been noted as particularly worrisome since pigs are thought to be a major potential future source of tissues and organs for transplant for infants and children (Günzburg & Salmons, 2000). These issues are discussed in the U.S. Public Health Service guideline on infectious disease issues in xenotransplantation (Centers for Disease Control and Prevention, 2001c). Human-to-human transplantation has been a method of spread for CJD (see chapter 17).

Emerging infectious diseases may belong to any of the classifications of infectious agents, and are transmitted to humans by a variety of mechanisms. The reasons for their emergence may be complex and are delineated in chapter 1. Often several factors converge so that conditions become favorable for an organism to emerge. The best ways to protect against the major consequences of such outbreaks is by having a good public health infrastructure with appropriate surveillance mechanisms and response plans. The chapters in part II highlight specific emerging infectious diseases that have affected or have the potential to have a significant impact on health care.

REFERENCES

Allain, J. P. (1998). Emerging viruses in blood transfusion. *Vox Sanguinis, 74*, 125–129.

Allain, J. P. (2000). Emerging viruses in blood transfusion. *Vox Sanguinis, 78*(Suppl. 2), 243–248.

Altekruse, S. F., Stern, N. J., Fields, P. I., & Swerdlow, D. L. (1999). *Campylobacter jejuni*—an emerging foodborne pathogen. *Emerging Infectious Diseases, 5*, 28–35.

Alter, M. (2000). How is Creutzfeldt-Jakob disease acquired? *Neuroepidemiology, 19*, 55- 61.

Atmar, R. L., & Estes, M. K. (2001). Diagnosis of noncultivatable gastroenteritis viruses, the human caliciviruses. *Clinical Microbiology Reviews, 14*, 15–37.

Aureli, P., Fiorucci, G. C., Caroli, D., Marchiaro, G., Novara, O., Leone, L., & Salmaso, S. (2000). An outbreak of febrile gastroenteritis associated with corn contaminated by *Listeria monocytogenes*. *New England Journal of Medicine, 342*, 1236–1241.

Barwick, R. S., Levy, D. A., Craun, G. F., Beach, M. J., & Calderon, R. L. (2000). Surveillance for waterborne-disease outbreaks—United States, 1997–1998. *Morbidity and Mortality Weekly Report, 49*(SS4), 1–35.

Breitschwerdt, E. B., & Kordick, D. L. (2000). *Bartonella* infection in animals: Carriership, reservoir potential, pathogenicity, and zoonotic potential for human infection. *Clinical Microbiology Reviews, 13*, 428–438.

Brown, P., Will, R. G., Bradley, R., Asher, D. M., & Detwiler, L. (2001). Bovine spongiform encephalopathy and variant Creutzfeldt-Jakob disease: Background, evolution, and current concerns. *Emerging Infectious Diseases, 7*, 6–16.

Butler, P., Parkinson, A. J., Funk, E., Beller, M., Hayes, G., & Hughes, J. M. (1999). Emerging infectious diseases in Alaska and the Arctic: A review and a strategy for the 21st century. *Alaska Medicine, 41*(2), 35–43.

Campins, M., Ferrer, A., Callis, L., Pelaz, C., Cortes, P. J., Pinart, N., et al. (2000). Nosocomial Legionnaires' disease in a children's hospital. *Pediatric Infectious Disease Journal, 19*, 228–234.

Centers for Disease Control and Prevention. (1997). Creutzfeldt-Jakob disease associated with cadaveric dura mater grafts—Japan, January 1979–May 1996. *Morbidity and Mortality Weekly Report, 46*, 1066–1069.

Centers for Disease Control and Prevention. (1999). Update: Multistate outbreak of listeriosis—United States, 1998–1999. *Morbidity and Mortality Weekly Report, 48*, 1117–1118.

Centers for Disease Control and Prevention. (2000a). Multistate outbreak of listeriosis—United States, 2000. *Morbidity and Mortality Weekly Report, 49*, 1129–1130.

Centers for Disease Control and Prevention. (2000b). Preliminary FoodNet data on the incidence of foodborne illnesses—selected sites, United States, 1999. *Morbidity and Mortality Weekly Report, 49*, 201–205.

Centers for Disease Control and Prevention. (2000c). Probable locally acquired mosquito-transmitted *Plasmodium vivax* infection—Suffolk county, New York, 1999. *Morbidity and Mortality Weekly Report, 49*, 495–498.

Centers for Disease Control and Prevention. (2000d). Update: *Clostridium novyi* and unexplained illness among injecting-drug users—Scotland, Ireland and England, April–June 2000. *Morbidity and Mortality Weekly Report, 49*, 543–545.

Centers for Disease Control and Prevention. (2001a). Diagnosis and management of foodborne illnesses: A primer for physicians. *Morbidity and Mortality Weekly Report, 50*(RR-02), 1–69.

Centers for Disease Control and Prevention. (2001b). "Norwalk-like viruses." Public health consequences and outbreak management. *Morbidity and Mortality Weekly Report, 50*(No. RR-9), 1–20.

Centers for Disease Control and Prevention. (2001c). U.S. Public Health Service guideline on infectious disease issues in xenotransplantation. *Morbidity and Mortality Weekly Report, 50*(No. RR-15), 1–50.

Chamberland, M. E., Alter, H. J., Busch, M. P., Nemo, G., & Ricketts, M. (2001). Emerging infectious disease issues in blood safety. *Emerging Infectious Diseases, 7*(3, Suppl.), 552–553.

Conrad, D. A. (2001). Treatment of cat-scratch disease. *Current Opinion in Pediatrics, 13*(1), 56–59.

Didier, E. (1998). Microsporidiosis. *Clinical Infectious Diseases, 27*, 1–8.

Dodd, R. Y. (2000). Transmission of parasites and bacteria by blood components. *Vox Sanguinis, 78*(Suppl. 2), 239–242.

Emmerson, A. M. (2001). Emerging waterborne infections in health-care settings. *Emerging Infectious Diseases, 7*, 272–276.

Engelthaler, D. M., Mosley, D. G., Cheek, J. E., Levy, C. E., Komatsu, K. K., Ettestad, P., et al. (1999). Climatic and environmental patterns associated with hantavirus pulmonary syndrome, Four Corners region, United States. *Emerging Infectious Diseases, 5*, 87–94.

File, T. M., Jr., & Tan, J. S. (2000). Group A streptococcus necrotizing fasciitis. *Comprehensive Therapy, 26*, 73–81.

Franzen, C., & Müller, A. (2001). Microsporidiosis: Human diseases and diagnosis. *Microbes and Infection, 3*, 389–400.

Gao, F., Bailes, E., Robertson, D. L., Chen, Y., Rodenburg, C. M., Michael, S. F., Cummins, L. B., et al. (1999). Origin of HIV-1 in the chimpanzee *Pan troglodytes troglodytes*. *Nature, 397*, 436–441.

Gilbert, L., & Blake, P. (1998). Outbreak of *Escherichia coli* O157:H7 infections associated with a water park. *Georgia Epidemiology Report, 14*, 1–2.

Glynn, S. A., Kleinman, S. H., Schreiber, G. B., Busch, M. P., Wright, D. J., Smith, J. W., et al. (2000). Trends in incidence and prevalence of major transfusion-transmissible viral infections in U.S. blood donors, 1991 to 1996. *Journal of the American Medical Association, 284*, 229–235.

Goddard, J. (1999). Arthropods, tongue worms, leeches, and arthropod-borne diseases. In R. L. Guerrant, D. H. Walker, & P. F. Weller (Eds.), *Tropical infectious diseases: Principles, pathogens, & practice* (pp. 1325–1342). Philadelphia: Churchill Livingstone.

Günzburg, W. H., & Salmons, B. (2000). Xenotransplantation: Is the risk of viral infection as great as we thought? *Molecular Medicine Today, 6*, 199–208.

Hahn, B., Shaw, G., De Cock, K., & Sharp, P. (2000). AIDS as a zoonosis: Scientific and public health implications. *Science, 287,* 607–614.

Hansen, G. R., Woodall, J., Brown, C., Jaax, N., McNamara, T., & Ruiz, A. (2001). Emerging zoonotic diseases. *Emerging Infectious Diseases,* 7(3, Suppl.), 537.

Hajjeh, R. A., Reingold, A., Weil, A., Shutt, K., Schuchat, A., & Perkins, B. A. (1999). Toxic shock syndrome in the United States: Surveillance update, 1979–1996. *Emerging Infectious Diseases,* 5, 807–810.

Hatta, M., Gao, P., Halfmann, P., & Kawaoka, Y. (2001). Molecular basis for high virulence of Hong Kong H5N1 influenza A viruses. *Science, 293,* 1840–1842.

Hennessey, T. W., Hedberg, C. W., Slutsker, L., White, K. E., Besser-Wiek, J. M., Moen, M. E., et al. (1996). A national outbreak of *Salmonella* enteritidis infections from ice cream. *New England Journal of Medicine, 334,* 1281–1286.

Horimoto, T., & Kawaoka, Y. (2001). Pandemic threat posed by avian influenza A viruses. *Clinical Microbiology Reviews, 14,* 129–149.

Jones, T. F., Kellum, M. E., Porter, S. S., Bell, M., & Schaffner, W. (2002). *Emerging Infectious Diseases, 8* [On-line]. Available: http://www.cdc.gov/ncidod/EID/eid.htm

Kerkhoff, F. T., Bergmans, A. M. C., Van der Zee, A., & Rothova, A. (1999). Demonstration of *Bartonella grahamii* DNA in ocular fluids of a patient with neuroretinitis. *Journal of Clinical Microbiology,* 37, 4034–4038.

Klein, H. G. (2000). Will blood transfusion ever be safe enough? *Journal of the American Medical Association, 284*(2), 238–240.

Koehler, J. E. (1998). *Bartonella*: An emerging human pathogen. In W. M. Scheld, D. Armstrong, & J. M. Hughes (Eds.), *Emerging infections 1* (pp. 147–163). Washington, DC: ASM Press.

Kolata, G. (2001). *Flu: The story of the great influenza pandemic of 1918 and the search for the virus that caused it.* New York: Simon and Schuster.

Lashley, F. R. (2000). The clinical spectrum of HIV infection and its treatment. In J. D. Durham & F. R. Lashley (Eds.), *The person with HIV/AIDS: Nursing perspectives* (3rd ed., pp. 167–269). New York: Springer Publishing Co.

Ling, A. E., Robbins, K. E., Brown, T. M., Dunmire, V., Thoe, S. Y. S., Wong, S. Y., et al. (2000). Failure of routine HIV-1 tests in a case involving transmission with preseroconversion blood components during the infectious window period. *Journal of the American Medical Association, 284,* 210–214.

Mackenzie, J. S. (1999). Emerging viral diseases: An Australian perspective. *Emerging Infectious Diseases,* 5, 1–8.

MacKenzie, W. R., Hoxie, N. J., Proctor, M. E., Gradus, M. S., Blair, K. A., Peterson, D. E., et al. (1994). A massive outbreak in Milwaukee of *Cryptosporidium* infection transmitted through the public water supply. *New England Journal of Medicine, 331,* 161–167.

MacLean, J. D. (1998). The North American liver fluke, *Metorchis conjunctus.* In W. M. Scheld, W. A. Craig, & J. M. Hughes (Eds.), *Emerging infections 2* (pp. 243–256). Washington, DC: ASM Press.

Maguiña, C., & Gotuzzo, E. (2000). Bartonellosis: New and old. *Infectious Disease Clinics of North America, 14,* 1–22.

Mandell, G. L., Bennett, J. E., & Dolin, R. (Eds.). (2000). *Mandell, Douglas, and Bennett's principles and practice of infectious diseases* (5th ed.). Philadelphia: Churchill Livingstone.

Mathis, A. (2000). Microsporidia: Emerging advances in understanding the basic biology of these unique organisms. *International Journal For Parasitology, 30*, 795–804.

Matsubayashi, N., Koike, T., Mikata, I., Takei, N., & Hagiwara, S. (1959). A case of *Encephalitozoon*-like body infection in man. *Archives of Pathology, 67*, 181–187.

McQuiston, J. H., Childs, J. E., Chamberland, M. E., & Tabor, E., for the Working Group on Transfusion Transmission of Tick-borne Diseases. (2000). Transmission of tick-borne agents of disease by blood transfusion: A review of known and potential risks in the United States. *Transfusion, 40*, 274–284.

Mead, P. S., Slutsker, L., Dietz, V., McCaig, L. F., Bresee, J. S., Shapiro, C., et al. (1999). Food-related illness and death in the United States. *Emerging Infectious Diseases, 5*, 207–225.

Mètènier, G., & Vivarès, C. P. (2001). Molecular characteristics and physiology of microsporidia. *Microbes and Infection, 3*, 407–415.

Moor, A. C. E., Dubbelman, T. M. A. R., VanSteveninck, J., & Brand, A. (1999). Transfusion-transmitted diseases: Risks, prevention and perspectives. *European Journal of Haematology, 62*, 1–18.

Mota, P., Rauch, C. A., & Edberg, S. C. (2000). Microsporidia and *Cyclospora*: Epidemiology and assessment of risk from the environment. *Critical Reviews in Microbiology, 26*, 69–90.

Mungai, M., Tegtmeier, G., Chamberland, M., & Parise, M. (2001). Transfusion-transmitted malaria in the United States from 1963 through 1999. *New England Journal of Medicine, 344*, 1973–1978.

Murray, K., Eaton, B., Hooper, P., Wang, L., Williamson, M., & Young, P. (1998). Flying foxes, horses, and humans: A zoonosis caused by a new member of the *Paramyxoviridae*. In W. M. Scheld, D. Armstrong, & J. M. Hughes (Eds.), *Emerging infections I* (pp. 43–58). Washington, DC: ASM Press.

Nichols, G. L. (2000). Food-borne protozoa. *British Medical Bulletin, 56*, 209–235.

Olsen, S. J., DeBess, E. E., McGivern, T. E., Marano, N., Eby, T., Mauvais, S., et al. (2001). A nosocomial outbreak of fluoroquinolone-resistant *Salmonella* infection. *New England Journal of Medicine, 344*, 1572–1579.

Paradisi, F., Corti, G., & Messeri, D. (2001). Antistaphylococcal (MSSA, MRSA, MSSE, MRSE) antibiotics. *Medical Clinics of North America, 85*, 1–16.

Parola, P., & Raoult, D. (2001). Ticks and tickborne bacterial diseases in humans: An emerging infectious threat. *Clinical Infectious Diseases, 32*, 897–928.

Phillips, R. S. (2001). Current status of malaria and potential for control. *Clinical Microbiology Reviews, 14*, 208–226.

Pozio, E. (2000). Is horsemeat trichinellosis an emerging disease in the EU? *Parasitology Today, 16*, 266.

Pretorius, A-M., & Kelly, P. J. (2000). An update on human bartonelloses. *Central African Journal of Medicine, 46*, 194–200.

Prusiner, S. B. (2001). Shattuck lecture—neurodegerative diseases and prions. *New England Journal of Medicine, 344*, 1516–1524.

Quiroz, E. S., Bern, C., MacArthur, J. R., Xiao, L., Fletcher, M., Arrowood, M. J., et al. (2000). An outbreak of cryptosporidiosis linked to a foodhandler. *Journal of Infectious Diseases, 181*, 695–700.

Rauolt, D., & Olson, J. G. (1999). Emerging rickettsioses. In W. M. Scheld, W. A. Craig, & J. M. Hughes (Eds.), *Emerging infections 3* (pp. 17–35). Washington, DC: ASM Press.

Reingold, A. L. (1998). Toxic shock syndrome (staphylococcal). In A. S. Evans & P. S. Brachman (Eds.), *Bacterial infections of humans* (3rd ed., pp. 759–775). New York: Plenum Medical Book Co.

Robinson, L. A. (1999). Aspergillus and other fungi. *Chest Surgery Clinics of North America, 9*, 193–225.

Rojas-Molina, N., Pedraza-Sanchez, S., Torres-Bibiano, B., Meza-Martinez, H., & Escobar-Gutierrez, A. (1999). Gnathostomosis, an emerging foodborne zoonotic disease in Acapulco, Mexico. *Emerging Infectious Diseases, 5*, 264–266.

Roos, R. P. (2001). Controlling new prion diseases. *New England Journal of Medicine, 344*, 1548–1551.

Schantz, P. M., Moore, A. C., Muñoz, J. L., Hartman, B. J., Schaefer, J. A., Aron, A. M., et al. (1992). Neurocysticercosis in an orthodox Jewish community. *New England Journal of Medicine, 327*, 692–695.

Schlech, W. F., III. (2000). Foodborne listeriosis. *Clinical Infectious Diseases, 31*, 770–775.

Schmidt, A. (Ed.). (1998). Bartonella *and* Afipia *species emphasizing* Bartonella henselae. Basel: Karger.

Selvey, L. A. R. M., Wells, J. G., McCormack, A. J., Ansford, K., Murray, R. J., Rogers, R. J., et al. (1995). Infection of humans and horses by a newly described morbillivirus. *Medical Journal of Australia, 162*, 642–645.

Shortridge, K. F., Gao, P., Guan, Y., Ito, T., Kawaoka, Y., Markwell, D., et al. (2000). Interspecies transmission of influenza viruses: H5N1 virus and a Hong Kong SAR perspective. *Veterinary Microbiology, 74*, 141–147.

Sirisanthana, T. (2001). *Penicillium marneffei* infection in patients with AIDS. *Emerging Infectious Diseases*, 7(3 Suppl.), 561.

Slutsker, L., Altekruse, S. F., & Swerdlow, D. L. (1998). Foodborne diseases: Emerging pathogens and trends. *Infectious Disease Clinics of North America, 12*, 199–214.

Stevens, D. L. (2000). Streptococcal toxic shock syndrome associated with necrotizing fasciitis. *Annual Review of Medicine, 51*, 271–288.

Stevens, D. L. (2001). Invasive streptococcal infections. *Journal of Infection and Chemotherapy, 7*, 69–80.

Stoler, M. H., Bonfiglio, T. A., Steigbigel, R. T., & Pereira, M. (1983). An atypical subcutaneous infection associated with acquired immune deficiency syndrome. *American Journal of Clinical Pathology, 80*, 714–718.

Strickland, G. T. (Ed.). (2000). *Hunter's tropical medicine and emerging infectious diseases*. Philadelphia: WB Saunders Co.

Tauxe, R. V. (1999). *Salmonella* Enteritidis and *Salmonella* Typhimurium DT104: Successful subtypes in the modern world. In W. M. Scheld, W. A. Craig, & J. M. Hughes (Eds.), *Emerging infections 3* (pp. 37–52). Washington, DC: ASM Press.

Todd, J., Fishaut, M., Kapral, F., & Welch, T. (1978). Toxic-shock syndrome associated with phage-group-I Staphlococci. *Lancet, 2,* 1116–1118.

van den Heuvel, J. F. J. M., Hogenhout, S. A., & van der Wilk, F. (1999). Recognition and receptors in virus transmission by arthropods. *Trends in Microbiology, 7,* 71–76.

Verhoef, J. (2001). Stopping short the spread of methicillin-resistant *Staphlococcus aureus. Canadian Medical Association Journal, 165,* 31–32.

Walsh, T. J. (1998). Emerging fungal pathogens: Evolving challenges to immunocompromised patients. In W. M. Scheld, D. Armstrong, & J. M. Hughes (Eds.), *Emerging infections 1* (pp. 221–232). Washington, DC: ASM Press.

Weiss, R. A. (2001). The Leeuwenhoek lecture 2001. Animal origins of human infectious disease. *Philosophical Transactions of the Royal Society of Medicine, 356,* 957–977.

White, A. C., Jr. (2000). Neurocysticercosis: Updates on epidemiology, pathogenesis, diagnosis and management. *Annual Review of Medicine, 51,* 187–206.

Will, R. G., Ironside, J. W., Zeidler, M., Cousens, S. N., Estibeiro, K., Alperovitch, A., et al. (1996). A new variant of Creutzfeldt-Jakob disease in the U.K. *Lancet, 347,* 921–925.

Windsor, J. J. (2001). Cat-scratch disease: Epidemiology, aetiology and treatment. *British Journal of Biomedical Sciences, 58,* 101–110.

World Health Organization. (2000.) Outbreak news. Legionellosis, Australia (update). *Weekly Epidemiological Record, 75,* 173.

Yuki, N. (2001). Infectious origins of, and molecular mimicry in, Guillain-Barré and Fisher syndromes. *Lancet Infectious Diseases, 1,* 29–37.

Zucker, J. R. (1996). Changing patterns of autochthonous malaria transmission in the United States: A review of recent outbreaks. *Emerging Infectious Diseases, 2,* 37–43.

Part II

Specific Diseases

4

Cholera

Laurie J. Singel and Felissa R. Lashley

As the red light above the luggage carousel began to flash, Michael Lee, a 34-year-old businessman, smiled in anticipation. He had just spent a week on a fishing trip to the Gulf Coast, and was returning with a well-established tan and a cooler, packed with Gulf shrimp and crabs. He planned to throw a party later that night, serving his Chicago friends the delicacies from the Gulf. Two days later, Mr. Lee was rushed by ambulance to a local hospital, after collapsing at home from loss of fluids and electrolytes, from what he thought was a simple case of "travelers' diarrhea."

Positive identification of a stool specimen from Mr. Lee revealed a surprising diagnosis: *Vibrio cholerae*, biotype El Tor, serogroup O1. The nursing staff were baffled as to how a healthy businessman, vacationing within the United States, could contract such a disease. Cholera cases are usually limited to developing countries without proper sanitation facilities and clean water. Mr. Lee received rapid, large-volume intravenous fluid replacement and was discharged to his home 3 days after admission without any complications. The cause of the outbreak was later traced to undercooking of the contaminated shellfish he had brought back from the Gulf.

Although this type of scenario is rare in the United States, cholera, the acute diarrheal disease caused by the bacterium *Vibrio cholerae*, is no longer restricted to developing countries, but is considered to have a worldwide distribution and is endemic in much of the world. In 2000, 56 countries officially reported cholera to the World Health

Organization (WHO), for a total of 137,071 cases worldwide, a decrease from 1999 when 61 countries reported cholera. The majority of the global cases were from Africa (87%), especially Madagascar, South Africa, Mozambique, Democratic Republic of the Congo, Tanzania, followed by Asia, especially Afghanistan, India, China, Iraq, and Iran. There was a decline from the Americas especially in the west coast of South America, and only four imported cases in the United States. In Europe, there were no locally acquired cases in contrast to the previous year when there were 7 such cases in the Russian Federation and the Ukraine (World Health Organization, 2000; 2001a). In late 2000 and early 2001, cholera outbreaks were much more severe than expected in South Africa, Zimbabwe, and Malawi although an upswing is usually anticipated during the rainy season.

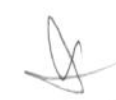

Vibrio cholerae is a highly motile, gram-negative anaerobic bacteria with a long, unipolar flagellum, that propels it through water. These bacteria prefer an alkaline environment. They thrive in brackish water, that is, water that contains elevated sodium levels and organic matter, but they can also survive in fresh water. The bacteria can also survive freezing. *V. cholerae* is classified into groups based on the O antigen of the organism by whether or not the isolate aggulutinates sera from patients who had cholera (Albert & Morris, 2000). There are 193 serogroups of *V. cholerae* that are now recognized (Basu, Garg, Datta, Chakraborty, Bhattacharya, Khan, et al., 2000). While until recently it was thought that only strains of the serogroup O1 could cause cholera, there are now two serogroups of *V. cholerae* known to cause cholera, O1 and O139 (also called Bengal after the site of its origin). The group that did not agglutinate sera were initially thought to be nonpathogenic, but it is now known that this is not the case. This non-agglutinating group may be collectively referred to as non-O1, non-O139 group or noncholera vibrios (Albert & Morris, 2000; Levine & Gotuzzo, 1999). *V. cholerae* O1 has two biotypes, the classic and El Tor, and each biotype has two major serotypes known as Ogawa and Inaba with a third intermediate one known as Hikojima. *V. cholerae* has the ability to essentially hibernate in less favorable environmental conditions, and while it is viable in this state, it may not be able to be cultured. It can survive up to 14 days in foods and can be shed by humans for months or even years (Seas & Gotuzzo, 2000). *V. cholerae* has a natural reservoir in warm estuarine waters where it may attach to plankton and other plant life as well as invade shellfish, or be free-living. Once humans are infected, pathogenic strains of *V. cholera* that cause cholera produce an enterotoxin known as the cholera toxin that results in the typical severe diarrhea and fluid and electrolyte loss described below (Albert & Morris, 2000).

Descriptions of what some historians believe was cholera were first noted in the writings of Hindu physicians about 400 BC (Cartwright, 1972), but there has been much debate among medical historians as to whether cholera is a disease of ancient populations or whether it emerged in the early 19th century as a new infectious disease of humans (Levine & Gotuzzo, 1999). Cholera outbreaks were historically associated with the industrial civilization of developing countries. Rapidly growing cities attracted large numbers of workers, who flooded into crowded slums and overwhelmed the available public health services. Breaks in sanitation led to contamination of food and water supplies, with resultant epidemics. The classic work of John Snow during the cholera epidemics in London in the 1850s regarding the Broad Street pump as the source of infection, and ultimately in establishing the importance of clean water in preventing cholera, is well known (Albert & Morris, 2000). The establishment of European empires in Asia helped cholera spread from its homeland in the Bengal basin, at the delta of the Ganges and Brahmaputra rivers, to other parts of the world, in repeated pandemic waves that affected virtually all of the inhabited world. Of the seven pandemics of cholera since the first was recorded in 1817, six have originated in the Ganges delta of India, an estuarine environment with ideal conditions for *V. cholerae* (Tauxe, 1998).

Cholera then went into an unexplained 50-year lull after the sixth pandemic, but emerged again in 1961 on the Celebes island of Sulawesi, Indonesia and had moved to Asia, parts of Europe, and Africa by the 1970s largely through trade, tourism, and religious pilgrimage routes (Albert & Morris, 2000; Tauxe & Barrett, 1998). This seventh pandemic, caused by *V. cholerae* O1, El Tor strain, has continued since then. At this time, cases of cholera were identified in the southern United States, and in northeastern Australia, but were cases determined not to be part of the pandemic (Tauxe & Barrett, 1998). In 1991, cholera outbreaks began in Peru, and by 1992, most of Central and South America had been affected. This was believed to have resulted from a ship carrying contaminated water from Asia in its ballast tanks to the coast of Peru where the tanks were discharged, contaminating shellfish beds. The contamination can occur because oysters feed by using their gills to filter water. If the water is contaminated with parasites, they can harbor the parasites in their gills. When humans eat the oysters raw or without adequate cooking, infection can result. In 1992, the then new strain of *V. cholerae*, O139, emerged in Madras, India, spreading quickly through Asia. Some refer to this as a possible eighth pandemic while others do not (Tauxe & Barrett, 1998; Levine & Gotuzzo, 1999). In many countries, cholera has become endemic after the pandemic has passed through the area. In addition to the Ganges delta in India, cholera is now endemic in the Philippines, a number of countries in Southeast Asia, sub-Saharan Africa, and several Latin American countries including Peru and Ecuador (Levine & Gotuzzo, 1999).

In the United States, from 1965 to 1991, the start of the epidemic in Latin America, only 136 cases of cholera were reported, while from 1992 to 1994, 160 cases were reported from 20 states and 1 territory. The vast majority of these people acquired cholera during travel—either U.S. residents who returned to their country of origin to visit, or non-U.S. residents who visited the U.S. from cholera-affected countries (Mahon, Mintz, Greene, Wells, & Tauxe, 1996). In 1992, an Aerolineas Argentina flight originating in Buenos Aires with a stop in Lima, Peru arrived in Los Angeles. One week later, 31 people, most dispersed to California or Nevada were found to have culture-confirmed *V. cholerae* infection, whereas 54 others had diarrheal illness (Centers for Disease Control and Prevention, 1992a). In another example, a man boarded a flight in the Philippines bound for Hawaii. He developed severe diarrhea while on board, which was later determined to be caused by *V. cholerae* O1 biotype El Tor (Centers for Disease Control and Prevention, 1992b). Other U.S. cases have been acquired through contaminated foods, often imported ones, including the following examples. In August, 1991, three cases of cholera resulted when people attending a party ate a homemade rice pudding topped with a topping containing frozen coconut milk. The milk, produced in Thailand and exported to the U.S., was the source of the outbreak (Centers for Disease Control and Prevention, 1991a). In two separate instances in 1991, visits by two persons to Ecuador included buying frozen crab meat there and bringing it back to the United States. It was then served cooked at their respective dinner parties resulting in eight cases of cholera in New Jersey and four in New York (Centers for Disease Control and Prevention, 1991b, 1991c). In March, 1994, a woman in California developed cholera after eating raw seaweed that a friend had brought back from the Philippines (Vugia, Shefer, Douglas, Greene, Bryant, & Werner, 1997).

In 1973, one case of cholera was reported in Texas—that of a fisherman who had the *V. cholerae* O1 El Tor strain, and 5 years later, an outbreak of an identical strain occurred in about 24 persons resulting from undercooked, contaminated seafood from the Gulf of Mexico, leading to identification of a focus of infection in the brackish Gulf waters that affected persons in Louisiana and Texas (Blake, Allegra, Snyder, Barrett, McFarland, Caraway, et al., 1980; Levine & Gotuzzo, 1999; Weissman, Dewitt, Thompson, Muchnick, Portnoy, Feeley, et al., 1974). Cases of cholera in the U.S. not associated with travel are most often due to eating contaminated shellfish such as crabs, shrimp, or oysters from the Gulf of Mexico, which hosts a persistent strain of *V. cholerae*. Mobile Bay oyster beds were found contaminated with the El Tor biotype of *V. cholerae* during a routine check in 1991, and were closed for a time. About 8 months after reopening, they were again found contaminated and were closed until August, 1992. Since then no new isolates have been found there (Centers for Disease Control and Prevention, 1993).

The major source for the transmission of cholera is contaminated water, especially when a common source is used for washing, bathing, and drinking. The fecal-oral route of transmission is the major one. Food that has been in contact with contaminated water is another major source, and foods known to have transmitted cholera have included shellfish, coconut milk, raw vegetables, and cooked rice, lentils, and other grains, especially when these are reheated. Acidifying condiments such as lemons, limes, tomatoes, or yogurt can help prevent the growth of the organism on grains. Nosocomial transmission is possible but is not a major source of infection. Cholera is not usually spread through person-to-person contact but in some instances this does occur (Albert & Morris, 2000). Transmission coincidental with sharing food with an infected person and eating food at a funeral feast in Africa for deceased cholera victims have been described. Methods of geographic spread have included travel-associated cases involving an asymptomatic infected person (Tauxe & Barrett, 1998). In one case, such an individual who became infected abroad transmitted *V. cholerae* to others via a dish of sliced fresh fruit she prepared in the U.S. (Ackers, Pagaduan, Hart, Greene, Abbott, Mintz, et al., 1997). Other methods of spread have been through commercial and recreational travel, and the Muslim pilgrimage to Mecca (Hajj) has played a role in several of the pandemics (Tauxe & Barrett, 1998). Other ways in which cholera enters a new geographic site include through contaminated foods from another country and from the ballast waters of ships. In these cases, ships had taken on ballast water in countries with cholera infections. They then exchanged the water in ports where cholera was not present previously, contaminating shellfish beds and washing to shore. It has been recommended that ships exchange ballast waters on the high seas before entry into U.S. ports (McCarthy & Khambaty, 1994).

Susceptibility and severity of illness are determined by many factors, including size of the inoculum, the biotype, any preexisting immunity, and other host and organism factors (Ryan & Calderwood, 2000). Persons with blood group O, and those with hypochlorhydria from causes such as malnutrition, medications that reduce acid in the stomach, atrophic gastritis, and chronic *Helicobacter pylori* infection appear to be particularly vulnerable. In regard to age, in endemic areas, a peak incidence is observed in children aged 2–9 years, while it is rare in children below 1 year (Albert & Morris, 2000). The elderly may be susceptible because of decreased immunity or less gastric acid (Tauxe, 1998). In non-endemic areas, cases may be distributed across age groups (Albert & Morris, 2000). Women of childbearing age may be particularly susceptible. Cases are rare among health staff caring for cholera patients, microbiologists, and undertakers preparing the bodies of cholera victims for burial, which highlights the effectiveness of simple hygienic measures in the prevention of cholera transmission (Tauxe & Barrett, 1998).

Seasonality is observed in endemic areas that are related in India and other parts of Asia to the monsoon onset and to warm weather (Albert & Morris, 2000). A role has been postulated for a relationship between cholera and the El Niño Southern Oscillation (ENSO) that is a source of interannual variation in climate in Bangladesh (Pascual, Rodó, Ellner, Colwell, & Bouma, 2000). Global warming is associated with floods and droughts, both of which can promote waterborne diseases such as cholera. When excess rains resulting from a warmed Indian Ocean to the Horn of Africa occurred in 1997–1998, epidemics of cholera resulted. A heated Caribbean sea resulted in Hurricane Mitch being stalled over Central America for 3 days resulting in thousands of cases of cholera in Honduras (Epstein, 2000).

In developing countries, a presumptive diagnosis of cholera is made when a report is received of two or more adults with severe watery diarrhea or an adult dying of watery diarrhea (Tauxe & Barrett, 1998). In the United States, anyone with a severe diarrheal illness, who has recently traveled to a developing country, is suspected to have been infected with *V. cholerae* and appropriate stool cultures are done. While the symptoms may be presumptively diagnostic, particularly during an epidemic, several commercial rapid tests are available that are based on monoclonal antibody agglutination, latex agglutination, or other techniques. PCR and DNA probe testing can be used in some circumstances as can cultures and microscopy (Albert & Morris, 2000). The incubation period for cholera may range from 12–72 hours, with 18–40 hours being the average, depending on the inoculum ingested and the susceptibility of the host (Levine & Gotuzzo, 1999). After ingestion, the bacteria pass through the stomach to the small intestine where they produce the cholera toxin, that causes the intestines to fill with an alkaline, salty fluid, greatly facilitating the growth of *V. cholerae* (Tauxe & Barrett, 1998).

Although the majority of cholera infections are either asymptomatic or mildly symptomatic, in the full clinically manifested cases, the first symptom is usually diarrhea that begins when the diarrheal fluid accumulates in the small intestine and causes distention, increased intestinal motility, and decreased transit time (Albert & Morris, 2000). This diarrhea progresses over several hours to assume a translucent rice-water appearance that is typical of cholera. The fluid loss through diarrhea can be as much as one liter per hour, leading rapidly to dehydration, tachycardia, hypotension, and vascular collapse. Patients may develop acidosis with Kussmaul breathing, and signs of severe dehydration such as lack of urine production, sunken eyes, raspy voices, and poor skin turgor. Vomiting may occur even before the diarrhea. As the severity of the illness increases, patients can become obtunded although they are usually conscious (Albert & Morris, 2000). Severe muscular cramping may occur, particularly in the legs. Rehydration is the cornerstone of treatment. If dehydration is not severe, oral rehydration using oral rehydration solution can be accomplished and is relatively inexpensive. If it is available intravenous fluid therapy may be needed to quickly restore fluid volume (Albert & Morris, 2000). Antibiotic therapy is generally secondary to the fluid replacement and typically consists of tetracycline or doxycycline, depending on the local pattern of resistance to *V. cholerae*. Cholera cots have been used for patients with severe diarrhea to facilitate stool collection and disposal. Often both diagnosis and treatment must take place under field conditions in developing countries during epidemics, and procedures for such conditions have been developed by WHO. Fortunately, "the disease is reversible to the moment of death" (Tauxe, 1998, p. 235). With rapid and appropriate rehydration and therapy, mortality commonly thought to be 25%–50% if untreated, is reduced to 1% or less (Tauxe, 1998).

Groups such as the World Health Organization and the Centers for Disease Control and Prevention have developed simple strategies for use in developing countries with increased potential for cholera outbreaks. Prevention of cholera transmission appears to be relatively clearcut for an individual: basic hygienic procedures such good hand washing; clean, chlorinated water sources with good pressure; avoidance of raw or undercooked shellfish; thorough cooking of all foods, avoiding shellfish from potentially contaminated waters; avoidance of food and beverages sold by street vendors; use of narrow-necked containers to store water so that the water is not contaminated by hands scooping water from it; and appropriate disposal of human waste. As *V. cholerae* are "exquisitely sensitive to acid," simple modifications in food preparation including the use of lemons, limes, tomatoes, tamarinds, and yogurt can acidify foods so that *V. cholerae* cannot survive (Levine & Gotuzzo, 1999; Rodrigues, Sandström, Cá, Steinsland, Jensen, & Aaby, 2000). Training of street vendors in appropriate sanitation, and educating consumers regarding food vendors is also important (Tauxe, 1998). Industrialized countries, such as the United States, have the resources to provide these basic services and a network of surveillance agencies to monitor public health concerns. In developing countries, building infrastructures to support delivery of clean water and proper elimination of waste products is often considered too expensive and complicated to implement, but is necessary for long-term prevention.

Although oral cholera vaccines are available in countries outside the United States, they only provide short-term protection and varying effects, and U.S. public health authorities have not been eager to recommend widespread use of such vaccines, although the WHO is more liberal about use recommendations (World Health Organization, 2000). Work continues on vaccine development and an important step toward this goal occurred when the *V. cholerae* DNA was sequenced (Fraser, Eisen, & Salzberg, 2000; Ryan & Calderwood, 2000). A review of cholera vaccines can be found in a WHO position paper where two oral vaccines are recommended under certain conditions (World Health Organization, 2001b). What is of particular concern is evidence from several studies of *Vibrio cholerae* that have shown a continued emergence of new clones of the bacteria in areas where epidemic cholera occurs, by such means as natural selection, host population immunity, and genetic reassortment (Basu et al., 2000). In the initial phases of the seventh pandemic most of the organisms were susceptible to the common antibiotics but resistance is increasingly seen. Cholera, an ancient disease, is still not conquered throughout the world. The knowledge is present for prevention, however, through sanitation and hygiene.

REFERENCES

Ackers, M., Pagaduan, R., Hart, G., Greene, K. D., Abbott, S., Mintz, E., et al. (1997). Cholera and sliced fruit: Probable transmission from an asymptomatic carrier in the United States. *International Journal of Infectious Disease, 1,* 212–214.

Albert, M. J., & Morris, J. G., Jr. (2000). Cholera and other vibrioses. In G. T. Strickland (Ed.), *Hunter's tropical medicine and emerging infectious diseases* (pp. 323–331). Philadelphia: WB Saunders Co.

Basu, A., Garg, P., Datta, S., Chakraborty, S., Bhattacharya, T., Khan, A., et al. (2000). *Vibrio cholerae* O139 in Calcutta, 1992–1998: Incidence, antibiograms and genotypes. *Emerging Infectious Diseases, 6,* 139–147.

Blake, P. A., Allegra, D. T., Snyder, J. D., Barrett, T. J., McFarland, L., Caraway, C. T., et al. (1980). Cholera—a possible endemic focus in the United States. *New England Journal of Medicine, 302,* 305–309.

Cartwright, F. (1972). *Disease and history.* New York: Dorset Press.

Centers for Disease Control. (1991a). Cholera associated with imported frozen coconut milk—Maryland, 1991. *Morbidity and Mortality Weekly Report, 40,* 844–845.

Centers for Disease Control. (1991b). Cholera—New Jersey and Florida. *Morbidity and Mortality Weekly Report, 40,* 287–289.

Centers for Disease Control. (1991c). Cholera—New York. *Morbidity and Mortality Weekly Report, 40,* 516–518.

Centers for Disease Control. (1992a). Cholera associated with an international airline flight, 1992. *Morbidity and Mortality Weekly Report, 41,* 134–135.

Centers for Disease Control. (1992b). Cholera associated with international travel, 1992. *Morbidity and Mortality Weekly Report, 41,* 664–667.

Centers for Disease Control. (1993). Isolation of *Vibrio cholerae* O1 from oysters—Mobile Bay, 1991-1992. *Morbidity and Mortality Weekly Report, 42,* 91–93.

Epstein, P. R. (2000). Is global warming harmful to health? *Scientific American, 283*(2), 50–57.

Fraser, C. M., Eisen, J. A., & Salzberg, S. L. (2000). Microbial genome sequencing. *Nature, 406,* 799–803.

Levine, M. M., & Gotuzzo, E. (1999). Cholera. In R. L. Guerrant, D. H. Walker, & P. F. Weller (Eds.), *Tropical infectious diseases: Principles, pathogens and practice* (pp. 326–335). Philadelphia: Churchill Livingstone.

Mahon, B. E., Mintz, E. D., Greene, K. D., Wells, J. G., & Tauxe, R. V. (1996). Reported cholera in the United States, 1992–1994: A reflection of global changes in cholera epidemiology. *Journal of the American Medical Association, 276*, 307–312.

McCarthy, S. A., & Khambaty, F. M. (1994). International dissemination of epidemic *Vibrio cholerae* by cargo ship ballast and other nonpotable waters. *Applied Environmental Microbiology, 60*, 2597–2601.

Pascual, M., Rodó, X., Ellner, S. P., Colwell, R., & Bouma, M. J. (2000). Cholera dynamics and El Niño-Southern Oscillation. *Science, 289*, 1766–1769.

Rodrigues, A., Sandström, A., Cá, T., Steinsland, J., Jensen, H., & Aaby, P. (2000). Protection from cholera by adding lime juice to food—results from community and laboratory studies in Guinea-Bissau, West Africa. *Tropical Medicine and International Health, 5*, 418–422.

Ryan, E. T., & Calderwood, S. B. (2000). Cholera vaccines. *Clinical Infectious Diseases, 31*, 561–565.

Seas, C., & Gotuzzo, E. (2000). *Vibrio cholerae.* In G. L. Mandell, J. E. Bennett, & R. Dolin (Eds.), *Mandell, Douglas, and Bennett's principles and practice of infectious diseases* (5th ed., pp. 2266–2272). Philadelphia: Churchill Livingstone.

Tauxe, R. V. (1998). Cholera. In A. S. Evans & P. S. Brachman (Eds.), *Bacterial infections of humans: Epidemiology and control* (3rd ed., pp. 223–242). New York: Plenum Medical Book Co.

Tauxe, R. V., & Barrett, T. J. (1998). Cholera and *Vibrio cholerae*: New challenges from a once and future pathogen. In W. M. Scheld, W. A. Craig, & J. M. Hughes (Eds.), *Emerging Infections 2* (pp. 125–144). Washington, DC: ASM Press.

Vugia, D., Shefer, A., Douglas, J., Greene, K., Bryant, R., & Werner, S. (1997). Cholera from raw seaweed transported from the Philippines to California. *Journal of Clinical Microbiology, 35*, 284–285.

Weissman, J. B., DeWitt, W. E., Thompson, J., Muchnick, C. M., Portnoy, B. L., Feeley, J. C., et al. (1974). A case of cholera in Texas, 1973. *American Journal of Epidemiology, 100*, 487–498.

World Health Organization. (2000). Cholera, 1999. *Weekly Epidemiological Record, 75*, 249–254.

World Health Organization. (2001a). Cholera, 2000. *Weekly Epidemiological Record, 76*, 233–240.

World Health Organization. (2001b). Cholera vaccines. *Weekly Epidemiological Record, 76*, 117–124.

5

Cryptosporidiosis

Jeanne B. Hewitt and Marlene W. Schmid

The largest known cryptosporidiosis outbreak occurred when an estimated 403,000 people were affected during a waterborne outbreak in late March and early April 1993, in Milwaukee, Wisconsin (MacKenzie, Hoxie, Proctor, Gradus, Blair, Peterson, et al., 1994). Officials at the Milwaukee Health Department noticed widespread absenteeism among students, teachers, and hospital personnel, which prompted them to notify the Wisconsin Division of Health on April 5. Subsequently, two laboratories confirmed the presence of *Cryptosporidium* oocysts in stool samples from seven adult residents of the Milwaukee area.

Two water-treatment plants supplied 800,000 Milwaukee residents and 10 other municipalities (MacKenzie et al., 1994). Water-quality records showed an increased turbidity at the South plant beginning around March 21, with much higher turbidity noted from March 23 through April 5. A boil-water advisory was issued April 7 and the South plant was temporarily closed on April 9. From March 1 through April 6, 12 of 42 (29%) specimens tested positive for *Cryptosporidium*; from April 8 through April 16, 331 of 1009 specimens (33%) tested positive. In a 2-year follow-up study, 54 death records in the Milwaukee area listed cryptosporidiosis as a contributing or underlying cause of death; 85% of these cases were associated with acquired immunodeficiency syndrome (AIDS) (Hoxie, Davis, Vergeront, Nashold, & Blair, 1997).

Although the gastrointestinal coccidian protozoan *Cryptosporidium* was first described in 1907 (Juranek, 2000), the first human cases of cryptosporidiosis were only reported in 1976 (Meisel, Perera, Meligro, & Rubin, 1976; Nime, Burek, Page, Holscher, & Yardley, 1976). Most *Cryptosporidium* species (spp) are infectious to a single host, although *C. parvum* is thought to be infectious in more than 150 mammalian spp including humans (Fayer, Morgan, & Upton, 2000). *Cryptosporidium* is widely distributed globally (Juranek, 2000). There are at least 10 species of *Cryptosporidium*. One, *C. parvium*, has two genotypes that are responsible for most human infection (Fayer et al., 2000; Xiao, Limor, Bern, & Lal, 2001). Other *Cryptosporidium* species, such as *C. felis* although uncommon causes of human infection, may be responsible for illness in HIV-infected persons more than in the immunocompetent host; however, they do occur, especially in children (Cacciò, Pinter, Fantini, Mezzaroma, & Pozio, 2002; Xiao, Bern, Limor, Sulaiman, Roberts, Checkley, et al., 2001).

Cryptosporidia have been found in a variety of biologic hosts: fish; amphibians; reptiles including snakes, lizards, and tortoises; wild and domesticated birds including chickens, turkeys, ducks, canaries, and cockatiels; and mammals including rodents, cats, dogs, sheep, goats, pigs, deer, cows, and humans (Fayer et al., 2000). *Cryptosporidium* spp may be transmitted via the fecal–oral route through oocyst-contaminated drinking water, recreational water, food, or through close contact with *C. parvum*-infected humans or other hosts such as animals in petting zoos, as well as contaminated surfaces. The incubation period for *Cryptosporidia* infections is estimated to range from 2–14 days with a median incubation period of 7 days (Fayer et al., 2000; Juranek, 2000; Saini, Ransom, & McNamara, 2000). Food sources implicated in outbreaks have included a variety of raw vegetables, basil, cilantro, fresh-pressed cider, unpasteurized apple juice, chicken salad, and shellfish (Centers for Disease Control and Prevention, 2001a; Fayer et al., 2000; Weber & Rutala, 2001). In one outbreak in Minnesota, a caterer changed an infant's diaper and later prepared chicken salad for a social event resulting in the infection of 50 people (Centers for Disease Control and Prevention, 1996).

National surveillance for *C. parvum* infection from 1995–1998 reported 11,612 laboratory confirmed cases in the United States. Although underreporting of cryptosporidiosis is a major problem, Mead and colleagues (1999) used multiple data sources to estimate that 300,000 cases occur annually, of which 90% are waterborne. Across the United States, cryptosporidiosis affects all age groups and is geographically widespread with a trend to more cases in the late summer among people below 20 years of age (Dietz & Roberts, 2000). The official number of cases of cryptosporidiosis reported to the Centers for Disease Control and Prevention (CDC) in 2000 was 2,573 (Centers for Disease Control and Prevention, http://www.cdc.gov/mmwr/preview/mmwrhtml/mm4952md.htm). With the widespread use of protease inhibitors to treat HIV infection (Durham & Lashley, 2000), the prevalence of cryptosporidiosis among HIV-infected persons is believed to have decreased (Miao, Awad-El-Kariem, Gibbons, & Gazzard, 1999). In addition to HIV-infected persons, others who have some degree of immunosuppression (such as those with malignancies or on immunosuppressive medications, the elderly, and to some degree those who are transplant recipients) are vulnerable to cryptosporidiosis, which may be harder to treat in them than in the immunocompetent person and result in more severe sequelae (Gerber, Green, Jaffe, Greenberg, Mazariegos, & Reyes, 2000).

Cryptosporidiosis may be a greater problem in developed countries than commonly acknowledged. It can be asymptomatic. A prevalence study of asymptomatic cryptosporidial infections in 169 immunocompetent persons undergoing endoscopy showed that 12.7% harbored oocysts in the duodenum and 46% had at least one out of three positive stool samples (Roberts, Green, Ma, Carr, & Ginsberg, 1989). Morris, Naumova, and Griffiths (1998) found that cryptosporidiosis may have been affecting Milwaukee residents for more than one year prior to being recognized in 1993. This was speculated retrospectively based on an analysis of water turbidity from the same water district and the number of emergency room visits for severe diarrhea during the same period.

The major symptom of cryptosporidiosis is diarrhea. In the 1993 Milwaukee outbreak, 100% of laboratory confirmed cases had diarrhea (MacKenzie et al., 1994). The median duration of the diarrhea was 9 days (range 1–53 days) with a median of 12 stools per day. Cryptosporidial diarrhea commonly is accompanied by the loss of copious amounts of fluids (Juranek, 2000). Other symptoms reported by persons with laboratory confirmed cryptosporidiosis in Milwaukee included fatigue (87%), abdominal cramps (84%), loss of appetite (81%), nausea (70%), fever (57%), chills (54%), sweats (53%), aching muscles or joints (53%), headache (52%), and vomiting (48%) (MacKenzie et al., 1994). In immunocompromised hosts, when CD4+ cells exceed 150–200/μl, cryptosporidiosis is more likely to be acute and resolve, than when fewer CD4+ cells are reported. In such cases, infection may be lifelong (Hewitt, Yiannoutsos, Higgs, Carey, Geiseler, Soave, et al., 2000).

In young persons (ages 7–27 years), presenting symptoms associated with *Cryptosporidum* infections confined to the intestinal tract included arthritis, tenosynovitis, conjunctivitis, urethritis, plantar fasciitis, and/ or erythema of the oral mucosa (Fayer, 1997). Extra-intestinal infections also occur, especially in the immunocompromised, accompanied by site-specific symptoms such as conjunctivitis, cholangitis, pancreatitis, hepatitis, and pulmonary infections. Symptoms associated with pulmonary cryptosporidiosis include coughing, wheezing, croup, hoarseness, and shortness of breath.

During the acute phase of cryptosporidiosis, the host may excrete 1×10^9 oocysts or more each day (Franzen & Muller, 1999). *Cryptosporidium* oocysts may be excreted for 1–4 weeks or longer after gastroenteritis symptoms subside (Arrowood, 1997). In both symptomatic and asymptomatic individuals, excretion of oocysts is intermittent. As a result, three independent stool samples (obtained on different days) should be evaluated to reduce the chance of false negatives (Arrowood, 1997).

In immunocompetent persons, cryptosporidiosis is self-limited and no chemotherapy is needed. In immunocompromised persons, such as those with HIV infection, chemotherapy may be indicated. While paromomycin initially showed promise in treatment, it has not been shown to be more effective than placebo but has not been completely rejected (Hewitt et al., 2000). Symptomatic treatment consists of oral rehydration and antimotility drugs (Juranek, 2000).

Primary prevention of cryptosporidiosis focuses on environmental controls in handling animal waste and prevention of human infection through contaminated water, food, and fomites. The best overall strategy to control this infection in domestic animal populations is to move the animals to uninfected areas (Fayer, 1997). For humans, the best strategies are to use good personal hygiene such as hand washing, institute procedures using appropriate disinfectants, and effectively decontaminate recreational and drinking water (Fayer et al., 2000). Flood control will aid in preventing runoff from contaminated soil—often from animals who may be asymptomatic but excrete *Cryptosporidium* oocysts—to surface waters and wells (Fayer et al., 2000; Skerrett & Holland, 2001). Maintenance and replacement of water and sewage distribution systems are important. Further ways to prevent waterborne and foodborne infections are listed in Appendix C, Tables C.1, C.2, and C.3.

Laboratory studies reviewed by Fayer (1997) showed that *Cryptosporidium* oocysts are resistant to many chemical disinfectants including chlorine, cidex, and lysol. Effective chemical disinfectants included formol saline (10% for 18 hours), ammonia (5% for 18 hours or 100% gas for 24 hours), and ethylene oxide gas (100% for 24 hours). Fayer concluded that high temperature (45° C for 20 minutes, 64.2° C for 5 minutes, or 72.4° C for 1 minute), low temperature (–20° C for 3 days), and desiccation (air-dried feces, 1–4 days) were the most effective and practical methods of environmental decontamination.

Heat-sensitive medical equipment, such as endoscopes, can serve as fomites for nosocomial transmission of *Cryptosporidium*. Endoscopic equipment can be disinfected using hydrogen peroxide gas plasma sterilization (Vassal, Favennec, Ballet, & Brasseur, 1998), or with ammonia, ethylene oxide, or methyl bromide gases (Fayer, Graczyk, Cranfield, & Trout, 1996). Glutaraldehyde solution (e.g., cidex) is ineffective (Wilson & Margolin, 1999).

Water filtration systems that meet or exceed regulatory requirements do not entirely prevent cryptosporidiosis outbreaks (Goldstein et al., 1996) or *Cryptosporidium* oocysts from entering drinking water supplies (LeChevallier, Norton, & Lee, 1991). These are discussed in detail in *Cryptosporidium and Water* (Working Group on Waterborne Cryptosporidiosis, 1997). Other measures to avoid cryptosporidiosis, particularly in high-risk individuals, include using reverse osmosis water filter systems (Addiss, Pond, Remshak, Juranek, Stokes, & Davis, 1996); or drinking bottled water exclusively (Goldstein et al., 1996). When the drinking water supply may be contaminated with bacteria, protozoa, or hepatitis A, the CDC (1994) and the Environmental Protection Agency recommend boiling water at a rolling boil for 1 minute and/or filtration through a submicron filter (Weber & Rutala, 2001). Haas (2000) notes that protecting the drinking water of the general public may not protect those who are more vulnerable due to immunosuppression.

Although the 1993 cryptosporidiosis outbreak in Milwaukee is the largest and most well known, a number of other outbreaks have been reported. These outbreaks include 64 cases among members of a U.S. Coast Guard cutter that docked in Milwaukee during the outbreak in 1993 (Moss, Bennet, Arrowood, Wahlquist, & Lammie, 1998); 55 cases in Lane county, Oregon, in 1992, associated with primary exposure to a local wave pool or secondary transmission (McAnulty, Fleming, & Gonzalez, 1994); 35 persons infected through the use of one of two swimming pools in Dane county, Wisconsin in 1993 (Centers for Disease Control and Prevention, 1994); 160 cases in Maine in 1993 that involved schoolchildren who drank fresh-pressed apple cider at a fair (Millard, Gensheimer, Addiss, Sosin, Beckett, Houck-Jankoski, et al., 1994); 78 confirmed cases in Las Vegas, Nevada, in 1994 attributed to drinking contaminated municipal water (Goldstein et al., 1996); and an estimated 2,070 persons affected by cryptosporidiosis due to exposure to contaminated recreational lake water in New Jersey in 1994 (Kramer, Sorhage, Goldstein, Dalley, Wahlquist, & Herwaldt, 1998). Approximately 1,000 cases were involved in two outbreaks associated with swimming pools in Ohio and Nebraska in the summer of 2000 (Centers for Disease Control and Prevention, 2001b). Oysters may also be infected with *Cryptosporidium* oocysts, as was found by Fayer and colleagues (1999). Nosocomial transmission, such as through the use of inadequately disinfected endoscopes, has not been addressed widely in the literature, but is a concern due to the resistance of *C. parvum* oocysts to many disinfectants (Fayer, 1997). Standard Precautions can be used for most hospitalized patients with cryptosporidiosis. Contact Precautions are recommended for children who are in diapers or incontinent younger than 6 years of age. Immunocompromised persons such as those with HIV infection should not share a room with someone infected with *Cryptosporidium* (Weber & Rutala, 2001).

Cryptosporidiosis has only been recognized as an infection in humans since 1976. Since that time it has been identified as the responsible agent in several large outbreaks of severe diarrheal illness in communities. In the immunocompetent, however, illness is usually self-limited, requiring only symptomatic relief. In HIV-infected persons and others who are immunosuppressed, including the elderly, illness may be long lasting, and result in fatality. No effective antimicrobial treatment is yet known. Ensuring the safety of drinking water is a major preventive endeavor.

REFERENCES

Addiss, D. G., Pond, R. S., Remshak, M., Juranek, D. D., Stokes, S., & Davis, J. P. (1996). Reduction of risk of watery diarrhea with point-of-use water filters during a massive outbreak of waterborne *Cryptosporidium* infection in Milwaukee, Wisconsin, 1993. *American Journal of Tropical Medicine and Hygiene, 54*, 549–553.

Arrowood, M. J. (1997). Diagnosis. In R. Fayer (Ed.), Cryptosporidium *and cryptosporidiosis* (pp. 43–62). Boca Raton, FL: CRC Press.

Cacciò, S., Pinter, E., Fantini, R., Mezzaroma, I., & Pozio, E. (2002). Human infection with *Cryptosporidium felis*: Case report and literature review. *Emerging Infectious Diseases, 8* [On-line]. Available: http://www.cdc.gov/nciod/EID/eid.htm

Centers for Disease Control and Prevention. (1994). Assessment of inadequately filtered public drinking water—Washington, D.C. *Journal of the American Medical Association, 272*, 1401–1402.

Centers for Disease Control and Prevention. (1996). Foodborne outbreak of diarrheal illness associated with *Cryptosporidium parvum*—Minnesota 1995. *Morbidity and Mortality Weekly Report, 45*, 783.

Centers for Disease Control and Prevention. (1997). Summary of notifiable diseases, United States, 1996. *Morbidity and Mortality Weekly Report, 45*, 1–87.

Centers for Disease Control and Prevention. (2001a). Diagnosis and management of foodborne illnesses: A primer for physicians. *Morbidity and Mortality Weekly Report, 50*(RR-02), 1–69.

Centers for Disease Control and Prevention. (2001b). Protracted outbreaks of cryptosporidiosis associated with swimming pool use—Ohio and Nebraska, 2000. *Morbidity and Mortality Weekly Report, 50*, 406–410.

Dietz, V. J., & Roberts, J. M. (2000). National surveillance for infection with *Cryptosporidium parvum*, 1995–1998: What have we learned? *Public Health Reports, 115*, 358–363.

Durham, J. D., & Lashley, F. R. (Eds.). (2000). *The person with HIV/AIDS: Nursing perspectives.* New York: Springer Publishing Co.

Fayer, R. (1997). The general biology of *Cryptosporidium*. In R. Fayer (Ed.), Cryptosporidium *and cryptosporidiosis* (pp. 2–42). Boca Raton, FL: CRC Press.

Fayer, R., Graczyk, T. K., Cranfield, M. R., & Trout, J. M. (1996). Gaseous disinfection of *Cryptosporidium parvum oocysts. Applied Environmental Microbiology, 62*, 3908–3909.

Fayer, R., Lewis, E. J., Trout, J. M., Graczyk, T. K., Jenkins, M. C., Higgins, J., et al. (1999). *Cryptosporidium parvum* in oysters from commercial harvesting sites in the Chesapeake Bay. *Emerging Infectious Diseases, 5*, 706–710.

Fayer, R., Morgan, U., & Upton, S. J. (2000). Epidemiology of *Cryptosporidium*: Transmission, detection and identification. *International Journal of Parasitology, 30*, 1305–1322.

Franzen, C., & Muller, A. (1999). *Cryptosporidia* and *Microsporidia*—waterborne diseases in the immunocompromised host. *Diagnosis in Microbiology and Infectious Disease, 34*, 245–262.

Gerber, D. A., Green, M., Jaffe, R., Greenberg, D., Mazariegos, G., & Reyes, J. (2000). Cryptosporidial infections after solid organ transplantation in children. *Pediatric Transplantation, 4*, 50–55.

Goldstein, S. T., Juranek, D. D., Ravenholt, O., Hightower, A. W., Martin, D. G., Mesnik, et al. (1996). Cryptosporidiosis: An outbreak associated with drinking water despite state-of-the-art water treatment. *Annals of Internal Medicine, 124*, 459–468.

Haas, C. N. (2000). Epidemiology, microbiology, and risk assessment of waterborne pathogens including *Cryptosporidium. Journal of Food Protection, 63*, 827–831.

Hewitt, R. G., Yiannoutsos, C. T., Higgs, E. S., Carey, J. T., Gieseler, P. J., Soave, R., et al. (2000). Paromomycin: No more effective than placebo for treatment of cryptosporidiosis in patients with advanced human immunodeficiency virus infection. *Clinical Infectious Diseases, 31*, 1084–1092.

Hoxie, N. J., Davis, J. P., Vergeront, J. M., Nashold, R. D., & Blair, K. A. (1997). Cryptosporidiosis-associated mortality following a massive waterborne outbreak in Milwaukee, Wisconsin. *American Journal of Public Health, 87*, 2032–2035.

Juranek, D. D. (2000). Cryptosporidiosis. In G. T. Strickland (Ed.), *Hunter's tropical medicine and emerging infectious diseases* (pp. 594–600). Philadelphia: WB Saunders.

Kramer, M. H., Sorhage, F. E., Goldstein, S. T., Dalley, E., Wahlquist, S. P., & Herwaldt, B. L. (1998). First reported outbreak in the United States of cryptosporidiosis associated with a recreational lake. *Clinical Infectious Diseases, 26*, 27–33.

LeChevallier, M. W., Norton, W. D., & Lee, R. G. (1991). *Giardia* and *Cryptosporidium* spp. in filtered drinking water supplies. *Applied and Environmental Microbiology, 57*, 2617–2621.

MacKenzie, W. R., Hoxie, N. J., Proctor, M. E., Gradus, M. S., Blair, K. A., Peterson, D. E., et al. (1994). A massive outbreak in Milwaukee of *Cryptosporidium* infection transmitted through the public water supply. *New England Journal of Medicine, 331*, 161–167.

McAnulty, J. M., Fleming, D. W., & Gonzalez, A. H. (1994). A community-wide outbreak of cryptosporidiosis associated with swimming at a wave pool. *Journal of the American Medical Association, 272*, 1597–1600.

Mead, P. S., Slutsker, L., Dietz, V., McCaig, L. F., Bresee, J. S., Shapiro, C., et al. (1999). Food-related illness and death in the United States. *Emerging Infectious Diseases, 5*, 607–625.

Meisel, J. L., Perera, D. R., Meligro, C., & Rubin, C. E. (1976). Overwhelming watery diarrhea associated with *Cryptosporidium* in an immunosuppressed patient. *Gastroenterology, 70*, 1156–1160.

Miao, Y. M., Awad-El-Kariem, F. M., Gibbons, C. L., & Gazzard, B. C. (1999). Cryptosporidiosis: Eradication or suppression with combination antiretroviral therapy. *AIDS, 13*, 734–735.

Millard, P. S., Gensheimer, K. F., Addiss, D. T., Sosin, D. M., Beckett, G. A., Houck-Jankoski, A., et al. (1994). An outbreak of cryptosporidiosis from fresh-pressed apple cider. *Journal of the American Medical Association, 272*, 1592–1596.

Morris, R. D., Naumova, E. N., & Griffiths, J. K. (1998). Did Milwaukee experience waterborne cryptosporidiosis before the large documented outbreak in 1993? *Epidemiology, 9*, 264–270.

Moss, D. M., Bennett, S. N., Arrowood, M. J., Wahlquist, S. P., & Lammie, P. J. (1998). Enzyme-linked immunoelectrotransfer blot analysis of a cryptosporidiosis outbreak on a United States Coast Guard cutter. *American Journal of Tropical Medicine, 58*(1), 110–118.

Nime, F. A., Burek, J. D., Page, D. L., Holscher, M. A., & Yardley, J. H. (1976). Acute enterocolitis in a human being infected with the protozoan *Cryptosporidium. Gastroenterology, 70*, 592–598.

Roberts, W. G., Green, P. H. R., Ma, J., Carr, M., & Ginsberg, A. M. (1989). Prevalence of cryptosporidiosis in patients undergoing endoscopy: Evidence for an asymptomatic carrier state. *American Journal of Medicine, 87*, 537–539.

Rust, M., & McArthur, K. (1998). *Slow sand filtration* [On-line]. Available: http://www.cee.vt.edu/program_areas/environmental/teach/wtprimer/slowsand/slowsand.htm

Saini, P. K., Ransom, G., & McNamara, A. M. (2000). Emerging public health concerns regarding cryptosporidiosis. *Journal of the American Veterinary Medicine Association, 217*, 658–663.

Skerrett, H. E., & Holland, C. V. (2001). Asymptomatic shedding of *Cryptosporidium* oocysts by red deer hinds and calves. *Veterinary Parasitiology, 94*, 239–246.

Timms, S., Slade, J. S., & Fridier, C. R. (1994). Removal of *Cryptosporidium* by slow sand filtration. *Water Science and Technology, 31*(5–6), 81–84.

Vassal, S., Favennec, L., Ballet, J.-J., & Brasseur, P. (1998). Hydrogen peroxide gas plasma sterilization is effective against *Cryptosporidium parvum* oocytes. *American Journal of Infection Control, 26*, 136–138.

Weber, D. J., & Rutala, W. A. (2001). The emerging nosocomial pathogens *Cryptosporidium, Escherichia coli* O157:H7, *Helicobacter pylori*, and hepatitis C: Epidemiology, environmental survival, efficacy of disinfection, and control measures. *Infection Control and Hospital Epidemiology, 22*, 306–315.

Wilson, J. A., & Margolin, A. B. (1999). The efficacy of three common hospital liquid germicides to inactivate *Cryptosporidium parvum* oocysts. *Journal of Hospital Infection, 42*, 231–237.

Working Group on Waterborne Cryptosporidiosis. (1997). *Cryptosporidium and water: A public health handbook*. Atlanta, Georgia: Author.

Xiao, L., Bern, C., Limor, J., Sulaiman, I., Roberts, J., Checkley, W., et al. (2001). Identification of 5 types of *Cryptosporidium* parasites in children in Lima, Peru. *Journal of Infectious Diseases, 183*, 492–497.

Xiao, L., Limor, J., Bern, C., & Lal, A. A. (2001). Tracking *Cryptosporidium parvum* by sequence analysis of small double-stranded RNA. *Emerging Infectious Diseases, 7*, 141–145.

6

Cyclospora cayetanensis: Arriving Via Guatemalan Raspberries

Felissa R. Lashley

In the spring and summer of 1996, newspaper headlines brought into the public consciousness awareness of a relatively new emerging pathogen causing severe diarrhea, known as *Cyclospora cayetanensis*: "Forbidding Fruit: How Safe is Our Produce?,"[1] "Red-Letter Berries,"[2] "Parasite Search Shifts to Raspberries,"[3], and finally, "Florida Officials Link Cyclospora to Raspberries."[4] In that time period, 1,465 cases of cyclosporiasis were reported in North America followed by more than 1,600 cases in 1997 (Guerrant & Thielman, 1998). Little was known about this organism, and the occurrence of multistate outbreaks in consecutive years emphasized the need to learn more about this parasite so that future outbreaks could be prevented or treated most effectively. At first, the vehicle for *Cyclospora cayetanensis* was believed to be strawberries. This belief had a monetary effect on that industry before Guatemalan raspberries were identified as the major culprit in these outbreaks. Before this time, *Cyclospora cayetanensis* was virtually unknown in North America.

[1]Boodman, S. G., *Washington Post*, Section W. H., p. 10, Col. 1, 1997, July 8
[2]Criswell, A., *Houston Chronicles*, Section F, p. 1, Col. 4, 1998, March 25
[3]Cohen, J. S., *USA Today*, Section D, p. 1, Col. 2, 1996, July 11
[4]*Washington Post*, Section A, p. 3, Col. 5, 1996, July 6

Cyclospora cayetanensis is a coccidian spore-forming protozoan parasite (Herwaldt, 2000). The species name was proposed after the Universidad Peruana Cayetano Heredia in Lima, Peru, where Y. R. Ortega did work on elucidating characteristics of the organism (Taylor, Davis, & Soave, 1997). *Cyclospora* share many similarities with *Isospora* and *Cryptosporidium*, other protozoan parasites causing diarrhea, and the clinical illnesses caused by the three are very similar. The oocysts of *Cyclospora* are spherical and measure 8–10 μm in diameter, which is larger than those of *Cryptosporidium* but smaller than those of *Isospora* (Taylor, Davis, & Soave, 1997). Infection occurs by ingesting sporulated oocysts (Herwaldt, 2000). During sporulation, each *Cyclospora* oocyst has two sporocysts, each containing two sporozoites, in contrast to *Isospora*, which has four sporozoites in two sporocysts, and *Cryptosporidium*, which has four sporozoites per oocyst (Taylor et al., 1997). In contrast to *Cryptosporidium*, which is immediately infectious to another host, it appears that a period of time (weeks or months) outside the human body is necessary for *Cyclospora* to sporulate and become infectious; thus direct transmission from person to person is unlikely, and secondary household cases have not been noted (Herwaldt, 2000; Koumans, Katz, Malecki, Kumar, Wahlquist, Arrowood, et al., 1998). The full life cycle is not yet completely known, and animal reservoirs have not been identified for *Cyclospora cayetanensis* (Brown & Rotschafer, 1999), although the participation of fowl in some way may be possible (García-López, Rodríguez-Tovar, & Medina-de la Garza, 1996). Many other aspects of its basic biology and related issues are not yet elucidated, such as the dose of the parasite needed for infection, the proportion of infected people who develop diarrhea, identification of an animal model, reasons for seasonal variation, its life cycle, development of protocols to detect *Cyclospora* on food, the range of hosts, the prevalence in non-outbreak settings in developed countries, and the minimum time and temperature needed to inactivate oocysts by heating and freezing (Bendall, Lucas, Moody, Tovey, & Chiodini, 1993; Centers for Disease Control and Prevention, 1997; Colley, 1996; Soave, Herwaldt, & Relman, 1998). Members of other *Cyclospora* species are found in other animals such as snakes, moles, rodents, and centipedes, but *Cyclospora cayetanensis* is the only species known to date to infect humans (Keystone & Kozarsky, 2000). It is resistant to chlorine and formalin (Taylor et al., 1997). Asymptomatic carriers may be reservoirs of infection since they may excrete oocysts without becoming ill (Bendall et al., 1993; Keystone & Kozarsky, 2000), and natives of endemic areas frequently are asymptomatic (Keystone & Kozarsky, 2000). Diagnosis is by identification of oocysts in stool samples using microscopy for measuring and characterizing oocysts. These exhibit bright blue autofluorescence under ultraviolet light and are acid-fast with variable appearance on staining. Polymerase chain reaction amplification may be used. Cost effective, accurate, rapid laboratory diagnosis is needed (Ortega, Sterling, & Gilman, 1998).

Identification of *Cyclospora* began to be made more often after acid-fast staining was modified for the detection of *Cryptosporidium* in the mid-1980s. Before *Cyclospora* had been characterized and named, it had been described in the literature in various ways, most commonly as coccidian-like, "big Crypto," *Cryptosporidium*-like, cyanobacterium-like body (CLB), a fungal spore, and blue-green alga-like body (Pape, Verdier, Boncy, Boncy, & Johnson, 1994; Soave et al., 1998). Thus, some cases of diarrheal illness attributed to *Cryptosporidium* may actually have been due to *Cyclospora*. Although first described in moles in 1870 (Ortega, Gilman, & Sterling, 1994), the first description of illness with *Cyclospora* in humans was in a 1979 publication describing it as an "undescribed coccidian" seen in human stool specimens "by chance" in Papua New Guinea in 1977 (Ashford, 1979). Other reports followed, and a worldwide distribution has been recognized across age groups (Taylor et al., 1997).

Much of the information on *Cyclospora* comes from Nepal, Haiti, and Peru, endemic areas where original research was performed early or in reports about illness in a small number of returning travellers. In 1986, diarrheal illness in returning travellers from Haiti and Mexico was associated with a "new intestinal pathogen" that was thought to be either a coccidian parasite or a fungus (Soave, Dubey, Ramos, & Tummings, 1986). In 1989, what is now known to be *Cyclospora* but which was described then as an "alga-like organism," was identified among 59 patients with prolonged diarrhea who attended a clinic for foreign tourists and foreign-born residents living in Katmandu, Nepal; the sickness occurred mainly during the monsoon season (Centers for Disease Control, 1991). In 1994, diarrhea due to *Cyclospora* was identified in British soldiers and dependants in a military detachment in Nepal due to contaminated chlorinated water, pointing out the need for additional water treatment (Rabold, Hoge, Shlim, Kefford, Rajah, & Echeverria, 1994). In Peru, among indigenous populations, 22% of children infected with *Cyclospora* had diarrhea, and the organism was recognized to cause mild disease that was asymptomatic (Madico, McDonald, Gilman, Cabrera, & Sterling, 1997). In Jakarta, Indonesia, *Cyclospora* was found to be the main protozoal cause of diarrhea in adult foreign residents in the wet season but rarely caused illness in the indigenous population (Fryauff, Krippner, Prodjodipuro, Ewald, Kawengian, Pegelow, et al., 1999). *Cyclospora* was reported as the second most frequent cause of diarrhea among foreigners with less than 2 years of residence in Nepal (Shlim, Hoge, Rajah, Scott, Pandy, & Echeverria, 1999). It is increasingly being recognized as a cause of diarrhea among international travelers to Caribbean destinations (Green, McKendrick, Mohsen, Schmid, & Prakasam, 2000).

The first reported outbreak in North America occurred in Chicago among 21 personnel (physician housestaff and 3 others) who drank chlorinated tap water supplied from an apparently contaminated storage tank in a physician's dormitory (Huang, Weber, Sosin, Griffin, Long, Murphy, et al., 1995). In the spring of 1993, three isolated cases of diarrhea in immunocompetent persons in Massachusetts who had not traveled outside the country were associated with *C. cayetanensis* (Ooi, Zimmerman, & Needham, 1995). An isolated case of explosive diarrhea due to *C. cayetanensis* in 1992 apparently resulted from exposure to sewage that backed up in the patient's basement in Utah (Hale, Aldeen, & Carroll, 1994). Other reports of infection detected in the United States were usually in returning travelers from countries such as Mexico and Thailand (Berlin, Novak, Porschen, Long, Stelma, & Schaeffer, 1994). In 1995, an outbreak of cyclosporiasis affecting 33 persons was linked to drinking from a water cooler at a New York golf course (Carter, Guido, Jacquette, & Rapoport, 1996; Herwaldt, 2000). Also in 1995, a laboratory in Florida identified cases of *Cyclospora*-associated diarrhea that were both sporadic and in clusters associated with separate social events. This identification occurred as a result of routine screening for the organism in stool specimens. Imported raspberries were implicated in most cases as the source of the infections but association with contact with soil such as during gardening could not be excluded as a cause in some instances (Koumans et al., 1998). These events are now considered to have been a harbinger of the large-scale events that occurred in 1996 and 1997.

In 1996 and 1997, major outbreaks called attention to *Cyclospora* and the need for considering this organism in the differential diagnosis of diarrhea. In 1996, ultimately 1,465 persons in 20 states of the U.S. (most east of the Rocky Mountains), the District of Columbia, and two Canadian provinces had cyclosporiasis (Centers for Disease Control and Prevention, 1997; Soave, 1998). Imported Guatemalan raspberries were identified as the major vehicle. Control measures were introduced at the end of 1996, and only those Guatemalan farms meeting certain standards in regard to water quality, employee hygiene, and sanitary conditions were allowed to export berries to the U.S. in 1997 (Centers for Disease Control and Prevention, 1997; Herwaldt, Beach, & the Cyclospora Working Group, 1999; Soave et al., 1998).

In 1997, U.S. health department surveillance systems were put on alert in anticipation of possible *Cyclospora* outbreaks. In the spring, outbreaks began to be reported in association with imported raspberries. Despite the identification of the association in early April, 1997, it was not until the end of May that the importation of raspberries into the U.S. from Guatemala was suspended (Osterholm, 1999). Epidemiologic investigation of the 1997 outbreaks in 18 states, the District of Columbia and two Canadian provinces, implicated not only Guatemalan raspberries but also mesclun (also known as spring mix, mixed baby lettuce, or field greens) and also was associated with fresh basil which, in one cluster, was served in a cold basil pesto pasta salad (Centers for Disease Control and Prevention, 1997; 1998b). How these were contaminated was not determined. Fresh basil was again linked to infection in an outbreak in Missouri in July, 1999 (López, Dodson, Arrowood, Orlandi, da Silva, Bier, et al., 2001).

The Food and Drug Administration (FDA) did not permit Guatemalan raspberries to be imported into the United States in the spring of 1998 but worked with the Guatemalan government and business community to allow importation under certain conditions in future years. Canada did not enact such a restriction. In the spring of 1998, in Toronto, Canada, clusters of cyclosporiasis were reported to be linked to fresh raspberries from Guatemala (Centers for Disease Control and Prevention, 1998a), and over 300 persons were affected ("Cyclosporiasis—Canada [Ontario]," 1999). In 1999, there were several outbreaks and Guatemalan blackberries were suggested but not proven to be the cause in two. In 2000, other outbreaks occurred, and in two of them Guatemalan raspberries were implicated as the source (Herwaldt, 2000).

How the berries were contaminated is not known. Possibilities investigated included fecal contamination of water used to spray fruit for irrigation or pests, contamination during the sorting and packing process through direct handling, and insect or bird dropping contamination occurring before picking (Bern, Hernandez, Lopez, Arrowood, de Mejia, de Merida, et al., 1999; Osterholm, 1999). Improvements related to sanitary practices and use of better quality water on berry farms in 1996 in Guatemala as a result of the 1996 outbreaks did not prevent the 1997 occurrences (Herwaldt et al., 1999). In developing countries, endemic infections with *Cyclospora* seem to fluctuate with the season, with a greater incidence in warm weather and rainy seasons; to display a higher frequency in children aged 18 months to 9 years; to be associated with certain variables such as fowl ownership, drinking untreated water, type of sewage and water systems; and to more frequently affect children under 2 years of age with exposure to soil (Bern et al., 1999). An epidemiological survey in Peru detected *Cyclospora* on the surfaces of vegetables sold in the marketplace, and while the numbers were reduced, the organism was not eliminated with washing (Ortega, Roxas, Gilman, Miller, Cabrera, Taquiri, et al., 1997).

Although identified in persons with HIV infection/AIDS, *Cyclospora* is not presently recognized as a common opportunistic pathogen in this population in developed countries, although it may be associated with chronic diarrhea in developing countries. Pape and colleagues (1994) identified *Cyclospora* as the third most frequent enteric protozoan in AIDS patients with diarrhea, in their series of 450 patients in Haiti. In HIV-infected persons, biliary infection with *Cyclospora* has been reported (Sifuentes-Osornio, Porras-Cortês, Bendall, Morales-Villareal, Reyes-Terán, & Ruiz-Palacios, 1995). In HIV-infected persons, the clinical manifestations are more prolonged and harder to treat (Lashley, 2000).

Clinically, *Cyclospora cayetanensis* infects both immunocompetent and immunocompromised hosts. It attacks the upper small intestine causing inflammation, villous atrophy, and crypt hyperplasia (Berlin et al., 1994). D-xylose absorption is impaired. Inflammatory changes may persist after *Cyclospora* has been eliminated, and a myelin-like material that is visible on electron microscopy may persist in the small intestine (Connor, Reidy, & Soave, 1999). The clinical features are very similar to syndromes caused by other parasitic organisms causing diarrhea. Watery diarrhea, often yellow or khaki green in color, without blood or inflammatory cells is the chief symptom. It may be explosive. Severe fatigue, anorexia, nausea, vomiting, increased flatus, abdominal bloating, weight loss, and stomach cramps often accompany the diarrhea. A small percentage may have fever, chills, and flu-like symptoms (Berlin et al., 1994; Centers for Disease Control and Prevention, 1997; Soave et al., 1998). There may be cycles of remission and relapse, and episodes of diarrhea may alternate with constipation (Centers for Disease Control and Prevention, 1997). Illness may occur as early as 1 day after exposure through 11 days, with an average of 1 week. In untreated immunocompetent adults the infection may last from up to 1 or 2 months or longer (Brown & Rotschafer, 1999). Reiter syndrome (ocular inflammation, oligoarthritis, and sterile urethritis), known to be a sequelae of other enteric infections, has been described following protracted *Cyclospora* infection (Connor, Johnson, & Soave, 2001).

Trimethoprim-sulfamethoxazole (TMP-SMX) is the treatment of choice and is very effective. No antibiotics have yet been shown to be effective for treatment, and this is a disadvantage for those who cannot tolerate sulfa drugs. TMP-SMX is recommended in a double-strength oral tablet (in adults, 160 mg TMP plus 800 mg SMX) twice a day for a week, although HIV-infected persons may require higher doses and longer treatment (Centers for Disease Control and Prevention, 1997; Lashley, 2000). Antidiarrheal agents, peristaltic regulators and histamine-receptor blockers do not appear effective in controlling symptoms. Oral instead of intravenous rehydration is usually adequate (Brown & Rotschafer, 1999). Precautions against acquiring *Cyclospora* during travel are the same as those for other intestinal parasites. Washing berries imported into the United States may or may not be effective in preventing illness, particularly because of the physical composition of raspberries; however, eating them can be avoided although it may be that their presence in a served dish such as fruit salad may be enough to allow infection without eating the actual contaminated fruit itself.

In summary, *Cyclospora cayetanensis* is a recently recognized emerging parasitic pathogen that is both food- and waterborne. Because it is resistant to chlorine, it may be necessary to boil water or use filters for better protection in endemic areas. Low levels of *C. cayetanensis* are sufficient to cause diarrhea. In the United States it has most often been associated with contaminated raspberries imported from Guatemala, mesclun lettuce, and fresh basil, although contaminated water has also been a source. It will be detected more often in coming years as laboratories develop better diagnostic methods and routinely screen for it. *Cyclospora* occurs in both immunocompetent and immunocompromised persons causing diarrhea, fatigue, anorexia, weight loss, and other symptoms, and may be seen in returning travelers and in community outbreaks. It has a worldwide distribution and is endemic in many developing countries. It should be considered in persons with prolonged or unexplained diarrhea, particularly if nonresponsive to therapy. *Cyclospora* responds readily to treatment with TMP-SMX, but other therapies need to be identified, especially for those allergic to sulfa drugs.

REFERENCES

Ashford, R. W. (1979). Occurrence of an undescribed coccidian in man in Papua New Guinea. *Annals of Tropical Medicine and Parasitology, 73*, 497–500.

Bendall, R. P., Lucas, S., Moody, A., Tovey, G., & Chiodini, P. L. (1993). Diarrhoea associated with cyanobacterium-like bodies: A new coccidian enteritis of man. *Lancet, 341*, 590–592.

Berlin, G. G. W., Novak, S. M., Porschen, R. K., Long, E. G., Stelma, G. N., & Schaeffer, F. W., III. (1994). Recovery of *Cyclospora* organisms from patients with prolonged diarrhea. *Clinical Infectious Diseases, 18*, 606–619.

Bern, C., Hernandez, B., Lopez, M. B., Arrowood, M. J., de Mejia, M. A., de Merida, A. M., et al. (1999). Epidemiologic studies of *Cyclospora cayetanensis* in Guatemala. *Emerging Infectious Diseases, 5*, 766–774.

Brown, G. H., & Rotschafer, J. C. (1999). Cyclospora: Review of an emerging parasite. *Pharmacotherapy, 19*, 70–75.

Carter, R. J., Guido, F., Jacquette, G., & Rapoport, M. (April, 1996). Outbreak of *Cyclospora* at a country club—New York, 1995 [abstract]. In *45th Annual Epidemic Intelligence Service (EIS) Conference* (p. 58). Atlanta, GA: U.S. Department of Health and Human Services, Public Health Service.

Centers for Disease Control. (1991). Outbreaks of diarrheal illness associated with cyanobacteria (blue-green algae)-like bodies—Chicago, Nepal, 1989 and 1990. *Morbidity and Mortality Weekly Report, 40*, 325–327.

Centers for Disease Control and Prevention. (1997). Update: Outbreak of cyclosporiasis—United States and Canada 1997. *Morbidity and Mortality Weekly Report, 46*, 521–523.

Centers for Disease Control and Prevention. (1998a). Outbreak of cyclosporiasis—Ontario, Canada, May, 1998. *Morbidity and Mortality Weekly Report, 47*, 806–809.

Centers for Disease Control and Prevention. (1998b). *Preventing emerging infectious diseases: A strategy for the 21st century*. Atlanta, GA: Author.

Colley, D. G. (1996). Widespread foodborne cyclosporiasis outbreaks present major challenges. *Emerging Infectious Diseases, 2*, 354–356.

Connor, B. A., Johnson, E. J., & Soave, R. (2001). Reiter syndrome following protracted symptoms of *Cyclospora* infection. *Emerging Infectious Diseases, 7*, 453–454.

Connor, B. A., Reidy, J., & Soave, R. (1999). Cyclosporiasis: Clinical and histopathologic correlates. *Clinical Infectious Diseases, 28,* 1216–1222.

Cyclosporiasis—Canada (Ontario). (1999). *ProMED Digest, 99*(157), unpaginated.

Fryauff, D. J., Krippner, R., Prodjodipuro, P., Ewald, C., Kawengian, S., Pegelow, K., et al. (1999). *Cyclospora cayetanensis* among expatriate and indigenous populations of West Java, Indonesia. *Emerging Infectious Diseases, 5,* 585–586.

Garcia-López, H. L., Rodríguez-Tovar, L. E., & Medina-de la Garza, C. E. (1996). Identification of *Cyclospora* in poultry. *Emerging Infectious Diseases, 2,* 356–357.

Green, S. T., McKendrick, M. W., Mohsen, A. H., Schmid, M. L., & Prakasam, S. F. (2000). Two simultaneous cases of *Cyclospora cayetanensis* enteritis returning from the Dominican Republic. *Journal of Travel Medicine, 7,* 41–42.

Guerrant, R. L., & Thielman, N. M. (1998). Emerging enteric protozoa: *Cryptosporidium, Cyclospora,* and microsporidia. In W. M. Schield, D. Armstrong, & J. M. Hughes (Eds.), *Emerging infections I* (pp. 233–245). Washington, DC: ASM Press.

Hale, D., Aldeen, W., & Carroll, K. (1994). Diarrhea associated with cyanobacterialike bodies in an immunocompetent host. *Journal of the American Medical Association, 271,* 144–145.

Herwaldt, B. L. (2000). *Cyclospora cayetanensis:* A review, focusing on the outbreaks of cyclosporiasis in the 1990s. *Clinical Infectious Diseases, 31,* 1040–1057.

Herwaldt, B. L., Beach, M. J., & the Cyclospora Working Group. (1999). The return of *Cyclospora* in 1997: Another outbreak of cyclosporiasis in North America associated with imported raspberries. *Annals of Internal Medicine, 130,* 210–220.

Huang, P., Weber, J. T., Sosin, D. M., Griffin, P. M., Long, E. G., Murphy, J. J., et al. (1995). The first reported outbreak of diarrheal illness associated with *Cyclospora* in the United States. *Annals of Internal Medicine, 123,* 409–414.

Keystone, J. S., & Kozarsky, P. (2000). *Isospora belli, Sarcocystis* species, *Blastocystis hominis,* and *Cyclospora.* In G. L. Mandell, J. E. Bennett, & R. Dolin (Eds.), *Mandell, Douglas, and Bennett's principles and practice of infectious diseases* (5th ed., pp. 2915–2920). Philadelphia: WB Saunders.

Koumans, E. H. A., Katz, D. J., Malecki, J. M., Kumar, S., Wahlquist, S. P., Arrowood, M., et al. (1998). An outbreak of cyclosporiasis in Florida in 1995: A harbinger of multistate outbreaks in 1996 and 1997. *American Journal of Tropical Medicine and Hygiene, 59,* 235–242.

Lashley, F. R. (2000). The clinical spectrum of HIV infection and its treatment. In J. D. Durham & F. R. Lashley (Eds.), *The person with HIV/AIDS: Nursing perspectives* (3rd ed., pp. 167–270). New York: Springer Publishing Co.

López, A. S., Dodson, D. R., Arrowood, M. J., Orlandi, P. A., Jr., da Silva, A. J., Bier, J. W., et al. (2001). Outbreak of cyclosporiasis associated with basil in Missouri in 1999. *Clinical Infectious Diseases, 32,* 1010–1017.

Madico, G., McDonald, J., Gilman, P. H., Cabrera, L., & Sterling, C. R. (1997). Epidemiology and treatment of *Cyclospora cayetanensis* infection in Peruvian children. *Clinical Infectious Diseases, 24,* 977–981.

Ooi, W. W., Zimmerman, S. K., & Needham, C. A. (1995). *Cyclospora* species as a gastrointestinal pathogen in immunocompetent hosts. *Journal of Clinical Microbiology, 33,* 1267–1269.

Ortega, Y. R., Gilman, R. H., & Sterling, C. R. (1994). A new coccidian parasite (Apicomplexa: Eimeriidae) from humans. *Journal of Parasitology, 80*, 625–629.

Ortega, Y. R., Roxas, R., Gilman, R. H., Miller, N. J., Cabrera, L., Taquiri, C., et al. (1997). Isolation of *Cryptosporidium parvum* and *Cyclospora cayetanensis* from vegetables collected in markets of an endemic region in Peru. *American Journal of Tropical Medicine and Hygiene, 57*, 683–686.

Ortega, Y. R., Sterling, C. R., & Gilman, R. H. (1998). *Cyclospora cayetanensis. Advances in Parasitology, 40*, 399–418.

Osterholm, M. T. (1999). Lessons learned again: Cyclosporiasis and raspberries. *Annals of Internal Medicine, 130*, 233–244.

Pape, J. W., Verdier, R-I, Boncy, M., Boncy, J., & Johnson, W. D., Jr. (1994). *Cyclospora* infection in adults infected with HIV. *Annals of Internal Medicine, 121*, 654–657.

Rabold, J. G., Hoge, C. W., Shlim, D. R., Kefford, C., Rajah, R., & Echeverria, P. (1994). *Cyclospora* outbreak associated with chlorinated drinking water. *Lancet, 344*, 1360–1361.

Shlim, D. R., Hoge, C. W., Rajah, R., Scott, R. M., Pandy, P., & Echeverria, P. (1999). Persistent high risk of diarrhea among foreigners in Nepal during the first two years of residence. *Clinical Infectious Diseases, 29*, 613–616.

Sifuentes-Osornio, J., Porras-Cortês, G., Bendall, R. P., Morales-Villarreal, F., Reyes-Terân, G., & Ruiz-Palacios, G. M. (1995). *Cyclospora cayetanensis* infection in patients with and without AIDS: Biliary disease as another clinical manifestation. *Clinical Infectious Diseases, 21*, 1092–1097.

Soave, R., Dubey, J. P., Ramos, L. J., & Tummings, M. (1986). A new intestinal pathogen? *Clinical Research, 34*(2), 533A.

Soave, R., Herwaldt, B. L., & Relman, D. A. (1998). *Cyclospora. Infectious Disease Clinics of North America, 12*, 1–12.

Taylor, A. P., Davis, L. J., & Soave, R. (1997). *Cyclospora. Current Clinical Topics In Infectious Diseases, 17*, 256–268.

7

Dengue Fever

Barbara J. Holtzclaw

In the summer of 1995, 12 male youths, ages 16 to 18 years, who were members of a community church in Brownsville, Texas, participated in a construction-assistance mission in Reynosa, a Mexican town across the border in Tamaulipas state. It was an unusually hot and rainy June in the area, and work was frequently interrupted by heavy showers and annoying bites from the resident mosquitoes. During this stay, two boys developed severe headache and fevers above 102° F, and were taken home by car and seen by their local physician. They were found to be leukopenic and were diagnosed with the "flu." A third boy developed similar but more severe symptoms during the next week, including vomiting, severe muscle and joint pain, and small petechiae on his face and extremities. His temperature rose to 104° F. It was clear that this was not the flu. He was transported by ambulance to the medical center in Brownsville. Healing mosquito bites on his skin, an enlarged liver, gradually worsening thrombocytopenia, and a history of recent travel to the Tamaulipas region were factors that led the attending physician to consult an expert in tropical diseases. A diagnosis of dengue fever was made when serological findings indicated DEN-4 viral isolates. His two other ill companions also tested positive for the same DEN serotype. Follow-up surveillance of the south Texas area during the next 2 months identified 29 persons with laboratory-diagnosed dengue, 7 of whom reported no travel outside Texas. Vector density studies found an abundance of the mosquito vector for dengue, *Aedes aegypti*, making it clear that a dengue outbreak was possible in south Texas. As measures to kill mosquitoes and destroy their habitats were taken, a dengue epidemic ensued in Tamaulipas state that lasted until December, with the largest numbers (2,706 cases) reported from the city of Reynosa (Centers for Disease Control and Prevention, 1996).

Dengue (pronounced "denghee") fever (DF), dengue hemorrhagic fever (DHF), and the complications of dengue shock syndrome (DSS) represent a complex of related conditions that rank high among new and newly emerging infectious diseases. Dengue is one of the most prevalent human viral diseases. While dengue began as an unpleasant but usually self-limiting disease, the infectious agent and the vector have evolved to induce more severe symptomatology and higher mortality. An ancient disease, dengue fever caused periodic epidemics in Asia, Africa, and North America as early as 1779, but these were usually infrequent and isolated to areas of endemic infections (Gubler, 1997, 1998), although outbreaks with signs similar to dengue fever were reported in 1635 in the French West Indies and Panama in 1699 (Istúriz, Gubler, & Brea del Castillo, 2000). Epidemics became more widespread and frequent in the 18th and 19th centuries with the rise of the shipping industry. Infected hosts and vectors were transported from one country to another by sea vessels. In the 20th century, wars and rapid transportation contributed to dengue outbreaks by returning infected military personnel from the Pacific tropics or Southeast Asia to regions where natural vectors exist. The number of dengue epidemics has risen dramatically since the early 1980s (Istúriz et al., 2000). These outbreaks and extensions to the Americas and Southeast Asia result from the increase in human and commercial traffic. Not only has the human population spread to sites where dengue is endemic, the mosquito vectors and viruses have widened their geographic range. The more serious outcome of this phenomenon, however, is the co-circulation of multiple virus serotypes in an area, termed *hyperendemicity* (Gubler, 1998). The newer hyperendemic pools of a more virulent infectious agent promote a resurgence of epidemics and the evolution of new strains.

The agent causing dengue is an RNA virus belonging to the family *Flaviviridae* and is considered to be an arbovirus (arthropod-borne). Four serotypes are known and designated by the names DEN-1, DEN-2, DEN-3, and DEN-4. The specific serotype is determined serologically by the number of antigens they have in common. One factor that influences the evolution of the disease in new regions is the ability of the virus to develop new strains. Despite the fact that infection with one dengue serotype confers lifelong immunity to that serotype, no cross-protective immunity exists against the other serotypes. All four dengue virus types have a number of features in common related to the way they initiate antibody responses. It is possible, however, for two or more virus serotypes to infect one host sequentially (secondary infections) and cause an antibody response in the sequential infection that is significantly different from that caused by primary infection. Therefore, the co-circulation of multiple viruses in a region increases the likelihood of this more severe reaction in a population. Immunization with a flavivirus outside the dengue complex also precipitates a secondary antibody response when the host develops a dengue virus infection.

The *Aedes aegypti* mosquito acquires and transmits the virus while probing and feeding on the blood of its host. Other mosquito species known to transmit the disease are *Aedes albopictus*, *Aedes polynesiensis*, and some forms of *Aedes scutellaris*. Humans are most often the original host, but in some regions monkeys have been found to be infected and are a potential source of infection. An infected mosquito harbors the virus throughout its life, and females are capable of passing the virus by transovarian transmission to offspring. This "vertical" transmission of virus in the mosquito has not been recognized as a significant source of dengue outbreaks but remains a source of potential problems in eradicating the vector. *Aedes aegypti* eggs can remain viable for long periods despite months of dry conditions. Inability to survive cool temperatures has kept *Aedes aegypti* confined to the warmer latitudes and lower altitudes nearest to the equator throughout history. Changing climatic conditions and unusually long warm seasons, however, have allowed the mosquito to stray as far as 45 degrees North (World Health Organization, 1997).

There are an estimated 50–100 million cases of DF and 400,000 cases of DHF each year globally. Dengue is endemic in more than 100 countries (World Health Organization, 2000). In the past decade, the incidence has risen in the western hemisphere with 250,000 cases of DF and 7,000 cases of DHF reported in Americas in 1995. Transmission of a virulent viral disease such as dengue fever depends on successful interaction of the infectious agent (the virus serotype), susceptible hosts (humans), and environmental conditions that harbor the vector (mosquitoes). Mosquitoes belonging to the tropical and subtropical species *Aedes aegypti* are the most common vectors of dengue virus transmission. Although *Aedes albopictus* and other mosquito types are potentially capable of carrying the virus, *Aedes aegypti* is particularly adapted to living easily in proximity of humans. The mosquito reproduces by laying larvae in standing water. As humans became more urbanized, the habitats for the mosquito increased (e.g., abandoned equipment, cooling vessels, waste containers, abandoned tires) (Gubler, 1998). International commerce in recycled goods also contributes as a source of mosquito transport (e.g., in 1985 larvae of the *Aedes albopictus* were found in water-logged used tires sent from Japan to Houston for retreading) (Moore & Mitchell, 1997). Within 2 years, the Centers for Disease Control and Prevention (CDC) reported that the mosquito species had invaded Texas, Kentucky, Delaware, Maryland, Ohio, California, Alabama, Arkansas, Florida, Illinois, Indiana, Louisiana, Mississippi, Missouri, North Carolina, and Tennessee.

The patterns of disease spread have changed significantly since the first reported DHF epidemic occurred in the Philippines in 1953–1955. By the mid-1970s, DHF reached epidemic proportions in Southeast Asia. Numbers grew in the 1980s and 1990s in Asia, moving east into China and westward to India, Pakistan, Sri Lanka, and Maldives. Epidemics had been kept in check in the Americas during the 1960s and 1970s by a strong eradication program against *Aedes aegypti*. When this program was discontinued in the early 1970s, a reinfestation of this species began. By the end of the 1990s, the geographic distribution of the mosquito was as wide as in the pre-eradication period. By the 1980s, major epidemics occurred, along with the development of hyperendemicity (Gubler, 1999). The United States has had documented sporadic cases of imported dengue over the past 20 years. Most have resulted from travel to the American and Asian tropics and have included all four virus serotypes. The potential for epidemic dengue transmission secondary to importation of the virus in humans is high in the United States. Although the species *Aedes aegypti* is found primarily in Gulf Coast states from Texas to Florida, new infestations have been reported in Tucson, Arizona (Gubler, 1999). Between 100 and 200 suspected cases are introduced into the United States each year by travelers (Centers for Disease Control and Prevention, 1997, 1999). A major problem for detection and control is the low index of suspicion for dengue among U.S. physicians, even if the patient has recent history of travel to a tropical area. Consequently, it is estimated that large numbers of dengue cases are never reported. After noting 11 confirmed and 49 suspected dengue cases in Laredo, Texas from July 23 to August 20, 1999, some not associated with travel outside the United States, aggressive public health activities resulted in no reports of cases in Laredo in 2000. Some of the cases were originally diagnosed as "viral syndrome" or "flu-like illness" (Centers for Disease Control and Prevention, 2001). In September 2001, an outbreak of dengue fever occurred in Hawaii, the first in more than 30 years (Dengue—USA Hawaii, 2001).

The spread of both vector and virus for dengue has been attributed to humans and is definitely a problem of urbanization. The urban environment is favorable for the breeding and survival of the mosquito. The increase of international travel has led to shorter intervals between epidemics and to recurrent epidemics involving multiple serotypes (Kuno, 1997). Return of an infected person to a region where mosquitoes are prevalent can create an outbreak in a fresh region. More serious is the returning traveler who brings a new dengue serotype to a region where others already exist. Vigorous attempts to eradicate the vector by insecticidal sprays may bring about a false sense of security. Most authorities agree that controlling or eliminating the breeding sites are the only effective means for controlling mosquitoes (Castle, Amador, Rawlins, Figueroa, & Reiter, 1999; Istúriz et al., 2000).

The environment is also significantly influenced by climatic changes that provide favorable milieu for the vector (such as unusually long warm and rainy seasons), thus raising concerns about changes in the environment brought about by even minimal global warming that allow vector mosquito species to survive northern latitudes as far north as Tokyo, Rome, and New York (Patz, Martens, Focks, & Jetten, 1998). The effects of El Niño and periodic changes in the environment have stimulated the study and prediction of changes and their influence on arboviral disease by environmentalists (Maelzer, Hales, Weinstein, Zalucki, & Woodward, 1999). Computer-based simulation analyses predict higher climate-related disease risks for hemorrhagic dengue by the year 2050 related to an average projected temperature elevation of 1.16° C (Patz et al., 1998). Use of new procedures for "climate-dengue modeling" with mathematical simulation models may improve the ability to predict future water and temperature conditions that favor dengue vectors (Cheng, Kalkstein, Focks, & Nnaji, 1998).

Infections with dengue virus serotypes encompass a spectrum of severity from asymptomatic to critical illness. A common general classification of these illnesses, in order of severity, includes mild dengue, classic dengue fever, and dengue hemorrhagic fever. Symptoms of classic DF include fever (rarely exceeding 40.5° C), severe headache, joint pains, weakness, and skin rashes. Mild dengue and classic dengue are similar in symptomatology, are not fatal, and rarely affect children. Incubation requires 5 to 8 days. Duration of the milder dengue is less than 72 hours while the patient with classic dengue is generally very ill for 7 days. Classic dengue is followed by intense weakness for many weeks. The more severe forms of the disease can affect nearly every organ system, either by direct viral invasion or by secondary sepsis, circulatory impairment, or coagulopathy. DHF is defined by the presence of high continuous fever (40°–41° C) for 2–7 days, platelet count $\leq$ 100,000/mm^3, hemorrhagic manifestations, and excessive vascular permeability (Centers for Disease Control and Prevention, 2001; Nimmannitya, 1997). Cough, headache, vomiting, and abdominal pain accompany fever and persist for 2–4 days. DHF has been classified by the World Health Organization into four grades of illnesses, based on severity. Grade I DHF includes fever with mild nonspecific symptoms and a positive tourniquet test (i.e., inflating a blood pressure cuff midway between the systolic and diastolic pressure for 5 minutes causes a shower of petechiae to appear below the cuff). Grade II has more severe symptoms and spontaneous hemorrhagic manifestations that include spontaneous petechiae, epistaxis, bleeding gums, and hematuria. Grade III is marked by circulatory failure with rapid weak pulse, narrowed pulse pressure, and hypotension. Grade IV is a severe form of the disease leading to dengue shock syndrome (DSS). While mild DHF may be treated successfully with fluid and electrolyte therapy, the onset of shock can lead quickly to death without appropriate management (McBride & Bielefeldt-Ohmann, 2000).

The exact pathogenesis of DHF remains unclear, although there is growing evidence that pro-inflammatory cytokines, such as interleukins (IL), may play a role (Mustafa, Elbishbishi, Agarwal, & Chaturvedi, 2001). Vascular permeability is a hallmark of DHF and DSS and can lower plasma volume more than 20% in severe cases (Gubler, 1999). Understanding the effects of altered microvascular permeability is an area of current research (Bethell, Gamble, Pham, Nguyen, Tran, Ha, et al., 2001). Leakage of plasma from capillaries contributes to hepatomegaly, pleural or abdominal effusions, hemoconcentration, or hypoproteinemia. The tendency toward hemorrhage involves vascular fragility, thrombocytopenia, and coagulopathy. Thrombocytopenia leads to abnormal blood clotting and disseminated intravascular coagulopathy. Autopsies on most patients who die from DHF reveal gastrointestinal hemorrhage. Extensive circulatory collapse and internal hemorrhaging may result in death or dengue shock syndrome. DSS typically occurs between the third and seventh day of the disease, concurrent with or shortly after the fall in temperature.

Neurologic involvement, ranging from headache and dizziness to the more severe manifestations of convulsions, paresis, and coma, is associated with both dengue fever and DHF which are generally more severe when the DEN-2 and DEN-3 serotypes are involved. The pathophysiology of dengue-related neurological manifestations has not been well defined. Most patients exhibit cerebral edema rather than the presence of inflammatory lesions or encephalitis. Evidence of dengue virus serotypes in the CSF of symptomatic patients suggests that the virus may cross the blood-brain barrier during viremic phases. Pathologic studies of brain tissue, however, fail to support this view (Kuno, 1997). Encephalographic disturbances may be seen (Angibaud, Luaute, Laille, & Gaultier, 2001).

Primary treatment of severe DHF involves fluid replacement of lost plasma with plasma, plasma expanders, or electrolyte solutions. Replacement of fluid must often be done rapidly, but with careful monitoring against overhydration to prevent pulmonary edema. Early replacement of fluid usually reverses DSS and can often prevent coagulopathy. The mortality rate of appropriately managed DHF is as low as 1% while the lack of health resources pushes mortality rates above 5% (McBride, 1999). Patients with mild DHF can usually be treated with oral fluids and non-salicylate antipyretic drugs. Aspirin and other salicylates are contraindicated because they may precipitate bleeding, acidosis, or Reye's syndrome. Acetaminophen should be used with caution for temperatures above 39° C (World Health Organization, 1997). There is a surprisingly short recovery period for patients with DHF, even those surviving shock, of 2 to 3 days (Gubler, 1999).

There is presently no available vaccine for protection from the dengue viruses, although considerable progress has been made in its development. Ideally, the vaccine should be effective against all serotypes to prevent the possibility of sequential infection and confer lifelong immunity. Experts determine that the ideal vaccine to achieve these goals would be a live, attenuated tetravalent vaccine (Jacobs, 2000). Despite impressive progress, the wide array of monovalent, trivalent, and tetravalent vaccines remain in animal and clinical trials. A safe and effective vaccine for dengue will probably not be available in the near future (Istûriz et al., 2000).

The primary mode of controlling dengue virus spread is through eliminating the mosquito vector in domestic sites where most transmission takes place. Early use of DDT in the late 1940s brought remarkable success but rapidly developing resistance to DDT and other insecticides point out the shortcomings of this approach. Neighborhood spraying programs and aerial application of insecticide have failed to reduce the mosquito population. The use of ultra low-volume sprays of malathion during the 1995 epidemic of DHF in Jamaica was found ineffective in preventing *Aedes aegypti* reproduction (Castle et al., 1999). Use of space insecticide sprays in homes is of little help, while the use of screens and elimination of water-holding containers are effective means of control. In tropical areas, travelers are recommended to use aerosol "bomb" type insecticides to kill indoor mosquitoes and to use diethyltoluamide (DEET) insect repellent on exposed skin and on protective clothing (Gubler, 1999). Larval source reduction remains a major effort of officials involved in vector control. Use of the larvicides VectoLex and Altosid in catch basins and car and truck waste tires in the U.S. is under study (Siegel & Novak, 1999). Attempts are underway to find organisms that are natural predators for controlling the mosquito *Aedes aegypti*. Field trials in northeastern Mexico and in Costa Rica tested the use of copepods, micro-crustacean predators, which were seeded into metal drums, discarded tires, cemetery flower vases, and bromeliad leaf axils. All were water collectors important as breeding sites for the mosquito (Gorrochotegui-Escalante, Fernandez-Salas, & Gomez-Dantes, 1998; Schaper, 1999). Despite the severe effects of drought and dry seasons on survival of the copepods in both study regions, the use of this natural predator reduced larvae and may hold promise for mosquito control.

Community-wide participation is needed for effective vector control to avoid excessive reliance on insecticides and for help in clearing neighborhoods of receptacles that hold water where mosquitoes breed. Experts in control and prevention are not optimistic about success in keeping dengue vectors from spreading unless surveillance and control are supported by individuals, communities, and governmental agencies (Reiter & Gubler, 1997). Educating and motivating the public to be active participants are important steps, while the cooperation of nations in prevention and control is crucial. Maintaining a balance between concern for the environment and intervention to control or eradicate insect vectors remains a key challenge to the control of dengue fever.

REFERENCES

Angibaud, G., Luaute, J., Laille, M., & Gaultier, C. (2001). Brain involvement in dengue fever. *Journal of Clinical Neurosciences, 8,* 63–65.

Bethell, D. B., Gamble, J., Pham, P. L., Nguyen, M. D., Tran, T. H., Ha, T. H., et al. (2001). Noninvasive measurement of microvascular leakage in patients with dengue hemorrhagic fever. *Clinical Infectious Diseases, 32,* 243–253.

Castle, R., Amador, M., Rawlins, S., Figueroa, J. P., & Reiter, P. (1999). Absence of impact of aerial malathion treatment on *Aedes aegypti* during a dengue outbreak in Kingston, Jamaica. *Panamerican Journal of Public Health, 5,* 100–105.

Centers for Disease Control and Prevention. (1996). Dengue fever at the U.S.-Mexico border. *Morbidity and Mortality Weekly Report, 45,* 841–842.

Centers for Disease Control and Prevention. (1997). Fact sheet: Dengue/dengue hemorrhagic fever. *DVBID home page* [On-line]. Available: http://www.cdc.gov/ncidod/dvbid/dhfacts.htm

Centers for Disease Control and Prevention. (1999). Imported dengue—Florida. *Morbidity & Mortality Weekly Report, 48,* 1150–1151.

Centers for Disease Control and Prevention. (2001). Underdiagnosis of dengue—Laredo, Texas, 1999. *Morbidity & Mortality Weekly Report, 50,* 57–59.

Cheng, S., Kalkstein, L. S., Focks, D. A., & Nnaji, A. (1998). New procedures to estimate water temperatures and water depths for application in climate-dengue modeling. *Journal of Medical Entomology, 35,* 646–652.

Dengue—USA (Hawaii). (September 28, 2001). ProMED Digest, 2001(234), unpaginated.

Gorrochotegui-Escalante, N., Fernandez-Salas, I., & Gomez-Dantes, H. (1998). Field evaluation of *Mesocyclops longisetus* for the control of larval *Aedes aegypti* in northeastern Mexico. *Journal of Medical Entomology, 35,* 699–703.

Gubler, D. J. (1997). Dengue and dengue hemorrhagic fever: Its history and resurgence as a global public health problem. In D. J. Gubler & G. Kuno (Eds.), *Dengue and dengue hemorrhagic fever* (pp. 1–22). New York: CAB International.

Gubler, D. J. (1998). Epidemic dengue and dengue hemorrhagic fever: A global public health problem in the 21st century. In W. M. Scheld, D. Armstrong, & J. M. Hughes (Eds.), *Emerging infections* (pp. 1–14). Washington, DC: ASM Press.

Gubler, D. J. (1999). Dengue and dengue hemorrhagic fever. In R. L. Guerrant, D. H. Walker, & P. F. Weller (Eds.), *Tropical infectious diseases: Principles, pathogens & practice* (pp. 1265–1274). Philadelphia: Churchill Livingstone.

Istúriz, R.W., Gubler, D. J., & Brea del Castillo, J. B. (2000). Dengue and dengue hemorrhagic fever in Latin America and the Caribbean. *Infectious Disease Clinics of North America, 14,* 121–140.

Jacobs, M. (2000). Dengue: Emergence as a global public health problem and prospects for control. *Transactions of the Royal Society of Typical Medicine and Hygiene, 94,* 7–8.

Kuno, G. (1997). Factors influencing the transmission of dengue viruses. In D. J. Gubler & G. Kuno (Eds.), *Dengue and dengue hemorrhagic fever* (pp. 61–88). New York: CAB International.

Maelzer, D., Hales, S., Weinstein, P., Zalucki, M., & Woodward, A. (1999). El Niño and arboviral disease prediction. *Environmental Health Perspectives, 107,* 817–818.

McBride, W. J. H. (1999). Dengue fever: An Australian perspective. *Australian Family Physician, 28,* 319–323.

McBride, W. J. H., & Bielefeldt-Ohmann, H. (2000). Dengue viral infections: Pathogenesis and epidemiology. *Microbes and Infection, 2,* 1041–1060.

Moore, C. G., & Mitchell, C. J. (1997). *Aedes albopictus* in the United States: Ten-year presence and public health implications. *Emerging Infectious Diseases, 3,* 329–334.

Mustafa, A., Elbishbishi, E., Agarwal, R., & Chaturvedi, U. (2001). Elevated levels of interleukin-13 and IL-18 in patients with dengue hemorrhagic fever. *FEMS Immunology and Medical Microbiology, 30,* 229–233.

Nimmannitya, S. (1997). Dengue hemorrhagic fever: Diagnosis and management. In D. J. Gubler & G. Kuno (Eds.), *Dengue and dengue hemorrhagic fever* (pp. 133–145). New York: CAB International.

Patz, J. A., Martens, W. J. M., Focks, D. A., & Jetten, T. H. (1998). Dengue fever epidemic potential as projected by general circulation models of global climate change. *Environmental Health Perspectives, 106,* 147–153.

Reiter, P., & Gubler, D. J. (1997). Surveillance and control of urban dengue vectors. In D. J. Gubler & G. Kuno (Eds.), *Dengue and dengue hemorrhagic fever* (pp. 425–462). New York: CAB International.

Schaper, S. (1999). Evaluation of Costa Rican copepods for larval *Aedes aegypti* control with special references to *Mesocyclops thermocyclopoides. Journal of the American Mosquito Control Association, 15,* 510–519.

Siegel, J. P., & Novak, R. J. (1999). Duration of activity of the microbial larvicide VectoLex CG (*Bacillus sphaericus*) in Illinois catch basins and waste tires. *Journal of the American Mosquito Control Association, 15,* 366–370.

World Health Organization. (1997). *Dengue haemorrhagic fever: Diagnosis, treatment, prevention and control* (2nd ed.). Geneva: Author.

World Health Organization. (2000). Dengue/dengue haemorrhagic fever. Situation in 2000. *Weekly Epidemiological Record, 75,* 193–196.

8

Ebola, Marburg, and Lassa Fevers

Wayne E. Ellis and Felissa R. Lashley

It began with a charcoal worker who brought more back from the forest than the charcoal he gathered. In January 1995, he died from Ebola hemorrhagic fever, but this and other cases occurring in this area of Zaire (now Democratic Republic of the Congo [DRC]) were not initially diagnosed as Ebola. Patients with bloody diarrhea were diagnosed as having *Shigella* infection, and treated with antibiotics. As the rainy season progressed, more persons became ill. In early April 1995, a small nosocomial cluster of Ebola cases occurred among the nursing staff at the Maternity hospital in Kikwit but were misdiagnosed as epidemic dysentery. A laboratory technician from this hospital was referred for surgery for a suspected bowel perforation at the Kikwit General Hospital in early April, and died 2 days later. After this surgery, the number of cases increased rapidly due to nosocomial transmission. A number of physicians and nurses involved in his care became ill with symptoms suggesting a viral hemorrhagic fever, and specimens were sent to Centers for Disease Control and Prevention (CDC) in early May, where it was determined that all cases were Ebola (Khan, Tshioko, Heymann, Le Guenno, Nabeth, Kerstiëns, et al., 1999).

International attention then focused on Kikwit, a town in the DRC a few hundred miles east of the capital of Kinshasha, as it became the site of a major and highly publicized outbreak of Ebola hemorrhagic fever. It was not until May 11, 1995 that an international commission was assembled to combat the epidemic and manage patient care, education, research, and the transport of cadavers. Many difficulties were encountered in the course of their work in the areas of public education and surveillance due to language and cultural differences, logistics such as lack of telephones and transportation, lack of local mass media, low literacy rates, school closures, concealing cases of illness to avoid social stigma, and conversely, reporting noncases in the belief that this would lead to some benefit for the person or village (Khan et al., 1999). In all, 317 people were affected and 245 died (Muyembe-Tamfun, Kipasa, Kiyungu, & Colebunders, 1999).

Although a number of hemorrhagic fever viruses have been identified worldwide, Ebola virus has become most notorious through popular media such as the book by Richard Preston, *The Hot Zone* (New York, Random House, 1994), and the movie, *Outbreak* starring Dustin Hoffman (Warner Brothers, 1995). Many of the hemorrhagic fever viruses have common themes in their pathology and clinical manifestations, and all are RNA viruses, but there are also differences. This chapter discusses the Ebola, Marburg, and Lassa viruses. Information about the hantaviruses is in chapter 10, dengue and dengue hemorrhagic fever in chapter 7, and other emerging hemorrhagic fever viruses such as Rift Valley Fever virus, and Machupo virus causing hemorrhagic fever are summarized in Appendix A, Table A.4. A detailed review of Ebola and Marburg viral infections including those that occurred in laboratories may be found in Schou and Hansen (2000).

EBOLA VIRUS

Ebola is a filovirus in the family *Filoviridae* which at this time has only two members: Marburg virus and Ebola virus. These are both RNA viruses. Ebola virus has four subtypes that have been identified to date: Zaire, Sudan, Reston, and Ivory Coast or Côte d'Ivoire. The Reston subtype is not known to cause severe disease in humans, but can be deadly to monkeys (Colebunders & Borchert, 2000). Ebola virus is rod-shaped with brushlike spikes protruding from the outer membrane, and branching forms, U-shapes and twisted rods may be seen. It is pleomorphic, changing shapes rapidly. The filamentous form is associated with high infectivity (Feldmann & Kiley, 2000). The hemorrhaging seen in severe disease appears to result from the adhesion of the virus to the endothelial lining of blood vessels, damaging them (Balter, 2000). A biosafety level of 4, or the highest level of biologic containment has been established for Ebola (and Marburg as well) because of high pathogenicity, ready transmission, high mortality rate, and the lack of effective treatment or vaccine (Feldmann & Kiley, 2000). Transmission is known to be person-to-person, but how the index case becomes infected presumably from an animal reservoir is not yet known. Airborne transmission of Ebola-Reston in the Reston, Virginia outbreak involving monkeys (discussed below) appeared likely as one method of spread (Richards, Murphy, Jobson, Mer, Zinman, Taylor, et al., 2000), the Zaire strain has been experimentally transmitted to monkeys by aerosol (Johnson, Jaax, White, & Jahrling, 1995), but airborne transmission from person to person is not known to occur. Transmission via semen may occur weeks after recovery (World Health Organization, December, 2000).

As Peters and LeDuc (1999) have phrased it, "humans meet Ebola virus in Africa in 1976" (p. ix). At that time, epidemics of a severe hemorrhagic fever occurred at nearly the same time in both Zaire and the Sudan ("After Marburg, Ebola," 1977). A filovirus, Ebola, was isolated from patients, and named after a river in northwest Zaire (now part of the Democratic Republic of Congo) near the town of Yambuku (Khan et al., 1999; Peters & LeDuc, 1999). Two different subtypes of the virus were responsible for these two outbreaks, and they were named respectively for the country in which they were found (Ebola-Zaire and Ebola-Sudan). The outbreak in Zaire was characterized by extensive transmission through reused needles and syringes and lack of barrier nursing techniques in the mission hospital, and affected about 318 persons, with 280 deaths (Khan et al., 1999; Peters & LeDuc, 1999). The following quote illustrates the problem:

> Five syringes and needles were issued to the nursing staff each morning for use at the outpatient department, the prenatal clinic and the inpatient wards. These syringes and needles were sometimes rinsed between patients in a pan of warm water. At the end of the day they were sometimes boiled. (Breman, Piot, & Johnson, White, Mbuyi, Sureau, et al., 1978, p. 105)

The Sudan outbreak appeared to originate among cotton factory workers in Nzara. A total of 284 cases with a 53% case fatality was documented. Following this, in 1977, a fatal case of Ebola hemorrhagic fever was identified in a child near Yambuku, and while this case was being investigated, a case was identified retrospectively from 1972 (Heymann, Weisfeld, Webb, Johnson, Cairns, & Berquist, 1980; Khan et al., 1999). These initial recognitions of the virus and the hemorrhagic fever it caused were soon followed by another outbreak in the southern Sudan in 1979 that affected 34 persons with a 65% case fatality (Baron, McCormick, & Zubeir, 1983; Khan et al., 1999). This outbreak was also linked to a hospital for spread, but the index case had apparently been a worker in the cotton factory that employed many of the people infected in the 1976 outbreak.

For a number of years, Ebola was relatively quiescent. Peters and LeDuc (1999) describe the next event as "Ebola visits the United States, the virus family grows" (p. ix). In 1989, an alarming event occurred which was the appearance of what became known as Ebola-Reston among macaque monkeys that were imported from the Philippines into the United States and housed at a primate facility in Reston, Virginia near Washington, D.C. (Peters & LeDuc, 1999). Four of their handlers had serologic evidence of recent infection by the development of antibody to Ebola but did not display symptoms (Centers for Disease Control, 1990; Sanchez, Ksiazek, Rollin, Peters, Nichol, Khan, et al., 1995). Antibody-positive persons were also identified in the Philippines (Miranda, White, Dayrit, Hayes, Ksiazek, & Burans, 1991). While it was subsequently determined that this subtype was not as pathogenic as the others, and that humans were minimally affected, for a time great concern was generated. An Asian origin for Ebola-Reston rather than African origin was confirmed. Other epidemics occurred in nonhuman primate facilities including in Italy in 1992 and in Texas in 1996 (Peters & LeDuc, 1999; World Health Organization, 1992). In 1994, a chimpanzee that was being necropsied because of an observed high death rate in a troop of chimpanzees that was being studied by ethologists in the Taï National Park in Côte d'Ivoire, suggested another link between nonhuman primates and humans in Ebola outbreaks. A single human case occurred in one of the scientists studying the chimpanzees—the one who had performed the autopsy. She was evacuated to Switzerland where she recovered. This incident led to the identification of a new subtype, Ebola-Côte d'Ivoire or Ivory Coast (Khan et al., 1999; Le Guenno, Formenty, Wyers, Gounon, Walker, & Boesch, 1995).

From 1994 to 1997, Ebola hemorrhagic fever outbreaks occurred in Gabon. The 1994 outbreak had a first wave that began in early December 1994 and a second wave in January and February of 1995. It was originally believed to be yellow fever. All of the patients in the first wave came from gold panning camps close to the edge of the rain forest, and it was anecdotally reported that prior to the outbreak there had been deaths occurring among the local chimpanzees and gorillas. The persons affected in the second waves were secondary patients. The first of these patients, who lived near the village healer, was probably infected because of contact with an Ebola-infected person who left the local hospital and returned to that village healer. People in the second wave had been in direct contact with relatives hospitalized at the local hospital where patients from the first wave had been taken, had slept in the home of the traditional healer, or had cared for patients. This outbreak, affecting 49, was declared over on February 17, 1995. In February 1996, 18 people who had "skinned and chopped" a dead chimpanzee for food preparation became ill and were admitted to the nearest general hospital. Six more were affected by secondary transmission of Ebola. The third epidemic began in October 1996 and was declared over in March 1997. It apparently began earlier with the death of a hunter in a logging camp. In all there were 60 cases and 45 deaths (Georges, Leroy, Renaut, Benissan, Nabias, Ngoc, et al., 1999; Leroy, Baize, Volchkov, Fisher-Hoch, Georges-Courbot, Lansoud-Soukate, et al., 2000). A physician who performed endoscopy on one of the Gabonese patients himself became ill. He sought care in South Africa where he was diagnosed with Ebola. A nurse involved in his care was a secondary case and died in Johannesburg (Georges et al., 1999).

An official statement from WHO in October 2000, described an Ebola outbreak in Uganda near the site of the previous Marburg outbreak. All schools were closed and a ban against funerals was put into effect (World Health Organization, 2001). The three most important means of transmission in this outbreak were attending funerals of those who died with Ebola hemorrhagic fever, where ritual contact occurred; intrafamilial; and nosocomial (Centers for Disease Control and Prevention, 2001). The outbreak occurred later in the Gulu and Masindi districts. By January 23, 2001, a total of 425 cases were reported, with 224 deaths (Centers for Disease Control and Prevention, 2001). In early January 2001, reports of Ebola cases from the Democratic Republic of the Congo in areas near the border with Uganda were reported. In 2001, a woman who had flown from Africa to Canada was admitted to a Canadian hospital with symptoms of hemorrhagic fever. Ebola was suspected, but it turned out not to be the diagnosis (Reuters, 2001). In November 2001, an Ebola outbreak occurred in Gabon close to sites of previous outbreaks.

Asymptomatic human Ebola infection has been found only recently. Formerly it was believed that symptomatic disease was the invariable consequence of Ebola infection. Whether or not symptomless Ebola carriers play a role in transmission remains to be determined (Baxter, 2000; Leroy et al., 2000). In the Gabon outbreak, seven persons were infected by Ebola virus but did not develop detectable blood antigens or symptoms of disease. Understanding immune responses to the Ebola virus may shed light on new approaches to protection (Leroy, Baize, Debre, Lansoud-Soukate, & Mavoungou, 2001). In Ebola hemorrhagic fever, the incubation period is typically 4–10 days (range 2–21 days). The onset of illness is abrupt, and initial symptoms such as fever, severe frontal headache, myalgia, and malaise may be nonspecific, delaying the diagnosis. Bradycardia and conjunctivitis may be present, along with pharyngitis, severe nausea, diarrhea, and vomiting. Obtunding may occur. A maculopapular rash appears around day 5 and survivors may experience desquamation. Blindness can occur. Hemorrhage occurs in about half the patients that is manifested as petechiae and ecchymoses, as well as conjunctival injection and uncontrolled bleeding from orifices and needle-puncture sites. The fatality rate is high, usually 65%–90%, and most who die are in a stupor with shock and tachypnea (Bwaka, Bonnet, Calain, Colebunders, De Roo, Guimard, et al., 1999). Convalescence is lengthy. Barrier-nursing techniques are needed to provide care with high-efficiency particulate air (HEPA) respirators if available (Centers for Disease Control and Prevention, 1995). No treatment is available and supportive care is indicated as described under Marburg hemorrhagic fever. Epidemics tend to burn out because of the high mortality rate.

Many mysteries regarding Ebola virus remain. Although, generally, index cases or clusters have been identified, the natural reservoir has not yet been. Most zoonoses have a natural host that maintains them in nature, and sometimes vectors as well. However, it is unknown how Ebola virus is maintained in nature and how the index case acquires it. Numerous investigations have been conducted and several animals have been postulated as reservoirs including monkeys, bats, and rodents. Fragments of the virus using newer techniques have been found in shrews and rodents in the Central African Republic. The reservoirs for Ebola virus, and vectors, if any, however, have not yet been identified (Morvan, Deubel, Gounon, Nakoune, Barriere, Murri, Perpete, et al., 1999). Of great concern is the possibility of the Ebola virus mutating into a form that has greater human-to-human transmissibility than has been observed to date.

MARBURG VIRUS

In 1967, commercial laboratory workers in Marburg, Germany, who were processing kidney tissue from imported African green monkeys for cell culture and vaccine production, began falling ill and were admitted to the hospital with a severe illness. There the "distinctive clinical picture" was recognized, and as additional cases were recognized, the monkeys were identified as the source. Other cases occurred at virtually the same time in Frankfurt, Germany and in what was then, Belgrade, Yugoslavia (now Serbia) (Peters & LeDuc, 1999). It was determined that the monkeys in all three sites were from the same imported batch from Uganda, and that on arrival in Belgrade the shipment had contained many dead monkeys (Garrett, 1994). In all 32 people (31 were identified immediately and 1 that was not universally accepted was added later based on seropositivity) were identified as infected, including 6 secondary cases, and 7 died (Feldmann, Slenczka, & Klenk, 1996; Rollin et al., 2000). The full investigation ultimately led to the recognition of a new family of viruses, the *Filoviridiae*, of which Marburg virus was the first to be identified (Feldmann & Kiley, 2000). It also led to recommendations about the quarantine and handling of imported animals to prevent further outbreaks, but these recommendations are not yet uniformly followed in various countries and sites, as was learned in the Ebola-Reston outbreak discussed above. Investigations in Uganda did not reveal a reservoir host or vector at that time and none have yet been found.

Marburg virus is also a filovirus. It, too, is an RNA virus, and is similar to Ebola both genetically and morphologically (Feldmann & Kiley, 2000). It is not known how the animal host of Marburg transmits the virus to humans initially; however, once a person or monkey is ill, Marburg virus can be spread through direct contact. This spread can be through direct contact with body fluids, secretions or excretions, cultures, and equipment or objects contaminated with infectious material, all of which are believed to also be sources of disease. In at least one instance, the disease was transmitted from a male to a female by sexual contact 3 months after his illness. The virus has been found in seminal fluid months after infection (Centers for Disease Control, 1988; Rollin et al., 2000; Slenczka, 1999).

Marburg virus was not recognized again until 1975 when three cases were reported from Johannesburg, South Africa. The index case was a young Australian man who had been on vacation doing a walkabout in what was then Rhodesia and is now Zimbabwe with a female companion. Apparently during this time, he noticed a red swelling on his leg, and he believed he had been bitten but did not know by what. His illness began nearly a week later after arrival in South Africa. His companion became ill about a week later, and the nurse caring for her, a week after that. The man died, and the two women survived. Investigations of the couple's travel route yielded many potential opportunities for contact with some source for the virus including handling raw meat, touching monkeys in the Great Zimbabwe ruins, and sleeping outdoors in zebra grazing land (Garrett, 1994; "Lassa or Marburg or Jo'burg," 1975), but no reservoir could be found.

In 1980, Marburg was next recognized when an index patient became ill in western Kenya, followed by the secondary illness of his physician who tried to resuscitate him (Smith, Johnson, Isaacson, Swanepoel, Johnson, Killey, et al., 1982). In 1982, another single case was identified in South Africa (Centers for Disease Control, 1988). The next report, in 1987, involved a single case—also in western Kenya—in a 15-year-old male who had visited a bat cave before becoming ill and dying, leading to extensive investigations of the possibility that bats could be a reservoir host. No evidence was found to support this, and many other animal species also inhabited this cave (Johnson, Johnson, Silverstein, Tukei, Geisbert, Sanchez, et al., 1996). In late 1998, an outbreak of Marburg hemorrhagic fever occurred in Durba in the Democratic Republic of the Congo. Many of those affected were illegal gold miners in abandoned mines. The remote location and local warfare prevented experts from CDC and WHO from arriving for months. New cases were still apparent in September, 2000, and the total number of cases was 99 with a mortality rate of over 80% (Balter, 2000).

Marburg hemorrhagic fever has affected many fewer persons than Ebola to date. Its clinical manifestations, however, are no less severe. The incubation period is typically 5–10 days, after which there is a sudden onset of symptoms such as fever, chills, headache, and myalgia. At about the fifth day after onset, a maculopapular rash typically appears on the trunk, along with other symptoms such as nausea, vomiting, chest pain, diarrhea, sore throat, and abdominal pain. Symptoms increase in severity and may include jaundice, pancreatititis, severe weight loss, delirium, shock, liver failure, massive hemorrhaging, and multiorgan dysfunction. Recovery is prolonged, and may be accompanied by orchititis (in men), hepatitis, transverse myelitis, and/or uveitis. The case-fatality rate is usually between 23% and 25%

but has been higher. Treatment is nonspecific and supportive, including maintenance of fluid and electrolytes, maintaining oxygenation and blood pressure, and treating any complicating conditions and infections. Sometimes transfusions of various blood components related to preventing consumption of clotting factors are used. It is extremely important to use proper barrier-nursing techniques to prevent secondary cases to caretakers and families, including wearing protective gowns, gloves, and masks, strict isolation techniques and the proper disposal or sterilization of needles, equipment, and patient excretions (Centers for Disease Control and Prevention, 1999b). Primary cases appear to be at a higher risk for death (Centers for Disease Control, 1988).

LASSA VIRUS

Lassa fever first came to attention in 1969, when two missionary nurses in Jos, Nigeria contracted a mysterious fever while caring for patients in the mission hospital, although it had been described in the 1950s in native populations of West Africa (Fisher-Hoch & McCormick, 2000). In contrast to Ebola and Marburg viruses, Lassa virus is a member of the virus family known as *Arenaviridae* or arenaviruses. Arenaviruses are divided into two groups: the New World or Tacaribe complex and the Old World or LCM/Lassa complex. Some of the other members of these that cause illness in humans include the lymphocytic choriomeningitis virus, and the Junín, Machupo, and Guanarito viruses (see Appendix A, Table A.4). Lassa virus is a ribonucleic (RNA) virus that is enveloped and single stranded. There are four genetically diverse strains: Josiah, Nigeria, LP, and AV (Günther, Emmerich, Laue, Kühle, Asper, Jung, et al., 2000). Lassa virus was named after a town in northeastern Nigeria. The natural host has been identified as a rodent known as the multimammate rat of the *Mastomys* genus. At least two species of this rat carry the virus in Sierra Leone, *M. huberti*, and *M. erythroleucus*. This genus of rodent produce large numbers of offspring and are numerous in the savannas and forests of west, central, and east Africa. Some of the species prefer to live in or around human residences. Transmission results through direct contact with the rodent urine or droppings, through touching objects or eating food contaminated by them, or through breaks in the skin as well as through inhalation of air contaminated with rodent excretion in an aerosol. Since these rodents are a food source in Africa, infection may occur during food preparation or direct contact with the rodent. Person-to-person spread also occurs when a person comes into contact with infected blood, tissue, secretions, or excretions or through breathing airborne particles of the virus. Within health care settings, contaminated medical equipment such as reused needles and syringes may also spread the virus (Centers for Disease Control and Prevention, 1999).

Lassa fever is considered an endemic disease in such west African nations as Guinea, Liberia, Sierra Leone, and Nigeria, and may be in other parts of Africa as well. It may also occasionally be epidemic, in which instance the case fatality rate can reach as high as 50%, and outbreaks have been recognized in Central African Republic, Liberia, Nigeria, and Sierra Leone (World Health Organization, April 2000). It is estimated that there are about 100,000–300,000 Lassa virus infections each year, with about 5,000 deaths. Because surveillance is not uniform, these estimates are considered crude. About 10%–16% of patients admitted to hospitals in some areas of Sierra Leone and Liberia have Lassa fever. Lassa fever tends to peak in March with the dry season's harvest which allows the rodents to flourish, and diminish with the rainy season, but in 2000, this dip did not occur, and was attributed to overcrowded populations of displaced people. The incubation period can be 21 days (World Health Organization, April 2000).

In about 80% of those infected, persons are either asymptomatic or show mild symptoms. In the other 20%, symptoms may be severe, consisting of fever, retrosternal pain, sore throat with white tonsillar patches, back pain, cough, abdominal pain, vomiting, diarrhea, conjunctivitis, facial swelling, and mucosal bleeding. Neurological symptoms such as hearing loss, tremors, and encephalitis may also occur and are not well understood (Günther, Weisner, Roth, Grewing, Asper, Drosten, et al., 2001). For both the Ebola and Marburg viruses, a cellular entry factor, folate receptor-alpha, facilitates the entry of these viruses into cells (Chan, Empig, Welte, Speck, Schmaljohn, Kreisberg, et al., 2001). This finding may lead to new approaches in treatment and in vaccine development. The antiviral drug ribavirin administered intravenously is effective in treatment, especially when given early (Fisher-Hoch & McCormick, 2000; World Health Organization, 2000). Supportive care as described under Marburg hemorrhagic fever is also needed. The most common complication is deafness that can occur in about one third of the cases, even in mild cases. Hair loss and loss of coordination can occur. Spontaneous abortion is another complication. Overall, about 1% of Lassa viral infections result in death, but in those hospitalized for Lassa fever, the death rate is between 15% and 20% (Centers for Disease Control and Prevention, 1999).

In the year 2000, four identified cases of imported Lassa fever, all of whom died, were reported from Europe. These cases illustrate how quickly a person carrying a deadly infectious disease can be transported from endemic sites to non-endemic areas where the disease may not be readily recognized. In one case, a 23-year-old female student had been in Côte d'Ivoire and Ghana in November and December, 1999, returning to Germany on January 7, 2000 via Lisbon. She was admitted to a hospital soon after arrival with fever and flu-like symptoms, and died on January 15. No secondary cases were reported ("Imported case of Lassa fever," 2000). In another instance, a 48-year-old surgeon who was working in Sierra Leone returned to the Netherlands on July 14th after being treated for "malaria" on July 11th. He actually had Lassa fever. Airline officials contacted passengers who sat near him on the plane from Abidjan to Amsterdam, as well as cabin attendants, but no secondary cases were identified (World Health Organization, 2000).

PREVENTION OF THE AFRICAN VIRAL HEMORRHAGIC FEVERS

Prevention of the transmission of cases is through the use of appropriate barrier nursing techniques and through proper disposal of excreta, secretions, and the like. Prevention of Lassa viral infections also involves preventing contact with the rodent reservoir. These methods are detailed in Appendix C, Table C.6. Nosocomial spread in Africa is particularly difficult to control. While vaccine development would be attractive, the variability of the viruses and the risk of working with them have made progress somewhat difficult; however some progress is being made (Balter, 2000). Sociocultural and behavioral practices also influence preventive strategies. For example, Ebola virus is known to have been spread during funeral rites that include the washing of the body by the family of the deceased. Traditionally, there may be eating and dining from shared utensils. Another method of spread is by eating contaminated monkeys or other animals. People who are hungry will eat dead monkeys that they find for food regardless of health warnings to the contrary. Guidelines exist for management of the hemorrhagic fevers, especially under field conditions (Centers for Disease Control and Prevention, 1995; Colebunders & Borchert, 2000). The CDC has a number of teaching materials related to the viral hemorrhagic fevers that are available on-line through the special pathogens branch. The material on "Infection Control for Viral Haemorrhagic Fevers in the African Health Care Setting" is also available on-line in French at http://www.cdc.gov/ncidod/dvrd/spb.

SUMMARY

Nearly every year there are suspected cases of African viral hemorrhagic fevers in North America. Certainly because of the ease of global travel from Africa to the rest of the world (see chapter 22), and because initially the characteristics of the clinical syndromes caused by the hemorrhagic fever viruses may be nonspecific, the potential for actual cases in the rest of the world is real. In the last 15 years, there has been an increased frequency of outbreaks of the viral hemorrhagic fevers noted. The reasons are complex and include urbanization and population growth, inadequate housing, lack of sterilization of medical supplies and equipment, civil unrest, and lack of public health infrastructures. Many logistical and cultural practices impede surveillance and care. There are still many unknowns regarding the virology, natural history, ecology, epidemiology, treatment, and prevention of Ebola and Marburg hemorrhagic fevers. Further research should help elucidate the most effective approaches for prevention and care.

REFERENCES

After Marburg, Ebola. (1977). *Lancet, 1*(8011), 581-582.

Balter, M. (2000). On the trail of Ebola and Marburg viruses. *Science, 290*, 923–925.

Baxter, A. G. (2000). Symptomless infection with Ebola virus. *Lancet, 355*, 2178–2179.

Baron, R. C., McCormick, J. B., & Zubeir, O. A. (1983). Ebola virus disease in southern Sudan: Hospital dissemination and intrafamilial spread. *Bulletin of the World Health Organization, 61*, 997–1003.

Borchert, M., Boelaert, M., Sleurs, S., Muyembe-Tamfum, J. J., Pirard, P., Colebunders, R., et al. (2000). Viewpoint: Filovirus haemorrhagic fever outbreaks: Much ado about nothing? *Tropical Medicine and International Health, 5*, 318–324.

Breman, J. G., Piot, P., Johnson, K. M., et al. (1978). The epidemiology of Ebola haemorrhagic fever in Zaire, 1976. In S. R. Pattyn (Ed.), *Ebola virus haemorrhagic fever* (pp. 103–121). Amsterdam: Elsevier.

Bwaka, M. A., Bonnet, M. J., Calain, P., Colebunders, R., De Roo, A., Guimard, Y., et al. (1999). Ebola hemorrhagic fever in Kikwit, Democratic Republic of the Congo: Clinical observations in 103 patients. *Journal of Infectious Diseases, 179*(Suppl. 1), S1–S7.

Centers for Disease Control. (1988). Management of patients with suspected viral hemorrhagic fever. *Morbidity and Mortality Weekly Report, 37*(No. S-3), 1–16.

Centers for Disease Control. (1990). Update: Filovirus infections among persons with occupational exposure to nonhuman primates. *Morbidity and Mortality Weekly Report, 39,* 266, 273.

Centers for Disease Control and Prevention. (1995). Update: Management of patients with suspected viral hemorrhagic fever—United States. *Morbidity and Mortality Weekly Report, 44,* 475–479.

Centers for Disease Control and Prevention. (1999a). *Fact sheet—Lassa fever* [On-line]. Available: http://www.cdc.gov/ncidod/dvrd/spb/mnpages/disinfo.htm

Centers for Disease Control and Prevention. (1999b). *Fact sheet—Marburg hemorrhagic fever* [On-line]. Available: http://www.cdc.gov/ncidod/dvrd/spb/mnpages/disinfo.htm

Centers for Disease Control and Prevention. (2001). Outbreak of Ebola hemorrhagic fever—Uganda, August 2000–January 2001. *Morbidity and Mortality Weekly Report, 50,* 73–77.

Chan, S. Y., Empig, C. J., Welte, F. J., Speck, R. F., Schmaljohn, A., Kreisberg, J. F., et al. (2001). Folate receptor-alpha is a cofactor for cellular entry by Marburg and Ebola viruses. *Cell, 106,* 117–126.

Colebunders, R., & Borchert, M. (2000). Ebola hemorrhagic fever—a review. *Journal of Infection, 40,* 16–20.

Ebola haemorrhagic fever in Uganda—update 38. Disease outbreaks reported. (January 9, 2001). *WHO Communicable Disease Surveillance and Response,* unpaginated.

Feldmann, H., & Kiley, M. P. (2000). Classification, structure, and replication of filoviruses. *Current Topics in Microbiology and Immunology, 235,* 1–19.

Feldmann, H., Slenczka, W., & Klenk, H. D. (1996). Emerging and reemerging of filoviruses. *Archives of Virology Supplement, 11,* 77–100.

Fisher-Hoch, S. P., & McCormick, J. B. (2000). Lassa fever. In G. T. Stickland (Ed.), *Hunter's tropical medicine and emerging infectious diseases, 42,* (8th ed., pp. 275–279). Philadelphia: WB Saunders Co.

Garrett, L. (1994). *The coming plague.* New York: Farrar, Strauss and Giroux.

Georges, A-J, Leroy, E. M., Renaut, A. A., Benissan, C. T., Nabias, R. J., Ngoc, M. T., et al. (1999). Ebola hemorrhagic fever outbreaks in Gabon, 1994–1997: Epidemiologic and health control issues. *Journal of Infectious Diseases, 179*(Suppl. 1), S65–S75.

Günther, S., Emmerich, P., Laue, T., Kühle, O., Asper, M., Jung, A., et al. (2000). Imported Lassa fever in Germany: Molecular characterization of a new Lassa virus strain. *Emerging Infectious Diseases, 6,* 466–476.

Günther, S., Weisner, B., Roth, A., Grewing, T., Asper, M., Drosten, C., et al. (2001). Lassa fever encephalopathy: Lassa virus in cerebrospinal fluid but not in serum. *Journal of Infectious Diseases, 184,* 345–349.

Heymann, D. L., Weisfeld, J. S., Webb, P. A., Johnson, K. M., Cairns, T., & Berquist, H. (1980). Ebola hemorrhagic fever: Tandala, Zaire, 1977–1978. *Journal of Infectious Diseases, 142,* 372–376.

Imported case of Lassa fever in Germany—update. Disease outbreaks reported. (January 18, 2000). *WHO Communicable Disease Surveillance and Response,* unpaginated.

Johnson, E., Jaax, N., White, J., & Jahrling, P. (1995). Lethal experimental infections of rhesus monkeys by aerosolized Ebola virus. *International Journal of Experimental Pathology, 76,* 227–236.

Johnson, E. D., Johnson, B. K., Silverstein, D., Tukei, P., Geisbert, T. W., Sanchez, A. N., et al. (1996). Characterization of a new Marburg virus isolated from a 1987 fatal case in Kenya. *Archives of Virology Supplement, 11*(1), 101–114.

Khan, A. S., Tshioko, F. K., Heymann, D. L., Le Guenno, B., Nabeth, P., Kerstiëns, B., et al. (1999). The reemergence of Ebola hemorrhagic fever, Democratic Republic of the Congo, 1995. *Journal of Infectious Diseases, 179*(Suppl. 1), S76–S86.

Lassa or Marburg or Jo'burg. (1975). *Lancet, 1*(7909), 732–733.

Le Guenno, B., Formenty, P., Wyers, M., Gounon, P., Walker, F., & Boesch, C. (1995). Isolation and partial characterisation of a new strain of Ebola virus. *Lancet, 345,* 1271–1274.

Leroy, E. M., Baize, S., Debre, P., Lansoud-Soukate, J., & Mavoungou, E. (2001). Early immune responses accompanying human asymptomatic Ebola infections. *Clinical Exploratory Immunology, 124,* 453–460.

Leroy, E. M., Baize, S., Volchkov, V. E., Fisher-Hoch, S. P., Georges-Courbot, S. P., Lansoud-Soukate, J., et al. (2000). Human asymptomatic Ebola infection and strong inflammatory response. *Lancet, 355,* 2210–2215.

Miranda, M. E., White, M. E., Dayrit, M. M., Hayes, C. G., Ksiazek, T. G., & Burans, J. P. (1991). Seroepidemiological study of filovirus related to Ebola in the Philippines. *Lancet, 337,* 425–426.

Morvan, J. M., Deubel, V., Gounon, P., Nakoune, E., Barriere, P., Murri, S., Perpete, O., et al. (1999). Identification of Ebola virus sequences present as RNA or DNA in organs of terrestrial small mammals of the Central African Republic. *Microbes and Infection, 1,* 1193–1201.

Muyembe-Tamfun, J. J., Kipasa, M., Kiyungu, C., & Colebunders, R. (1999). Ebola outbreak in Kikwit, Democratic Republic of the Congo: Discovery and control measures. *Journal of Infectious Diseases, 179*(Suppl. 1), S259–S262.

Peters, C. J., & LeDuc, J. W. (1999). An introduction to Ebola: The virus and the disease. *Journal of Infectious Diseases, 179*(Suppl. 1), ix–xvi.

Reuters. (2001, February 8). Doctors say flier's illness was not Ebola. *New York Times* [On-line]. Available: http://www.nytimes.com/2001/02/08/health/08EBOL.html

Richards, G. A., Murphy, S., Jobson, R., Mer, M., Zinman, C., Taylor, R., et al. (2000). Unexpected Ebola virus in a tertiary setting: Clinical and epidemiologic aspects. *Critical Care Medicine, 28,* 240–244.

Rollin, P. E., Calain, P., & Ksiazek, T. E. (2000). Ebola and Marburg virus infections. In G. T. Strickland (Ed.), *Hunter's tropical medicine and emerging infectious diseases* (8th ed., pp. 281–284). Philadelphia: WB Saunders.

Sanchez, A., Ksiazek, T. G., Rollin, P. E., Peters, C. J., Nichol, S. T., Khan, A. S., et al. (1995). Reemergence of Ebola virus in Africa. *Emerging Infectious Diseases, 1,* 96–97.

Schou, S., & Hansen, A. K. (2000). Marburg and Ebola virus infections in laboratory non-human primates: A literature review. *Comparative Medicine, 50,* 108–123.

Slenczka, W. G. (1999). The Marburg virus outbreak of 1967 and subsequent episodes. *Current Topics in Microbiology and Immunology, 235,* 49–75.

Smith, D. H., Johnson, B. K., Isaacson, M., Swanepoel, R., Johnson, K. M., Killey, M., et al. (1982). Marburg-virus disease in Kenya. *Lancet, 1*(8276), 816–820.

World Health Organization. (1992). Viral haemorrhagic fever in imported monkeys. *Weekly Epidemiologic Record, 67,* 142–143.

World Health Organization. (2000). Outbreak news. Lassa fever, imported case, Netherlands. *Weekly Epidemiologic Record, 75,* 265.

World Health Organization. (April, 2000). Lassa fever. *Fact sheet* (No. 179), unpaginated.

World Health Organization (December, 2000). Ebola haemorrhagic fever. *Fact sheet* (No. 103), unpaginated.

World Health Organization. (2001). Outbreak news. Ebola, Uganda (update). *Weekly Epidemiologic Record, 76,* 1.

9

Escherichia coli O157:H7

Donna Tartasky

At the beginning of September 1999, the New York State Department of Health received at least 10 reports of children hospitalized with bloody diarrhea or *E. coli* O157:H7 infection near Albany, New York (Centers for Disease Control and Prevention, 1999). All cases had attended the Washington County Fair, that was held during the last week in August. By the middle of September, 921 persons had reported diarrhea after attending the fair. Stool cultures yielded *E. coli* O157:H7 from 116 persons. Sixty-five persons were hospitalized; 11 children developed hemolytic uremic syndrome (HUS); and 2 persons died: a 3-year-old girl from HUS and a 79-year-old man from HUS/thrombotic thrombocytopenic purpura. An environmental investigation determined that most of the fair was supplied with chlorinated water. A shallow well supplied unchlorinated water, however, to several food vendors in at least one area who used the water to make drinks and ice. Initial cultures of this water yielded high levels of coliforms and *E. coli*. DNA "fingerprints" demonstrated that isolates from the well, the water distribution system and most patients were similar. This confirmed the fact that the 116 persons whose stool cultures yielded *E. coli* O157:H7 were infected from the unchlorinated well water. While the source of the well's contamination was not established with certainty, it might have resulted from runoff from cow manure or from a septic system serving a 4-H dormitory on the fairgrounds near the well (Centers for Disease Control and Prevention, 1999; State of New York Department of Health, 2000).

Escherichia coli are gram-negative, non-spore forming, rod shaped bacteria of the Enterobacteriaceae family. They are one of the major normal organisms in the intestine (Levine & Nataro, 2000). They are capable of surviving in soil and in food for long periods (Weber & Rutala, 2001). Pathogenic strains that can cause diarrhea are categorized in various ways—enterohemorrhagic, enterotoxigenic, enteroinvasive, enteropathogenic, enteroaggregative, and diffuse-adherent based on virulence mechanisms (Levine & Nataro, 2000). Serotypes are designated on the basis of their O (somatic), and H (flagellar) antigens (Griffin & Boyce, 1998). Analysis of the decoded genome of *E. coli* O157:H7 may ultimately lead to new therapeutic approaches (Schubert, 2001). This chapter will focus on *E. coli* O157:H7, an emerging pathogen that has stimulated worldwide interest due to several large foodborne outbreaks in the United States (U.S.), Europe, and Japan. *E. coli* O157:H7 has the ability to produce two toxins called Shiga-like or Shiga toxins because of their similarity to toxins produced by *Shigella dysenteriae*. It also has two virulence factors, the first being its ability to produce Shiga toxins (Stx) and the second is the ability to adhere closely to mucosa. *E. coli* O157:H7 has been referred to as verocytotoxic (a term no longer recommended for use), and is classified as enterohemorrhagic (EHEC). It is also sometimes referred to as one of the Shiga-like *E. coli* (STEC) (Griffin & Boyce, 1998).

E. coli O157:H7 is the STEC strain that will be discussed in this chapter; however, other non-O157 strains have emerged, and although underreported are believed to be new pathogens also causing outbreaks of disease (López, Prado-Jimênez, O'Ryan-Gallardo, & Contrini, 2000). Both sporadic and epidemic gastrointestinal infections are caused by *E. coli* O157:H7 (Wong, Jelacic, Habeeb, Watkins, & Tarr, 2000). Transmission is foodborne, waterborne, and through animal-to-human and person-to-person contact, largely through the fecal-oral route. Nosocomial transmission has been described (Weightman & Kirby, 2000). Relatively few organisms are needed for infection from as few as 10 to around 100–200 (López et al., 2000; Schubert, 2001). In a 1994 outbreak of *E. coli* O157:H7 involving salami, the infectious dose was estimated to be lower than 50 organisms (Tilden, Young, McNamara, Custer, Boesl, Lambert-Fair, et al., 1996). Asymptomatic carriage of *E. coli* O157:H7 can occur and is important in secondary spread of this pathogen (Coia, 1998). Person-to-person transmission is the predominant mode of infection in outbreaks of *E. coli* O157:H7 in group settings such as day care facilities and in nursing homes and institutions (Belongia, Osterholm, Soles, Ammend, Braun, & MacDonald, 1993; López et al., 2000). Household transmission rates have been estimated at 4% to 15% (Weber & Rutala, 2001).

E. coli O157:H7 was first described as a human pathogen in 1982, when it was implicated as the causative agent in two outbreaks of hemorrhagic colitis, a clinical entity characterized by abdominal cramps, bloody stools, and little or no fever (Centers for Disease Control, 1982). The following year, researchers described an association between *E. coli* and Shiga toxins (Stx) and a post-diarrheal hemolytic uremic syndrome (HUS)—a clinical condition marked by acute renal injury, thrombocytopenia, and microangiopathic hemolytic anemia (Karmali, Steele, Petric, & Lim, 1983).

The incubation period from time of exposure to *E. coli* O157:H7 to presentation of symptoms is 1–14 days after exposure. The most common clinical presentation is bloody or non-bloody diarrhea accompanied by severe, cramping abdominal pain. Fever is uncommon but vomiting occurs in about half of people who are infected (Coia, 1998). Most people have symptoms that subside in about a week; but sequelae can include HUS, thrombotic thrombocytopenic purpura, and even death (Griffin & Boyce, 1998).

HUS is the most significant clinical complication of *E. coli* O157:H7 infection, occurring in about 6%–7% of patients. *E. coli* O157:H7 infection is the most common cause of HUS in children—especially under 5 years of age, and the elderly, but can occur at any age. Manifestations of HUS include microangiopathic anemia, thrombotic thrombocytopenic purpura (TTP), acute renal failure, and central nervous system manifestations (Centers for Disease Control and Prevention, 1999, 2001a; Coia, 1998; Grabowski, 2002; Griffin & Boyce, 1998). Complications related to manifestations of HUS may occur and include stroke, blindness, seizures and coma as well as chronic kidney failure. Some patients who regain renal function may develop end-stage kidney disease or other long-term sequelae such as colonic stricture, chronic pancreatitis, and cognitive impairment (Mead & Griffin, 1998). Hypertension, diabetes mellitus, and cardiomyopathy have also been described as long-term sequelae (Green, Murphy, & Uttley, 2000). TTP, mostly occurring in adults, tends to have less renal manifestations and more neurologic involvement. Approximately 3%–5% of persons who develop HUS die (Centers for Disease Control and Prevention, 1999). Risk factors for HUS have been bloody diarrhea, fever, elevated blood leukocytes, and treatment with antimotility agents (Griffin & Boyce, 1998). Antibiotic treatment has been shown to have an association with the development of HUS in children with *E. coli* O157:H7 infection, and therefore it is not recommended until the pathogen causing the diarrhea is known and antibiotic treatment is appropriate (Wong et al., 2000). In general, supportive measures are recommended for the treatment of *E. coli* O157:H7, including correcting and maintaining fluid and electrolyte balance, particularly in children (López et al., 2000). Treatment with antibiotics has not been shown to improve the course of illness or prevent complications (Griffin & Boyce, 1998) and may actually cause harm (Schubert, 2001). Therapy for HUS consists mainly of supportive care. Transfusion of packed red blood cells is recommended if the hemoglobin concentration falls below 6.0 g/dL or symptomatic anemia is present. Peritoneal or kidney dialysis may also be indicated with HUS.

E. coli O157:H7 appears mainly to be a disease reported in industrialized countries and has been reported in over 30 countries in six continents (Cody, Glynn, Farrar, Cairns, Griffin, Kobayashi, et al., 1999; Mead & Griffin, 1998). Yet, several countries in Europe have reported no outbreaks of *E. coli* O157:H7. FoodNet data for 1999, reported 530 *E. coli* O157:H7 infections and a 22% decline in the incidence of this pathogen from 1996–1999 (Centers for Disease Control and Prevention, 2000). No data specific to the H7 serotype were mentioned in this report. In Argentina, where more cases of HUS have been reported than anywhere else, STEC has been identified in fecal samples of cattle used for meat and milk production (López et al., 2000). A wide variety of foods have been implicated in *E. coli* O157:H7 infections. Typically they are of bovine origin such as undercooked ground beef, roast beef, yogurt, and unpasteurized milk. Foods such as apple cider, apple juice, fruits, salad vegetables, and alfalfa sprouts, however, have also been linked to infection (Centers for Disease Control and Prevention, 1997, 2001a).

The largest U.S. outbreak of *E. coli* O157:H7, which affected several hundred persons in Washington, Idaho, California, and Nevada was due to undercooked hamburgers served at a restaurant chain. Although the outbreak began in November, 1992, it came to the attention of the CDC in January, 1993 when a physician in Washington recognized a cluster of children with HUS and an increase in bloody diarrhea in the emergency room (Centers for Disease Control and Prevention, 1993). Outbreaks have also been associated with drinking unpasteurized commercial apple juice in several western states and British Columbia, and with drinking unpasteurized apple cider where some of the cider was made from apples that had dropped to the ground (Centers for Disease Control and Prevention, 1996; Centers for Disease

Control and Prevention, 1997). Additional outbreaks have been associated with produce including lettuce, potatoes, and fresh apple cider, that were presumably contaminated by animal manure (Ackers, Mahon, Leahy, Goode, Damrow, Hayes, et al., 1998; Cody et al., 1999). Fourteen separate clusters of *E. coli* O157:H7 were reported in Japan from May through August of 1996 (Watanabe, Ozasa, Mermin, Griffin, Masuda, Imashuku, et al., 1999). An investigation of one outbreak among Japanese factory workers linked eating radish sprout salad during lunch to illness (Watanabe et al., 1999). Similarly, an outbreak of infection in the United States related to eating alfalfa sprouts has also been reported (López et al., 2000). It is often the sprout seeds that are contaminated, and it is difficult to decontaminate the seeds (Mohle-Boetani, Farrar, Werner, Minassian, Bryant, Abbott, et al., 2001). Another source of infection may be through contact between animals and humans at farms or petting zoos (Centers for Disease Control and Prevention, 2001b).

Although reports of waterborne outbreaks of *E. coli* O157:H7 are relatively uncommon, they have been reported. The appearance of *E. coli* O157:H7 has been documented in unchlorinated swimming water and lakes (Griffin & Boyce, 1998; Wang & Doyle, 1998). And an outbreak of swimming-associated transmission of *E. coli* O157:H7 in freshwater was recently reported in Finland (Paunio, Pebody, Keskimaki, Kokki, Ruutu, Oinonen, et al., 1999). Surveillance of *E. coli* O157:H7 has demonstrated that over 60% of cases occur between May and September. Although the reason for this increased incidence in the summer is unknown, it is speculated that it may be related to increased ambient temperature (Michel, Wilson, Martin, Clarke, McEwen, & Gyles, 1999). Others have conjectured that the seasonal variation may reflect factors related to farming practices, variations in ground beef consumption or cooking practices (Griffin & Boyce, 1998).

Overall, *E. coli* O157:H7 is estimated to cause 21,000 infections in the U.S. annually (Griffin & Boyce, 1998). In a multicenter study, the rate of isolation of this pathogen from stool specimens with visible blood was higher than that of any other pathogen (Slutsker, Ries, Greene, Wells, Huttwagner, & *Escherichia coli* O157:H7 Study Group, 1997). While the numbers of infections are relatively small compared with other enteric pathogens, *E. coli* O157:H7 has the potential to produce severe, life-threatening illness. Unfortunately, natural infection with *E. coli* O157:H7 does not confer immunity and no vaccination is available to protect against this pathogen and specific Stx producing strains.

Shiga toxin *Escherichia coli* (STEC) O157:H7 lack rapid sorbitol fermentation and β-glucuronidase production. These phenotypic characteristics have been used to distinguish this serotype from other *E. coli* strains (March & Ratnam, 1986). The first of these is SMAC supplementation with fluorogenic and chromogenic methods (Thompson, Hodge, & Borczyk, 1990). Reports of chromogenic media targeting the beta-glucuronidase activity of *E. coli* O157:H7 suggest this may be better than SMAC for selective isolation of this pathogen (Goldwater & Bettelheim, 1998). Additionally, enyzme-linked immunosorbent assay (ELISA) kits are commercially available for rapid screening of the O157 antigen; however, positive screening results by ELISA still need to be confirmed by culture.

The importance of quick and accurate laboratory diagnosis of an *E. coli* O157:H7 outbreak is underscored by the need for case finding to define the extent of the outbreak, investigate the source of the contamination, examine specimens from suspected reservoirs of infection, and provide appropriate treatment measures. Once an isolate of *E. coli* O157:H7 is identified, the local public health department should be notified immediately. Exclusion of infected children from day care is necessary until two consecutive stool cultures are negative for *E. coli* O157:H7.

Reports from some well-publicized *E. coli* O157:H7 outbreaks document the virulence of this pathogen in terms of related morbidity and mortality. In 1996, a small cluster of *E. coli* O157:H7 was linked to a brand of unpasteurized apple juice in the western U.S. and British Columbia, Canada. Seventy people were infected due to exposure to the unpasteurized apple juice. Of these, 25 (36%) were hospitalized, 14 (20%) developed HUS, and 1 (1%) died (Cody et al., 1999). Aggregated U.S. data from 1982–early 1993 reported that 23% of patients with *E. coli* virus infection were hospitalized, 6% developed HUS or TTP, and 1.2% died (Griffin, 1995). A large outbreak that involved almost 8,000 schoolchildren in Sakai City, Japan, in 1996 has also been documented. In this outbreak, 758 children were hospitalized and 121 developed HUS. No statistics were given on mortality (Yoshioka, Yagi, & Moriguchi, 1999).

Primary prevention of *E. coli* O157:H7 is the most important way to prevent infection and HUS, as well as other complications. Such prevention requires multiple interventions that address cultural, behavioral, and societal factors. Since most preventative measures necessitate behavioral changes, they are often difficult to accomplish.

Educating people about the need to thoroughly cook meat and to drink pasteurized milk and juices would help decrease outbreaks related to this cause. Of parallel importance, people need to not only be educated about prevention of *E. coli* O157:H7 but also be aware of the relationship between their health practices and the health of others. For example, individuals who handle food either in restaurants or the home need to understand how improper food handling can affect the health of others. In other words, in order to prevent contamination or spread of *E. coli* O157:H7, individuals need to think of what is often labeled in public health as "the greater good." Measures to prevent this and other foodborne infections are given in Appendix C, Table C.1.

REFERENCES

Ackers, M. L., Mahon, B. E., Leahy, E., Goode, B., Damrow, T., Hayes, P. S., et al. (1998). An outbreak of *Escherichia coli* O157:H7 infections associated with leaf lettuce consumption. *Journal of Infectious Diseases, 177,* 1588–1593.

Belongia, E. A., Osterholm, M. T., Soler, J. T., Ammend, D. A., Braun, J. E., & MacDonald, K. L. (1993). Transmission of *Escherichia coli* O157:H7 infection in Minnesota child day-care facilities. *Journal of the American Medical Association, 269,* 2217–2220.

Centers for Disease Control. (1982). Isolation of *E. coli* O157:H7 from sporadic cases of hemorrhagic colitis—United States. *Morbidity and Mortality Weekly Report, 34,* 581–585.

Centers for Disease Control and Prevention. (1993). Update: Multistate outbreak of *Escherichia coli* O157:H7 infections from hamburgers—Western United States, 1992–1993. *Morbidity and Mortality Weekly Report, 42,* 258–263.

Centers for Disease Control and Prevention. (1996). Outbreak of *Escherichia coli* O157:H7 infections associated with drinking unpasteurized commercial apple juice—British Columbia, California, Colorado, and Washington, October, 1996. *Morbidity and Mortality Weekly Report, 45,* 975.

Centers for Disease Control and Prevention. (1997). Outbreaks of *Escherichia coli* O157:H7 infection and cryptosporidiosis associated with drinking unpasteurized apple cider—Connecticut and New York, October 1996. *Morbidity and Mortality Weekly Report, 46,* 4–8.

Centers for Disease Control and Prevention. (1999). Outbreak of *Escherichia coli* O157:H7 and *Campylobacter* among attendees of the Washington County Fair—New York. *Morbidity and Mortality Weekly Report, 48,* 803–805.

Centers for Disease Control and Prevention. (2000). Preliminary FoodNet data on the incidence of foodborne illnesses—selected sites, United States, 1999. *Morbidity and Mortality Weekly Report, 49,* 201–205.

Centers for Disease Control and Prevention. (2001a). Diagnosis and management of foodborne illnesses: A primer for physicians. *Morbidity and Mortality Weekly Report, 50*(RR-02), 1–69.

Centers for Disease Control and Prevention. (2001b). Outbreaks of *Escherichia coli* O157:H7 infections among children associated with farm visits—Pennsylvania and Washington, 2000. *Morbidity and Mortality Weekly Report, 50*, 293–297.

Cody, S. H., Glynn, M. K., Farrar, J. A., Cairns, K. L., Griffin, P. M., Kobayashi, J., et al. (1999). An outbreak of *Escherichia coli* O157:H7 infection from unpasteurized commercial apple juice. *Annals of Internal Medicine, 130*, 202–209.

Coia, J. E. (1998). Clinical, microbiological and epidemiological aspects of *Escherichia coli* O157 infection. *FEMS Immunology and Medical Microbiology, 20*, 1–9.

Goldwater, P. N., & Bettelheim, K. A. (1998). New perspectives on the role of *Escherichia coli* O157:H7 and the other enterohaemorrhagic *E. coli* serotypes in human disease. *Journal of Medical Microbiology, 47*, 1039–1045.

Grabowski, E. F. (2002). The hemolytic–uremic syndrome—Toxin, thrombin, and thrombosis. *New England Journal of Medicine, 346*, 58–61.

Green, D. A., Murphy, W. G., & Uttley, W. S. (2000). Haemolytic uraemic syndrome: Prognostic factors. *Clinical Laboratory Haematology, 22*, 11–14.

Griffin, P. M. (1995). *Escherichia coli* O157:H7 and other enterohemorrhagic *Escherichia coli*. In M. J. Blaser, P. D. Smith, J. I. Ravdin, H. B. Greenberg, & R. L. Guerrant (Eds.), *Infections of the gastrointestinal tract* (pp. 739–761). New York: Raven Press.

Griffin, P. M., & Boyce, T. G. (1998). *Escherichia coli* O157:H7. In W. M. Scheld, D. Armstrong, & J. M. Hughes (Eds.), *Emerging infections I* (pp. 137–145). Washington, DC: ASM Press.

Karmali, M. A., Steele, B. T., Petric, M., & Lim, C. (1983). Sporadic cases of haemolytic-uraemic syndrome associated with faecal cytotoxin and cytotoxin-producing *Escherichia coli* in stools. *Lancet, 1*(8325), 619–620.

Levine, M. M., & Nataro, J. P. (2000). Diarrhea caused by *Escherichia coli*. In G. T. Strickland (Ed.), *Hunter's tropical medicine and emerging infectious diseases, 42* (8th ed., pp. 334–338). Philadelphia: WB Saunders Co.

López, E. L., Prado-Jiménez, V., O'Ryan-Gallardo, M., & Contrini, M. M. (2000). Shigella and shiga toxin-producing *Escherichia coli* causing bloody diarrhea in Latin America. *Infectious Disease Clinics of North America, 14*, 41–65.

March, S. B., & Ratnam, S. (1986). Sorbitol-MacConkey medium for detection of *Escherichia coli* O157:H7 associated with hemorrhagic colitis. *Journal of Clinical Microbiology, 23*, 869–872.

Mead, P. S., & Griffin, P. M. (1998). *Escherichia coli* O157:H7. *Lancet, 352*, 1207–1212.

Michel, P., Wilson, J. B., Martin, S. W., Clarke, R. C., McEwen, S. A., & Gyles, C. L. (1999). Temporal and geographical distributions of reported cases of *Escherichia coli* O157:H7 infection in Ontario. *Epidemiology and Infection, 122*, 193–200.

Mohle-Boetani, J. C., Farrar, J. A., Werner, S. B., Minassian, D., Bryant, R., Abbott, S., et al. (2001). *Escherichia coli* O157:H7 and *Salmonella* infections associated with sprouts in California, 1996–1998. *Annals of Internal Medicine, 135*, 239–247.

Paunio, M., Pebody, R., Keskimaki, M., Kokki, M., Ruutu, P., Oinonen, S., et al. (1999). Swimming-associated outbreak of *Escherichia coli* O157:H7. *Epidemiology and Infection, 122*, 1–5.

Schubert, C. (2001). Busting the gut busters. Virulent *E. coli* are revealing some weaknesses. *Science News, 160*, 74–76.

Slutsker, L., Ries, A. A., Greene, K. D., Wells, J. G., Hutwagner, L., Griffin, P. M., & *Escherichia coli* O157:H7 Study Group. (1997). *Escherichia coli* O157:H7 diarrhea in the United States: Clinical and epidemiologic features. *Annals of Internal Medicine, 126*, 505–513.

State of New York Department of Health. (2000). *Health commissioner releases* E. coli *outbreak report* [On-line]. Available: http://www.health.state.ny.us/nysdoh/commish/2000/ecoli.htm

Thompson, J. S., Hodge, D. S., & Borczyk, A. A. (1990). Rapid biochemical test to identify verocytotoxin-positive stains of *Escherichia coli* serotype O157. *Journal of Clinical Microbiology, 28*, 2165–2168.

Tilden, J., Young, W., McNamara, A. M., Custer, C., Boesl, B., Lambert-Fair, M. A., et al. (1996). A new route of transmission for *Escherichia coli*: Infection from dry fermented salami. *American Journal of Public Health, 86*, 1142–1145.

Wang, G., & Doyle, M. P. (1998). Survival of enterohemorrhagic *Escherichia coli* O157:H7 in water. *Journal of Food Protection, 61*, 662–667.

Watanabe, Y., Ozasa, K., Mermin, J. H., Griffin, P. M., Masuda, K., Imashuku, S., et al. (1999). Factory outbreak of *Escherichia coli* O157:H7 infection in Japan. *Emerging Infectious Diseases, 5*, 424–428.

Weber, D. J., & Rutala, W. A. (2001). The emerging nosocomial pathogens *Cryptosporidium*, *Escherichia coli* O157:H7, *Helicobacter pylori*, and hepatitis C: Epidemiology, environmental survival, efficacy of disinfection, and control measures. *Infection Control and Hospital Epidemiology, 22*, 306–315.

Weightman, N. C., & Kirby, P. J. G. (2000). Nosocomial *Escherichia coli* O157 infection. *Journal of Hospital Infection, 44*, 107–111.

Wong, C. S., Jelacic, S., Habeeb, R. L., Watkins, S. L., & Tarr, P. I. (2000). The risk of the hemolytic-uremic syndrome after antibiotic treatment of *Escherichia coli* O157:H7 infections. *New England Journal of Medicine, 342*, 1930–1935.

Yoshioka, K., Yagi, K., & Moriguchi, N. (1999). Clinical features and treatment of children with hemolytic uremic syndrome caused by enterohemorrhagic *Escherichia coli* O157:H7 infection: Experience of an outbreak in Sakai City, 1996. *Pediatrics International, 41*, 223–227.

10

Hantavirus Pulmonary Syndrome

Amy V. Groom and James E. Cheek

In 1993, a young, previously healthy, athletic Navajo man died shortly after collapsing at the funeral of his fiancee in New Mexico. The two deaths signaled the beginning of an intense search for a mysterious killer of young, healthy adults living in sparsely populated rural areas of the American West. Both young people had died of adult respiratory distress syndrome (ARDS), a condition resulting from multiple etiologies including trauma, severe infections, and some environmental toxins. Particularly worrisome to clinicians was the rapid course of the illness; both victims had succumbed within 24 hours. Because plague was known to be endemic in the region, pneumonic plague was the first diagnosis to be ruled out. At that point, clinicians and public health authorities began to systematically work through a long list of known infectious agents and environmental toxins, such as phosphene gas, a toxin produced in World War I and still routinely used in the area to control prairie dogs; however, phosphene turned out to be nothing more than a tantalizing hypothesis as no evidence could be found that the two victims had been exposed.

The initial response of public health authorities in the region was to search for additional cases of the illness while simultaneously gathering information to develop working hypotheses on the etiology. Within a week of the first two cases, four additional cases of severe respiratory illness in young, previously healthy adults were identified. These cases occurred within the previous 6 months and were spread over an area of 40,000 square miles and 12 medical facilities. Epidemiologists immediately began to develop a case-control study to help identify the etiology of this mysterious disease, but the etiology remained elusive. Although pathologic changes found in tissues of victims were consistent with some viral infections, a specific causative agent was not readily identified.

A breakthrough finally came 2 weeks into the investigation when scientists at the Special Pathogens Branch at the Centers for Disease Control and Prevention (CDC) observed a consistently positive test result while testing patients' serum samples against a panel of known viral hemorrhagic fever agents. Surprisingly, the samples tested positive for two strains of hantavirus, an agent found in Eurasia, but previously not thought to cause illness in the Americas. Acute and convalescent titers from one of the few surviving patients confirmed the diagnosis as a hantavirus. The causative hantavirus, eventually named Sin Nombre Virus (SNV), was isolated in culture from small mammal carriers. Ultimately, 17 people were affected in this outbreak and 14 died.

Named for the Hantaan River in South Korea where the prototype virus (Hantaan) was first isolated in 1976 (Lee, Lee, & Johnson, 1978), the genus *Hantavirus* contains at least 30 viruses that are found worldwide (Peters, Mills, Spiropoulou, Zaki, & Rollin, 1999). A member of the *Bunyaviridae* family, hantaviruses are icosahedral, lipid-enveloped, tri-segmented negative sense RNA viruses. The length of time the virus can survive in the environment is unknown. Each hantavirus strain has one primary rodent reservoir. Transmission within rodent populations occurs horizontally via scratching and biting, resulting in a lifelong, asymptomatic infection (Butler & Peters, 1994; Peters, 1998). Vertical transmission of hantavirus has not been demonstrated in rodents or in humans (Howard, Doyle, Koster, Zaki, Khan, Petersen, et al., 1999; Mills, Ksiazek, Ellis, Rollin, Nichol, Yates, et al., 1997). Hantaviruses are not associated with illness in their rodent hosts, though infectious virus is shed through an infected rodent's saliva, urine, and feces. Virus transmission to humans occurs when aerosols of rodent excreta are inhaled. It may also be spread through the bite of an infected rodent, contamination of broken skin with infected rodent saliva and excreta, and possibly through the ingestion of contaminated food or water (Centers for Disease Control and Prevention, 1993a; Khan & Ksiazek, 2000). Transmission to humans can result in a range of illnesses depending on the particular hantavirus, including hemorrhagic fever with renal syndrome (HFRS) and HPS (Khan & Ksiazek, 2000). Although possible human-to-human transmission of a hantavirus pulmonary syndrome (HPS) causing hantavirus has been documented in Argentina (Wells, Sosa Estani, Yadon, Enria, Padula, Pini, et al., 1997), a review of HPS cases in the U.S. found no evidence to suggest that this has occurred in the United States (Wells, Young, Williams, Armstrong, Busico, Khan, et al., 1997). Hantaviruses associated with HFRS have been isolated in rodent species worldwide, though most commonly in Asia and Europe. Hantaviruses associated with HPS, however, have only been found in the Americas, with more than 800 cases identified throughout North, Central, and South America as of December 31st, 2000.

HANTAVIRUSES IN THE U.S.

Prior to 1993, hantaviruses found in indigenous rodent populations in the U.S., such as the Prospect Hill virus carried by meadow voles (*Microtus pennslyvanicus*) were not linked to human disease (Yanagihara, 1990). In 1993, however, environmental conditions in the southwest U.S. set the stage for the recognition of a previously unidentified hantavirus that caused a newly described syndrome: hantavirus pulmonary syndrome (Nichol, Spiropoulou, Morzunov, Rollin, Ksiazek, Feldmann, et al., 1993). The causative hantavirus was subsequently named Sin Nombre Virus (SNV). Since then, other hantaviruses that cause HPS have been identified in the United States: Black Creek Canal virus (Khan, Gaviria, Rollin, Hlady, Ksiazek, Armstrong, et al., 1996), Bayou virus (Morzunov, Feldmann, Spiropoulou, Semenova, Rollin, Ksiazek, et al., 1995), Monogahela virus (Rhodes, Huang, Sanchez, Nichol, Zaki, Ksiazek, et al., 2000), and New York virus (Hjelle, Krolikowski, Torrez-Martinez, Chavez-Giles, Vanner, & Laposata, 1995).

Distinct from one another, all of these HPS-causing viruses are part of the same clade (a group that shares a common ancestor) and are found among members of the Muridae subfamily Sigmodontinae. Sigmodontine rodents are found exclusively in the New World, which may explain why HPS is unique to the Americas (Peters, 1998). In the United States, SNV is responsible for the majority of HPS cases. The rodent host for SNV is the deer mouse (*Peromyscus maniculatus*), and is found extensively throughout Canada and the U.S. (Khan, Ksiazek, &

Peters, 1996). A largely rural species, *P. maniculatus* can invade suburban and urban dwellings (Khan, Graves, Fritz, Young, Metzger, Humphreys, et al., 2001).

ENVIRONMENTAL FACTORS

Environmental determinants of risk for hantavirus infection primarily reflect factors associated with an abundance of small mammal carriers of the virus. Clearly, risk of acquiring SNV increases with increasing numbers of *Peromyscus maniculatus* in the environment. Increases in rodent populations, called rodent blooms, appear to occur cyclically, and are one of many factors that contribute to increased risk of hantavirus infection in humans. Indeed, the initial case-control study of HPS in the southwestern U.S. found an elevated risk for households with more mice present (Zeitz, Butler, Cheek, Samuel, Childs, Shands, et al., 1995). Factors affecting rodent population density may be biotic in the form of predation and competition, or abiotic, such as weather. Predictive models of changing patterns of risk over large geographic areas can be developed for abiotic factors. Much of the variation in vegetation in the U.S. southwest, for example, is thought to reflect the influence of the El Niño Southern Oscillation (ENSO) phenomenon, which has an effect on rodent populations (Glass, Cheek, Patz, Shields, Doyle, Throughman, et al., 2000). ENSO, a recurring, cyclical oceanic/atmospheric disruption in the tropical Pacific, affects weather patterns around the world. In the southwestern U.S. this disruption causes an increase in precipitation, resulting in more vegetation. The abundant shelter and food provided by this vegetation improve rodent habitat, creating ideal conditions for a rodent population increase (Engelthaler, Mosley, Cheek, Levy, Komatsu, Ettestad, et al., 1999). The relationship between this phenomenon and human risk, however, is a more complex one. Predicting human risk spatially and temporally may not be a simple linear correlation, with more rain equaling more mice, and therefore more human risk (Mills, Yates, Ksiazek, Peters, & Childs, 1999). Concomitant with fluctuations in population density, seroprevalence in rodent populations can vary dramatically over time and geographical location.

To date, most predictive studies of HPS seek to define the mathematical relationship among remotely sensed satellite variables and human risk. Such studies are relatively large scale, using changes in landscape features visible by high altitude satellites such as LANDSAT or NOAA's Advanced Very High Resolution Recorder. One study linked rainfall and temperature to HPS cases (Engelthaler et al., 1999). Glass and colleagues (2000) developed a model using LANDSAT data to predict high-risk areas for HPS transmission in the Southwest up to 1 year before an outbreak may occur. This could be useful in hantavirus prevention activities.

The majority (96%) of HPS cases in the United States are caused by SNV and are inextricably linked to the ecology of its rodent host, *P. maniculatus. Peromyscus* species have a wider range of habitats compared to other U.S. hantavirus hosts. They also tend to favor peridomestic settings and have a higher population density than these other species, and as a result, are more likely to come into contact with humans (Khan et al., 1996). Although most (95%) of HSP cases have occurred west of the Mississippi River, cases have been identified in the eastern United States including New England (Centers for Disease Control and Prevention, 2001a, 2001b).

As of April 2001, 283 confirmed HPS cases in 31 states had been identified. About 60% of these cases occurred in men. The mean age for HPS cases is 37 years (range 10–75 years), with more cases occurring among adults than children (Centers for Disease Control and Prevention, 2001). Whether this pattern reflects suboptimal case identification among pediatric populations due to inherent biases in current surveillance, milder disease in this population, or lower incidence of hantavirus infection is unclear (Bryan, Doyle, Moolenaar, Pflieger, Khan, Ksiazek, et al., 1997). Although the majority of HPS cases in the United States have occurred in Whites, HPS cases have disproportionately affected American Indians, who account for about 20% of HPS cases. The case fatality rate across all groups is 41% (Centers for Disease Control and Prevention, 2001).

RISK FACTORS

HPS cases occur year-round with seasonal peaks in the spring and summer. As mentioned earlier, this observation is likely attributable to environmental factors that favor increases in rodent populations, combined with seasonal activities that increase human/rodent contact. Specific activities identified with increased risk of HPS include peridomestic cleaning and agricultural activities (Zeitz et al., 1995). In particular, cleaning or entering seldom-used, rodent-infested structures has been found to put people at increased risk of hantavirus infection (Centers for Disease Control and Prevention, 1993a). Occupational and recreational exposures have also been reported among HPS case patients, although less frequently. Persons living in manufactured homes such as mobile homes may be particularly vulnerable to exposure.

CLINICAL PICTURE

HPS cases are defined by the CDC as those that meet the following clinical criteria: 1) a febrile illness (temperature greater than 101° F) occurring in a previously healthy person, characterized by bilateral, diffuse interstitial pulmonary infiltrates that radiographically may resemble acute/adult respiratory distress syndrome (ARDS) that develops within 72 hours of hospitalization, with respiratory compromise requiring supplemental oxygen, or 2) an unexplained respiratory illness resulting in death with an autopsy examination demonstrating noncardiogenic pulmonary edema without an identifiable cause. In order to be confirmed, cases must also have confirmed serologic evidence (presence of hantavirus specific IgM or IgG), positive RT-PCR results for hantavirus RNA, or positive immunohistochemical results for hantavirus antigen in tissues (Centers for Disease Control and Prevention, 1993b). The clinical course of hantavirus pulmonary syndrome (HPS) is characterized by three phases (prodromal, cardiopulmonary, and convalescent), thought to reflect the effects of immune-mediated tissue injury. The incubation period is unclear, but appears to be between 5 days and 4 weeks, with most cases averaging 14–17 days (Young et al., 2001). The ensuing prodromal stage lasts for 3 to 4 days and is characterized by a nonspecific influenza-like illness consisting of fever, chills, malaise, and often severe myalgias affecting the large muscle groups (i.e., legs, shoulders, thighs, and lower back) (Peters, 1998). Other frequent symptoms include nausea, vomiting, diarrhea, headache, malaise, and, in later stages, cough. Less frequently, patients have abdominal pain, shortness of breath, dizziness, and arthralgias. Rarely do patients complain of sore throat, or show signs of rhinorrhea or otitis (Centers for Disease Control and Prevention, 1999). Patients often are sent home only to return within 24–48 hours, sometimes in florid respiratory failure. Thrombocytopenia (platelet count less than 150,000) is usually present at this stage, and is an important clue to suspecting HPS (Peters, 1998).

After the prodrome, a shock stage (cardiopulmonary phase) begins that lasts for several days until recovery or death ensue. It is characterized by ever-increasing respiratory and cardiovascular system compromise, the latter resulting from a direct myocardial depressant effect. Patients exhibit severe shortness of breath with development of tachypnea and tachycardia. In addition, as fluid leaves the vascular space there is hemoconcentration, seen as an elevated hematocrit, and a marked decline in O_2 saturation. Eighty-four percent of the first one hundred HPS patients required intubation with mechanical ventilation for a median of 4 days (Khan, Khabbaz, Armstrong, Holman, Bauer, Graber, et al., 1996). Chest radiographs reveal diffuse interstitial pulmonary infiltrates, that may progress to bibasilar infiltrates (Peterson, Bastian, & Tatton, 1996). The final stage (called diuretic or convalescent) is signaled by a return of the cardiac index to normal. A relatively rapid resolution of symptoms occurs over 1 to 2 days, with most patients taken off mechanical ventilation. Residual pulmonary deficits and cognitive impairment consistent with anoxic brain injury have been described (Hopkins, Larson-Lohr, Weaver, & Bigler, 1998). Renal impairment may be a component of infection with Sin Nombre and related viruses (Centers for Disease Control and Prevention, 2001b).

Milder cases of HPS associated with SNV have been reported in the United States. Although prodromal symptoms and thrombocytopenia and hemoconcentration appear as they do in classic HPS cases, these infections typically do not include severe pulmonary involvement (Kitsutani, Denton, Fritz, Murray, Todd, Pape, et al., 1999). In contrast to hantaviruses in the United States, hantaviruses in Central and South America are more frequently associated with flushing of the head and neck; hemorrhagic manifestations; and mild renal impairment causing proteinuria, hematuria, and casts, as well as classic HPS. In addition, disease may be milder than HPS based on the high seropositivity found in some South American rural populations (Ferrer, Jonsson, Esteban, Galligan, Basombrio, Peralta-Ramos, et al., 1998).

Diagnosis of HPS in the prodromal stage may be difficult due to the nonspecific symptoms and may be confused with influenza, pneumonia, and unexplained ARDS. Early distinguishing features of HPS patients are the presence of myalgias and the usual absence of sore throat, rhinorrhea, otitis, sinusitis, nasal congestion, or lobar infiltrates on chest X ray (Centers for Disease Control and Prevention,

1999). Nausea, vomiting, and abdominal pain may be severe. Thrombocytopenia is the only consistent (and often the earliest) laboratory sign, with the rapidly falling platelet count useful in distinguishing HPS from other infectious diseases such as bacterial sepsis, plague, tularemia, and borreliosis (Peters, Simpson, & Levy, 1999). Diagnosis is by serologic testing such as Western blot assay, or a RIBA strip immunoblot assay (Peters, 1998). Diagnosis may also be made from viral identification using RT-PCR from clots, biopsies, or postmortem tissues (Zaki, Khan, Goodman, Armstrong, Greer, Coffield, et al., 1996).

Treatment of HPS has been primarily supportive, with antiviral agents playing a minimal role. Supportive care of HPS is based on early detection and treatment of shock and hypoxia (Centers for Disease Control and Prevention, 1999). Intensive care unit management is most successful with early use of careful hemodynamic monitoring, preferably with pulmonary artery catheterization, judicious intravascular volume resuscitation, mechanical ventilation, and early use of inotropic agents such as dobutamine and amrinone (Centers for Disease Control and Prevention, 1999). Volume replacement requires careful administration of fluids to avoid exacerbating pulmonary edema. The nursing management of critically ill patients with HPS has been described by Goodman and Griego (1998). In some patients with elevated lactate levels (greater than 4 mmol/L) and other signs correlated with death, salvage therapy using extracorporeal membrane oxygenation (ECMO) has been successful. At the University of New Mexico medical facilities, of nine patients with a profile of lethal infection treated with ECMO, five survived (Centers for Disease Control and Prevention, 1999).

No vaccine is currently available. Prevention guidelines developed by the CDC (1993a) in cooperation with state health departments and others focus on reducing contact between humans and rodents and limiting human contact with rodent excreta by addressing three key areas: preventing rodents from entering the home, preventing rodents from living around the home, and taking appropriate precautions when cleaning out rodent-infested structures. These guidelines stress the importance of limiting rodent access to food, water, and shelter both inside and outside the home, and sealing off buildings. The guidelines also suggest methods to safely trap rodents and clean out rodent-infested areas. Measures for avoiding contact with rodents are in Appendix C, Table C.6.

EMERGING INFECTION?

The question may be asked that since hantaviruses have been known about for years in Eurasia, is HPS really an emerging infection? Clearly, it is a newly recognized disease, and SNV and other American hantaviruses are newly recognized pathogens, just as *Legionella*, *Bartonella*, *Ehrlichia* (see chapters 13, 3, and 22, respectively) and others are. But is HPS a new disease? Probably not, based on genetic evidence that suggests SNV is not the result of recent genetic mutation, but rather is a virus that has coevolved with its rodent host over many years (Khan, Khabbaz, et al., 1996; Nichol et al., 1993). Furthermore, serological evidence from as early as 1959 (Frampton, Lanser, & Nichols, 1995) indicates that HPS has been causing disease in humans for many years. This idea is further supported by the oral history of the Navajo, that cautions against human/rodent contact and describes the ill effects of such interaction (Bryan et al., 1997). Most likely, HPS has always been a rare disease, appearing in sparsely populated rural areas. Because a chance clustering of two cases in patients seen by the same physicians occurred in 1993, the disease was investigated rather than being ascribed to a nonspecific viral pneumonia. Without such clustering, cases would have been widely separated, geographically and temporally, with little likelihood of detection.

THE FUTURE

The key to preventing hantavirus infection is to begin unraveling the complex relationship between the ecology of rodents, the environment, and human risk. To this end, ongoing longitudinal rodent studies on factors affecting infection among carrier species are an important area of research (Mills et al., 1999). Information gathered from these rodent studies, combined with information gathered from satellite images, may help in developing predictive models to determine the level of human risk, and ultimately assist in prevention efforts (Glass et al., 2000). Research into the development of a human vaccine is also ongoing. Trials for a human vaccine against HFRS are underway in Asia, although to date no SNV vaccine has been developed.

Finally, supporting and expanding current surveillance of HPS is critical. Recent evidence of acute SNV infection with mild or no HPS suggests that subclinical cases of SNV infection may be occurring in the population (Kitsutani et al., 1999). Monitoring these infections, as well as the more severe HPS cases, may be crucial in identifying factors that contribute to mild and severe HPS, and lead to a better understanding of the pathogenic mechanisms of hantaviruses.

REFERENCES

Bryan, R. T., Doyle, T. J., Moolenaar, R. L., Pflieger, A. K., Khan, A. S., Ksiazek, T. G., et al. (1997). Hantavirus pulmonary syndrome. *Seminars in Pediatric Infectious Diseases, 8*, 44–49.

Butler, J. C., & Peters, C. J. (1994). Hantaviruses and hantavirus pulmonary syndrome. *Clinical Infectious Disease, 19*, 387-394.

Centers for Disease Control and Prevention. (1993a). Hantavirus infection—Southwestern United States. Interim recommendations for risk reduction. *Morbidity and Mortality Weekly Report, 43*, 1–13.

Centers for Disease Control and Prevention. (1993b). Update: Hantavirus pulmonary syndrome—United States, 1993. *Morbidity and Mortality Weekly Report, 42*, 816–820.

Centers for Disease Control and Prevention. (1999). *Hantavirus pulmonary syndrome clinical update*. Atlanta, GA: Author.

Centers for Disease Control and Prevention. (2001a). *Hantavirus* [Online]. Available: http://www.cdc.gov/ncidod/diseases/hanta/hps/index.htm

Centers for Disease Control and Prevention. (2001b). Hantavirus pulmonary syndrome—Vermont, 2000. *Morbidity and Mortality Weekly Report, 50*, 603–605.

Engelthaler, D. M., Mosley, D. G., Cheek, J. E., Levy, C. E., Komatsu, K. K., Ettestad, P., et al. (1999). Climatic and environmental patterns associated with hantavirus pulmonary syndrome, Four Corners region, United States. *Emerging Infectious Diseases, 5*, 87–94.

Ferrer, J. F., Jonsson, C. B., Esteban, E., Galligan, D., Basombrio, M. A., Peralta-Ramos, M., et al. (1998). High prevalence of hantavirus infection in Indian communities of the Paraguayan and Argentinean Gran Chaco. *American Journal of Tropical Medical and Hygiene, 59*, 438–444.

Frampton, J. W., Lanser, S., & Nichols, C. R. (1995). Sin Nombre virus infection in 1959. *Lancet, 346*, 781–782.

Glass, G. E., Livingstone, W., Mills, J. N., Hlady, W. G., Fine, J. B., Biggler, W., et al. (1998). Black Creek Canal Virus infection in *Sigmodon hispidus* in southern Florida. *American Journal of Tropical Medicine and Hygiene, 59*, 699–703.

Glass, G. E., Cheek, J. E., Patz, J. A., Shields, T. M., Doyle, T. J., Thoroughman, D. A., et al. (2000). Using remotely sensed data to identify areas at risk for hantavirus pulmonary syndrome. *Emerging Infectious Diseases, 6*, 238–247.

Goodman, D., & Griego, L. (1998). Hantavirus pulmonary syndrome: Implications for critical care nurses. *Critical Care Nurse, 18*(1), 23–30.

Hjelle, B. J., Krolikowski, J., Torrez-Martinez, N., Chavez-Giles, F., Vanner, C., & Laposata, E. (1995). Phylogenetically distinct hantavirus implicated in a case of hantavirus pulmonary syndrome in the northeastern United States. *Journal of Medical Virology, 46,* 21–27.

Hopkins, R. O., Larson-Lohr, V., Weaver, L. K., & Bigler, E. D. (1998). Neuropsychological impairments following hantavirus pulmonary syndrome. *Journal of International Neuropsychology and Sociology, 4,* 190–196.

Howard, M. J., Doyle, T. J., Koster, F. T., Zaki, S. R., Khan, A. S., Petersen, E. A., et al. (1999). Hantavirus pulmonary syndrome in pregnancy. *Clinical Infectious Diseases, 29,* 1538–1544.

Khan, A. S., Gaviria, M., Rollin, P. E., Hlady, W. G., Ksiazek, T. G., Armstrong, L. R., et al. (1996). Hantavirus pulmonary syndrome in Florida: Association with the newly identified Black Creek Canal virus. *American Journal of Medicine, 100,* 46–48.

Khan, A. S., Graves, T. K., Fritz, C. L., Young, J. C., Metzger, K. B., Humphreys, J. G., et al. (2001). The incubation period of hantavirus pulmonary syndrome. *American Journal of Tropical Medicine and Hygiene, 62,* 714–717.

Khan, A. S., Khabbaz, R. F., Armstrong, L. R., Holman, R. C., Bauer, S. P., Graber, J., et al. (1996). Hantavirus pulmonary syndrome: The first 100 U.S. cases. *Journal of Infectious Diseases, 173,* 1297–1303.

Khan, A. S., & Ksiazek, T. G. (2000). Diseases caused by hantaviruses. In G. T. Strickland (Ed.), *Hunter's tropical medicine and emerging infectious diseases* (8th ed., pp. 288–293). Philadelphia: WB Saunders Co.

Khan, A. S., Ksiazek, T. G., & Peters, C. J. (1996). Hantavirus pulmonary syndrome. *Lancet, 347,* 739–741.

Kitsutani, P. T., Denton, R. W., Fritz, C. L., Murray, R. A., Todd, R. L., Pape, W. J., et al. (1999). Acute Sin Nombre hantavirus infection without pulmonary syndrome, United States. *Emerging Infectious Diseases, 5,* 701–705.

Lee, H. W., Lee, P. W., & Johnson, K. M. (1978). Isolation of the etiologic agent of Korean hemorrhagic fever. *Journal of Infectious Diseases, 137,* 298–308.

Mills, J., Ksiazek, T., Ellis, B., Rollin, P., Nichol, S., Yates, T., et al. (1997). Patterns of association with host and habitat: Antibody reactivity with Sin Nombre virus in small mammals in the major biotic communities of the southwestern United States. *American Journal of Tropical Medicine and Hygiene, 56,* 273–284.

Mills, J. N., Yates, T. L., Ksiazek, T. G., Peters, C. J., & Childs, J. E. (1999). Long-term studies of hantavirus reservoir populations in the southwestern United States: Rationale, potential, and methods. *Emerging Infectious Diseases, 5,* 95–101.

Morzunov, S. P., Feldmann, H., Spiropoulou, C. F., Semenova, V. A., Rollin, P. E., Ksiazek, T. G., et al. (1995). A newly recognized virus associated with a fatal case of hantavirus pulmonary syndrome in Louisiana. *Journal of Virology, 69,* 1980–1983.

Nichol, S. T., Spiropoulou, C. F., Morzunov, S., Rollin, P. E., Ksiazek. T. G., Feldmann, H., et al. (1993). Genetic identification of a hantavirus associated with an outbreak of acute respiratory illness. *Science, 262,* 914–917.

Peters, C. J. (1998). Hantavirus pulmonary syndrome in the Americas. In W. M. Scheld, W. A. Craig, & J. M. Hughes (Eds.), *Emerging infections 2* (pp. 17–64). Washington, DC: ASM Press.

Peters, C. J., Mills, J. N., Spiropoulou, C., Zaki, S. R., & Rollin, P. E. (1999). Hantaviruses. In R. L. Guerrant, D. H. Walker, & P. F. Weller (Eds.), *Tropical infectious diseases: Principles, pathogens, & practice*. Philadelphia: Churchill Livingstone.

Peters, C. J., Simpson, G. L., & Levy, H. (1999). Spectrum of hantavirus infection: Hemorrhagic fever with renal syndrome and hantavirus pulmonary syndrome. *Annual Review of Medicine, 50*, 531–545.

Peterson, M. C., Bastian, B. V., & Tatton, J. A. (1996). Radiologic findings of the hantavirus pulmonary syndrome. *Western Journal of Medicine, 164*, 76–77.

Rhodes, L. V., III, Huang, C., Sanchez, A. J., Nichol, S. T., Zaki, S. R., Ksiazek, T. G., et al. (2000). Hantavirus pulmonary syndrome associated with Monongahela virus, Pennsylvania. *Emerging Infectious Diseases, 6*, 616–621.

Wells, R. M., Sosa Estani, S., Yadon, Z. E., Enria, D., Padula, P., Pini, N., Mills, J. N., et al. (1997). An unusual hantavirus outbreak in southern Argentina: Person-to-person transmission? Hantavirus Pulmonary Syndrome Study Group for Patagonia. *Emerging Infectious Diseases, 3*, 171–174.

Wells, R. M., Young, J., Williams, R. J., Armstrong, L. R., Busico, K., Khan, A. S., et al. (1997). Hantavirus transmission in the United States. *Emerging Infectious Diseases, 3*, 361–365.

Yanagihara, R. (1990). Hantavirus infection in the United States: Epizootiology and epidemiology. *Review of Infectious Diseases, 12*, 449–457.

Zaki, S. R., Khan, A. S., Goodman, R. A., Armstrong, L. R., Greer, P. W., Coffield, L. M., et al. (1996). Retrospective diagnosis of hantavirus pulmonary syndrome, 1978–1993: Implications for emerging infectious diseases. *Archives of Pathology and Laboratory Medicine, 120*, 134–139.

Zeitz, P. S., Butler, J. C., Cheek, J. E., Samuel, M. C., Childs, J. E., Shands, L. A., et al. (1995). A case-control study of hantavirus pulmonary syndrome during an outbreak in the southwestern United States. *Journal of Infectious Diseases, 171*, 864–870.

11

Hepatitis C

Victoria Davey

Mr. W, a muscular 40-year-old African American man, presented to an academic clinical research unit to be screened for a paid observational study that was recruiting healthy individuals. He was a currently unemployed construction worker with a history of gastrointestinal hemorrhage 10 years earlier. He was hospitalized for treatment of severe cellulitis after a human bite sustained in an altercation 2 years earlier. He reported use of injected and intranasal heroin and cocaine from his teens through his 20's. He had stopped all injection-drug use more than 10 years prior to this clinic visit but stated that he had last used intranasal cocaine approximately 1 month ago. He reported consumption of two quarts of beer per day since his teens and had been arrested twice for alcohol-related incidents. He reported approximately 40 lifetime heterosexual partners and currently lived with a female partner who had tested positively for human immunodeficiency virus (HIV), and who was positive for hepatitis B surface antigen. Mr. W had tested negatively for HIV at that time. He stated that he and his partner used condoms.

His physical complaints included yellowing of the whites of his eyes after particularly heavy alcohol ingestion, mild fatigue, and periodic headaches for which he took an over-the-counter analgesic. A physical examination and laboratory studies were done to establish eligibility for the clinical study. These included a complete blood count, blood chemistries, and liver function tests. Because of the risk factors of injected and intranasal drug use, multiple sexual partners, alcoholism, and potential recent or ongoing exposure to HIV and hepatitis B, serologic studies for HIV and hepatitis B and C were ordered.

The physical examination was normal except for mild tenderness in the epigastric region, and palmar erythema. There was no spleen tip felt; the liver was 11 cm by percussion. Results of the laboratory tests were normal except for an elevated serum alanine aminotransferase (ALT) of 345 units/L (laboratory normal 6–41 units/L), aspartate aminotransferase (AST) of 139 units/L (laboratory normal 9–34 units/L), and positive serology for antibodies to hepatitis C by enzyme-linked immunosorbent assay (ELISA or EIA) and confirmed by recombinant immunoblot assay (RIBA). HIV serology and hepatitis B surface antigen were negative.

Mr. W is typical of many hepatitis C patients. He lacked major symptoms; although he had noticed periodic scleral icterus and some degree of fatigue, these were not disturbing enough to cause him to seek medical attention. The positive hepatitis C serology was discovered, as it often is, when an individual seeks medical care for an unrelated event. Mr. W did not qualify for the clinical research study because of the positive hepatitis C serology and abnormal liver function tests. Interventions were initiated for his complex and interrelated list of medical and psychosocial problems. Mr. W attended prevention counseling with his partner to review their respective current and potential risks for HIV, hepatitis B, and hepatitis C. He was referred to the social services department for assistance in locating community resources for primary medical care, drug and alcohol treatment, and employment issues. He was scheduled for an appointment with a hepatologist for further evaluation of the hepatitis C infection.

After the causative agents of two transmissible types of hepatitis, A and B, were identified in the 1960s and 1970s, it was evident that at least one other agent, initially called "non-A, non-B" was responsible for disease in a large number of transfusion recipients and injection drug users (DiBisceglie & Bacon, 1999). This third agent, hepatitis C virus (HCV), is a single-stranded RNA virus of the *Flaviviridae* family (Lauer & Walker, 2001), that includes several viruses important in causing human disease: dengue (see chapter 7), West Nile fever (see chapter 20), Japanese encephalitis, yellow fever, and St. Louis encephalitis. It was isolated and sequenced in 1989, and an assay for detection in serum was developed shortly thereafter (Alter, Purcell, Shih, Melproder, Houghton, Choo, et al., 1989; Choo, Kuo, Weiner, Overby, Bradley, & Houghton, 1989). HCV is genetically diverse, existing as at least 6 major genotypes each with more than 50 subtypes designated as 1a, 1b, etc. While some HCV genotypes have worldwide distribution, there are distinct differences in prevalence as well as regional distribution (Zein, 2000).This genetic variability is one reason HCV may avoid detection and disposition by the immune system and also may help explain its varied clinical course and treatment responsiveness (Cheney, Chopra, & Graham, 2000; Zein, 2000). Coinfection with more than one genotype may occur (Cheney et al., 2000).

The overall prevalence of positive hepatitis C serology is 1.8% of the U.S. population, or an estimated 4 million people (Lawrence, 2000). Males in the 30–49 year-old age group have the highest prevalence (Cheney et al., 2000). Worldwide, more than 1 million cases are reported each year, and HCV may be more prevalent than hepatitis B virus (Zein, 2000). The worldwide prevalence is estimated at 170 million persons (Lauer & Walker, 2001). High prevalence rates are found in several areas. For example, in Egypt, prevalence rates in the population have been found to range from 10%–30%, and in Baltimore, Maryland, HCV prevalence was found to be 15%–18% in patients attending a clinic for sexually transmitted diseases and an urban emergency room respectively (Thomas, 2000). It is estimated that 30,000 new infections occur each year in the United States, although there has been a decline in the incidence of infection since 1989, when the virus was identified and serologic tests developed, leading in July, 1992, to a safer blood supply and better understanding of risk behaviors. However, 8,000–10,000 people die annually of the consequences of the disease, and hepatitis C is now the leading cause of chronic liver disease such as cirrhosis, end-stage liver disease, and liver cancer. It is the major reason for liver transplantation in the United States (Centers for Disease Control and Prevention, 1998; Cheney et al., 2000). Moreover, the number of chronic infections recognized is expected to increase (Catalina & Navarro, 2000). Many persons who received blood transfusions before 1990 could be unknowingly at risk for hepatitis C. Direct notification programs for those who received transfusions from donors who later tested positive for hepatitis C are being conducted (Buffington, Rowel, Hinman, Sharp, & Choi, 2001). The Third National Health and Nutrition Examination (NHANES III) survey among noninstitutionalized U.S. civilians detected higher HCV prevalence rates in African-American men; however when data were adjusted for transmission risk factors and socioeconomic variables, racial/ethnic and gender differences were not seen (Cheney et al., 2000).

The major route of transmission is by direct percutaneous exposure to the blood of an infected person. This may occur via transfusion of blood and blood products, through injected drug use via exposure to contaminated drug apparatus, or through transplantation (Thomas, 2000; Weber & Rutula, 2001). Once screening of blood donations by multiantigen tests was begun in July 1992, HCV infection decreased. The incidence of posttransfusion HCV infection is now less than 1 per 100,000 units of transfused blood (Sulkowski, Mast, Seeff, & Thomas, 2000). Intranasal cocaine use is associated with positive HCV serology, perhaps because of shared equipment/straws that are contaminated with blood from epistaxis (Bonkovsky & Mehta, 2001; Conry-Cantilena, VanRaden, Gibble, Melpolder, Shakh, Viladomiu, et al., 1996). About half of new cases of HCV in the U.S. currently occur in those who are injecting drug users, and hemodialysis patients show a high prevalence of HCV, up to 50%. The risk for hemophiliacs who received multiple transfusions is decreasing due to new preparation methods for clotting factors, although prevalence was as high as 75% (Lawrence, 2000). As many as one third of HIV-infected persons may be co-infected with HCV (Sulkowski et al., 2000). HCV transmission from patient to health care worker via needlestick, or exposure to blood via mucous membranes and conjunctiva have been reported (Sartori, La Terra, Aglietta, Manzin, Navino, & Verzetti, 1993; Thomas, 2000), and the risk after needlestick exposure to a HCV-infected patient has been reported to range from 2%–8% (Thomas, 2000). Transmission from health care providers to patients have also been described, including one case of 6 patients and their infected surgeon (Esteban, Gômez, Martell, Cabot, Quer, Camps, et al., 1996). Nosocomial transmission has been described. For example, a colonscope was implicated in the transmission of HCV from one patient to others (Bronowicki, Venard, Botté, Monhoven, Gastin, Choné, et al., 1997). Inadvertent transmission during preventive health campaigns, for example, has also been described, such as in injection therapy for schistosomiasis in Egypt. Tattooing, acupuncture, human bites, and medical folk practices including scarification rituals have been associated with HCV transmission (Habib, Mohamed, Abdel-Aziz, Magder, Abdel-Hamid, Gamil, et al., 2001; Thomas, 2000).

HCV may be transmitted sexually, and HCV-RNA has been detected in saliva and semen. In addition, high HCV prevalence is found in commercial sex workers and those with multiple sex partners, especially 50 and more (Centers for Disease Control and Prevention, 1998; Thomas, 2000). Unprotected sexual intercourse between long-term steady partners demonstrated HCV seroprevalence rates of 4.4% in the partner, with risk of infection increasing with the length of the relationship (Tong, Lai, Hwang, Lee, Co, Chien, et al., 1995). Perinatal transmission from a HCV-infected mother to her infant is known and rates average from 0%–8% (Tajiri, Miyoshi, Funada, Etani, Abe, Onodera, et al., 2001; Thomas, 2000). There is an increased risk for transmitting HCV perinatally in those women with high viral loads, viremia at delivery, and/or HIV co-infection. There are conflicting data on the risk of transmission from breast milk, and there are no recommendations to restrict breast feeding in HCV-infected mothers (Cheney et al., 2000; Tajiri et al., 2001).

The incubation period for HCV infection ranges from 2 weeks to 6 months with an average of 7 weeks (Catalina & Navarro, 2000; Cheney et al., 2000; Lauer & Walker, 2001). The majority of those who become infected remain asymptomatic. Such individuals may be asymptomatic for decades, not realizing that they are infected and can transmit HCV (Catalina & Navarro, 2000). Others may experience a nonspecific illness with symptoms such as malaise, fatigue, anorexia, right-sided abdominal pain, and weight loss with or without jaundice which may or may not be diagnosed. The jaundice appears in about 30% of symptomatic adults (Cheney et al., 2000). Hepatitis C infection may present as acute hepatitis in 20% of patients.

Only about 15% of persons with acute HCV infection experience resolution. About 85%–90% of persons who have had acute HCV infection develop chronic hepatitis C, which is characterized by persistent presence of HCV in the blood and fluctuations in levels of serum ALT, reflecting slow but inexorable liver damage, for as long as 10–20 years (Cheney et al., 2000). Extrahepatic manifestations may be associated with chronic HCV including essential mixed cryoglobulinemia as well as manifestations in other symptoms. For a review see Cheney and associates (2000). Interestingly, the liver damage caused by HCV is caused not by direct effects of the virus, but from the cellular immune response to it—immune system cells attacking liver cells displaying HCV markers (DiBisceglie & Bacon, 1999). In those with chronic HCV infection, 20%–30% develop cirrhosis, usually over a long period of time, as long as 20–30 years after initial infection (Cheney et al., 2000). Manifestations may include portal hypertension with ascites, edema, esophageal varices and bleeding; jaundice, prothrombin time prolongation, hypoalbuminemia, and hepatic encephalopathy (Catalina & Navarro, 2000). Hepatocellular carcinoma may develop in those with HCV-related cirrhosis, and the annual rate of progression is estimated at 1%–4% annually (Cheney et al., 2000). Risk factors for those who will develop progressive liver disease after HCV infection include: 40 years of age and older at the time of infection; longer duration of infection; males; fibrosis on liver biopsy; co-infection with HIV or other hepatitis virus; genotype 1, especially 1b, of HCV; iron overload; and alcohol use (Cheney et al., 2000).

The long quiescent period of hepatitis C infection, coupled with the presence of infectious HCV in the blood, allows this disease both to go unrecognized and to be readily transmitted by its apparently healthy host. Health care providers must recognize persons at risk and recommend testing for them. Risk factors for hepatitis C overlap with those of other bloodborne virus infections like HIV and hepatitis B. Persons with longstanding HIV or hepatitis B may not have been tested for hepatitis C since the serologic test for HCV was developed after that of hepatitis B or HIV, and the high rates of prevalence of HCV have only recently been recognized. Table 11.1 lists persons at risk for HCV infection.

Early diagnosis allows for implementation of practices to reduce transmission and to provide early treatment to limit disease progression before significant liver damage occurs. Serologic tests for presence of antibody to hepatitis C are reliable and accurate. These tests include enzyme-immunoassay (EIA) for use in screening and a recombinant immunoblot assay (RIBA), the latter usually employed as a confirma-

TABLE 11.1 Persons Who Should Consider Testing for Hepatitis C

- Persons who ever injected illegal drugs, including those who injected once or a few times many years ago and do not consider themselves drug users
- Persons who received clotting factor concentrates produced before 1987
- Persons who were ever on chronic (long-term) hemodialysis
- Persons with persistently abnormal alanine aminotransferase (ALT) levels
- Persons who were notified that they received blood from a donor who later tested positive for HCV infection
- Persons who received a transfusion of blood or blood components before July 1992
- Persons who received an organ transplant before July 1992
- Health care, emergency medical, and public safety workers who have had needlesticks, sharps, or mucosal exposures to HCV-positive blood
- Children born to HCV-positive mothers

Source: Centers for Disease Control and Prevention, 1998.

tory test. Diagnostic tests that directly detect HCV-RNA include both quanitative and qualitative PCR and branched DNA signal amplification assay (bDNA) (Lauer & Walker, 2001; Lawrence, 2000). HCV-RNA measurement is a useful technique to follow the response to therapy or to diagnose HCV in an immunocompromised patient who does not mount a measurable antibody response, thus leading to false-negative serologic tests.

Current approved treatments for hepatitis C are interferon monotherapy or interferon in combination with ribavirin. Interferon alfa-2b has been recommended for treatment to prevent chronic infection (Jaeckel, Cornberg, Wedemeyer, Santantonio, Mayer, Zankel, et al., 2001). Others are in clinical trials such as recombinant interleukins, amantadine, and pegylated interferon alfa-2a or peginterferon alfa (Cheney et al., 2000; Lauer & Walker, 2001). Treatment is recommended for those whose disease is most likely to progress and includes those with persistent abnormal alanine aminotransferase levels, circulating HCV-RNA, and moderate to severe hepatitis and fibrosis on biopsy (Catalina & Navarro, 2000). Viral genotype as well as host factors may also predict treatment success, and sustained response appears greater in genotypes 2 and 3, which also seem to require a shorter treatment time (Foster & Thomas, 2000; Hu, Vierling, & Redeker, 2001). A recent report indicates that using interferon alfa-2b to treat acute hepatitis C can prevent the development of chronic infection (Jaeckel et al., 2001). Liver transplantation may be recommended, but often, HCV infection will recur in the transplanted liver.

Many people currently living with hepatitis C acquired it through infected blood products. The discovery of the virus, the development of sensitive tests to detect it, and efficient and thorough means to eliminate it in plasma-derived products (such as blood-clotting factors and immunoglobulin) mean that this is no longer a major transmission consideration, in countries where these measures are used. Because of ongoing transmission among the other high-risk groups, there is a great need for all frontline health care providers to know and teach risk reduction measures for prevention of HCV infection (see Table 11.2).

SUMMARY

Hepatitis C virus frequently results in serious liver disease. An estimated 4 million Americans may be infected with hepatitis C. The

TABLE 11.2 Primary Prevention of Hepatitis C Infection

- Exclude HCV-positive donors, or persons at high risk for HCV, from donating blood, plasma, tissue, organs, or semen.
- Inactivate viruses in clotting factor concentrates and other plasma-derived products.
- Counsel clients to discontinue use of illegal drugs.
- If drugs are used: counsel clients never to share or reuse needles, syringes, water, or any part of "works," including straws used intranasally.
- Counsel clients not to share razors, toothbrushes, or manicure equipment items that might be contaminated with blood.
- Counsel patients that the best way to avoid sexually transmitted diseases including HIV, hepatitis B, and to an extent, hepatitis C, is to not have sex or to have sex with one faithful partner.
- Counsel patients to use male or female condoms correctly, every time they engage in sex.
- For persons who have hepatitis C, the best ways to protect the liver from further damage are to:

  not drink any alcohol;
  not use illegal drugs;
  not take medicines including over-the-counter, herbal, or alternative medicines without the recommendation of their health care provider;
  get vaccinated for hepatitis A and B; and
  get tested for HIV.

Source: Centers for Disease Control and Prevention, 1998.

disease develops without many symptoms over a long period of time, so that many people are often not aware that they are infected until they develop severe liver disease. HCV is transmitted by contact with blood of an infected person through transfusion of blood or blood products, sharing of needles or drug equipment, and, less frequently, through high-risk sex practices and from an infected mother to her child. Nosocomial transmission can occur. Many of the risk factors for hepatitis C overlap those of other bloodborne diseases, like HIV. Those coinfected with HCV and HIV have a more rapid progression and a poorer response to therapy (Lauer & Walker, 2001). Since 1992, blood and blood products in the U.S. are considered safe from hepatitis C virus. Transmission through sharing of needles or illegal drug equipment continues to be a major means of HCV transmission. Health care providers of every discipline need to know the risk factors for hepatitis C and to consider hepatitis C risk in every patient. The best way to reduce transmission and prevent progression of hepatitis C virus infection is to know what the risks are, to test for it, to educate persons at risk in prevention and lifestyle alteration, to treat those eligible, and to facilitate research in all facets of the disease.

REFERENCES

Alter, H. J., Purcell, R. H., Shih, J. W., Melpolder, J. C., Houghton, M., Choo, Q.-L., & Kuo, G. (1989). Detection of antibody to hepatitis C in prospectively followed transfusion recipients with acute and chronic non-A, non-B hepatitis. *New England Journal of Medicine, 321*, 1494–1500.

Bonkovsky, H. L., & Mehta, S. (2001). Hepatitis C: A review and update. *Journal of the American Academy of Dermatology, 44*, 159–182.

Bronowicki, J. P., Venard, V., Bottê, C., Monhoven, N., Gastin, I., Chonê, L., et al. (1997). Patient-to-patient transmission of hepatitis C virus during colonoscopy. *New England Journal of Medicine, 337*, 237–240.

Buffington, J., Rowel, R., Hinman, J. M., Sharp, K., & Choi, S. (2001). Lack of awareness of hepatitis C risk among persons who received blood transfusions before 1990. *American Journal of Public Health, 91*, 47–48.

Catalina, G., & Navarro, V. (2000). Hepatitis C: A challenge for the generalist. *Hospital Practice, 35*(1), 97–118.

Centers for Disease Control and Prevention. (1998). Recommendations for prevention and control of hepatitis C virus (HCV) infection and HCV-related chronic disease. *Morbidity and Mortality Weekly Report, 47*(RR-19), 1–39.

Cheney, C. P., Chopra, S., & Graham, C. (2000). Hepatitis C. *Infectious Disease Clinics of North America, 14*, 633–655.

Choo, Q.-L., Kuo, G., Weiner, A. J., Overby, L. R., Bradley, D. W., & Houghton, M. (1989). Isolation of a cDNA clone derived from a blood-borne non-A, non-B viral hepatitis genome. *Science, 244*, 359–362.

Conry-Cantilena, C., VanRaden, M. A., Gibble, J., Melpolder, J., Shakh, O., Viladomiu, L., et al. (1996). Routes of infection, viremia, and liver disease in blood donors found to have hepatitis C infection. *New England Journal of Medicine, 334*, 1691–1696.

DiBisceglie, A. M., & Bacon, B. R. (1999). The unmet challenges of hepatitis C. *Scientific American, 281*(4), 80–85.

Esteban, J. I., Gômez, J., Martell, M., Cabot, B., Quer, J., Camps, J., et al. (1996). Transmission of hepatitis C virus by a cardiac surgeon. *New England Journal of Medicine, 334*, 550–560.

Foster, G. R., & Thomas, H. C. (2000). Therapeutic options for HCV—management of the infected individual. *Baillières Best Practices and Research in Clinical Gastroenterology, 14*, 255–264.

Habib, M., Mohamed, M. K., Abdel-Aziz, F., Magder, L. S., Abdel-Hamid, M., Gamil, F., et al. (2001). Hepatitis C virus infection in a community in the Nile delta: Risk factors for seropositivity. *Hepatology, 33*, 248–253.

Hu, K. Q., Vierling, J. M., & Redeker, A. G. (2001). Viral, host and interferon-related factors modulating the effect of interferon therapy for hepatitis C virus infection. *Journal of Viral Hepatitis, 8,* 1–18.

Jaeckel, E., Cornberg, M., Wedemeyer, H., Santantonio, T., Mayer, J., Zankel, M., et al. (2001). Treatment of acute hepatitis C with interferon alfa-2b. *New England Journal of Medicine, 345,* 1452–1457.

Lauer, G. M., & Walker, B. D. (2001). Hepatitis C virus infection. *New England Journal of Medicine, 345,* 41–52.

Lawrence, S. P. (2000). Advances in the treatment of hepatitis C. *Advances in Internal Medicine, 45,* 65–105.

Sartori, M., La Terra, G., Aglietta, M., Manzin, A., Navino, C., & Verzetti, G. (1993). Transmission of hepatitis C via blood splash into conjunctiva. *Scandinavian Journal of Infectious Diseases, 5,* 270–271.

Sulkowski, M. S., Mast, E. E., Seeff, L. B., & Thomas, D. L. (2000). Hepatitis C virus infection as an opportunistic disease in persons infected with human immunodeficiency virus. *Clinical Infectious Diseases, 30,* S77–S84.

Tajiri, H., Miyoshi, Y., Funada, S., Etani, Y., Abe, J., Onodera, T., et al. (2001). Prospective study of mother-to-infant transmission of hepatitis C virus. *Pediatric Infectious Diseases Journal, 20,* 10–14.

Thomas, D. L. (2000). Hepatitis C epidemiology. *Current Topics in Microbiology and Immunology, 242,* 25–41.

Tong, M. J., Lai, P. P. C., Hwang, S.-J., Lee, S.-Y., Co, R. L., Chien, R. N., et al. (1995). Evaluation of sexual transmission in patients with hepatitis C infection. *Clinical and Diagnostic Virology, 3,* 39–47.

Weber, D. J., & Rutala, W. A. (2001). The emerging nosocomial pathogens *Cryptosporidium, Escherichia coli* O157:H7, *Helicobacter pylori,* and hepatitis C: Epidemiology, environmental survival, efficacy of disinfection, and control measures. *Infection Control and Hospital Epidemiology, 22,* 306–315.

Zein, N. N. (2000). Clinical significance of hepatitis C genotypes. *Clinical Microbiology Reviews, 13,* 223–233.

12

HIV/AIDS

Inge B. Corless

An emerging disease has all the drama of a good mystery—in some cases, an unknown assailant, one or more "victims" and various clues as to the mode and method of assault. HIV/AIDS was and, to some extent remains, a mystery and cause of continuing debate. In this chapter the evidence and debate on the cause of AIDS, how it arose in humans and subsequently became a pandemic will be examined, along with a brief review of the current epidemiology, pathogenicity, approaches to therapy, vaccine development efforts, and the political and economic ramifications of HIV/AIDS.

In the United States, the condition that came to be known as HIV/AIDS (or more recently as "HIV disease") was first recognized by physicians who noted uncommon presentations of disease such as *Pneumocystis carinii* pneumonia (PCP) and Kaposi's sarcoma in young homosexual men, and by a clerk at the Centers for Disease Control (CDC) who observed frequent requests for pentamidine, a drug used to treat *Pneumocystis carinii* pneumonia, a formerly rare condition (Centers for Disease Control, 1981a, 1981b; Friedman-Kien, 1981; Gottlieb, Schroff, Schanker, Weisman, Fan, Wolf, et al., 1981; Masur, Michelis, Greene, Onorato, Stouwe, Holzman, et al., 1981; Shilts, 1987). These observations marked the beginning of awareness of the HIV/AIDS epidemic in the United States.

Clinicians and scientists hypothesized early on that the disease, which induced severe immunosuppression, followed a transmission pattern similar to that of hepatitis B, a belief verified by the identification of transfusion-related infection in 1982 (Centers for Disease Control, 1982). The cause of the immunosuppression was first identified by the Pasteur Institute's Luc Montagnier (Barré-Sinoussi, Chermann, Rey, Nugeyre, Chamaret, Gruest, et al., 1983) as lymphadenopathy virus (LAV), thereafter by Gallo (Popovic, Sarngadharan, Read, & Gallo, 1984; Sarngadharan, Popovic, Bruch, Schupbach, & Gallo, 1984) as human T-lymphotropic virus type III (HTLV III), and by Levy (Levy, Hoffman, Kramer, Landis, Shimabukuro, & Oshiro, 1984) as AIDS-associated retrovirus (ARV). The differing nomenclature was resolved by a special committee designated to determine one name for the newly identified organism. The organism was named "human immunodeficiency virus" (HIV) and the resultant disease "acquired immunodeficiency syndrome" or AIDS (Coffin, Haase, Levy, Montagnier, Oroszlan, Teich, et al., 1986). HIV is a retrovirus that has two types, HIV-1 and HIV-2. HIV-1 has three "groups": M for main; N for non-M, non-O; and O for outlier. There are subtype designations within the groups. In group M, there are subtype or clade designations A–K (Hahn, Shaw, De Cock, & Sharp, 2000; Robertson, Anderson, Bradac, Carr, Foley, Funkhouser, et al., 2000).

Although the virus had a name, HIV as the cause of AIDS was challenged by Duesberg (1988) who argued that HIV did not comply with all of Koch's postulates, the ground rules of whether an organism causes a disease. In particular, Duesberg (1989, 1991, 1994) argued that HIV could not be isolated from all individuals who are immunosuppressed, thereby violating one of Koch's postulates. Advances in technology and the resultant identification of the presence of HIV refute this claim. Scientists have examined the evidence regarding "myths" about HIV as the cause of AIDS and have overwhelmingly concluded that HIV is the cause of AIDS (Ascher, Sheppard, Winkelstein, & Vittinghoff, 1993; Delaney, 2000; Hillis, 2000; Joint United Nations Programme on HIV/AIDS, 2000b; Kurth, 1990; National Institute of Allergy and Infectious Diseases, 2000a, 2000b).

Although the cause of AIDS has been scientifically established, questions about how HIV became established in humans still exist since humans are not the natural host. Apparently HIV became established in humans through cross-species transmission and thus AIDS is a zoonosis (Hahn et al., 2000). The simian lentivirus, simian immunodeficiency virus (SIV) of sooty mangabeys (SIVsm), was the source of HIV-2, and HIV-1 arose from the simian immunodeficiency virus from chimpanzees (SIVcpz), the *Pan troglodytes troglodytes* subspecies. Through elaborate analyses, it is believed that HIV-1 and HIV-2 have been transmitted to humans on multiple occasions (Hahn et al., 2000).

HIV-2 is particularly associated with areas in West Africa such as Senegal, Guinea-Bissau, Guinea "Conakry," Côte d'Ivoire, Sierra Leone, and Liberia. HIV-1 group N infections have been found primarily in Cameroon. Groups M, N, and O have all been found in Gabon, Equatorial Guinea, Cameroon, and the Republic of the Congo (Congo-Brazzaville) (Hahn et al., 2000). The clades of Group M have been found worldwide with clade B predominant in North America and Europe, clades A, B, and C in Africa, and clades B and E in Thailand. This picture of regional clade dominance is likely to change with time and the travel of HIV-infected individuals.

The manner in which transspecies crossover of HIV occurred is still debated. Hahn and colleagues (2000) have outlined two competing hypotheses. The one Hahn and her colleagues favor is that exposure to animal blood in the course of hunting, butchering, and ingestion of raw bushmeat accounts for the transmission of HIV from primate to human. The point of initial transmission that must have occurred multiple times to result in epidemic spread is accounted for through a combination of factors, including urbanization, disruption of family life through jobs at a distance from families leading to risky sexual behaviors, prostitution, cultural mores that promote men having numerous sexual partners, and the use of unsterilized needles for both medicinal and recreational drug injections. While these sociocultural factors pertain and help transmit an infection that has already gotten a toe-hold, the factors in and of themselves are necessary but not sufficient.

The other hypothesis noted by Hahn and associates (2000) has been proposed by a number of individuals including Curtis (1992), Elswood and Stricker (1994) and Hooper (1999). This hypothesis is that SIVcpz was present in the kidney substrate used in the propagation of oral polio virus (OPV) for vaccination trials in the Belgian Congo in the 1950s. Elswood and Stricker (1994) focused on SV40 contamination of early polio vaccine and view this as a means of transmitting a simian precursor of HIV to man. Hooper (1999) investigated the various clues, interviewed key informants who were present at the conduct of the oral polio vaccine trials in Africa or who had knowledge of them, examined the travels of various armies and other migrations and consulted with world-renowned scientists. He listed 27 arguments for the OPV contamination thesis and 4 against the hypothesis. In his view, the argument against the OPV connection boils down to the lack of definitive evidence. Specifically against the hypothesis is that most of the animals used for the oral polio vaccine were from different species than the ones from which HIV originated, and that the M group of HIV-1 is believed to have originated 10–50 years before the vaccine trials began (Hahn et al., 2000; Korber, Theiler, & Wolinsky, 1998). Additional data from four groups of researchers found no evidence of chimpanzee DNA in an analysis of multiple oral polio vaccine samples, and thus there appears to be no support for the introduction of HIV to humans through OPV (Poinar, Kuch, & Pääbo, 2001).

At the end of 2000, an estimated 36.1 million persons were living with HIV/AIDS, most of them in developing nations. More than 5 million persons were infected with HIV in 2000 alone and an estimated 5.3 million died from HIV disease in that year. Since the onset of the pandemic, almost 22 million persons worldwide have died from the disease (Joint United Nations Programme on HIV/AIDS, 2000a). In the U.S., an estimated 317,000 persons were living with AIDS in 2000, more than half in just five states and in metropolitan areas. Most (79%) were male and most (62%) were from ethnic minority groups (Centers for Disease Control and Prevention, 2001). Through December 2000, 774,467 cases of AIDS had been reported among Americans, with more than half (54%) among ethnic minority populations. More than 58% of these individuals had died from AIDS by December 2000.

Transmission of HIV occurs by sexual contact; blood, including transfusions, contaminated injection equipment and needles; and from an infected mother to her child during the perinatal period including breastfeeding (Durham & Lashley, 2000). The hallmark of HIV infection is immunosuppression leading to decreased CD4+ cells and derangements of the immune system. Opportunistic illnesses, infections, and neoplasms result. Many of these infections were not seen or seen only rarely in humans, especially in developed countries, before the AIDS epidemic. Thus, they can be considered as emerging. Since their initial recognition, some of them have been increasingly noticed, sometimes in the immunocompetent person. These include infections with such organisms and diseases as *Cryptosporidium* (see chapter 5), microsporidia (see chapter 3), West Nile virus (see chapter 20), multidrug-resistant tuberculosis (see chapter 16), Kaposi's sarcoma (see chapter 21), cervical intraepithelial neoplasia, *Rhodococcus equi*, *Penicillium marneffei*, hepatitis C (see chapter 11), *Bartonella*, unusual forms of *Candida*, atypical mycobacteria, *Cyclospora* (see chapter 6), and others. Many of these are discussed in tables in Appendices A and B. These infections may have the following characteristics in persons with HIV infection: more likely to be disseminated, have an atypical presentation, be more severe, have atypical locations, rapidly progress, and be difficult to treat (Durham & Lashley, 2000). Emerging infectious diseases often appear disproportionately in those with HIV infection. The surveillance definition and clinical categories of AIDS may be found at the Centers for Disease Control and Prevention Internet site (http://www.cdc.gov).

Although drug therapy with antiretroviral drugs and protease inhibitors as well as protocols for prophylaxis of infections has reduced HIV-related morbidity and mortality, debate continues about when to initiate this treatment (see Panel on Clinical Practices [2001] for most recent HIV infection treatment guidelines). While agreement exists on the treatment of symptomatic individuals, those with a high viral load, and those experiencing acute retroviral syndrome, when to initiate therapy for those not fitting into these categories is not clear. Some clinicians support treating those with very early or primary HIV infection as a means of preserving the immune architecture. There is general consensus that HIV-infected persons should be monitored and treated by HIV disease specialists.

The standard of care for initiation of therapy earlier in the pandemic was based on CD4+ count. As the understanding about HIV disease has improved, drug treatment also takes into account such factors as level of plasma HIV RNA and drug resistance, the latter influenced by inadequate treatment, and poor adherence. The need for strict adherence to sometimes complex drug regimens remains a key challenge to successful antiretroviral treatment of HIV-infected persons. Because persons living with HIV disease may take numerous drugs simultaneously, the potential for drug interactions and adverse reactions is significant.

Various government agencies have issued and updated guidelines for treatment. These guidelines are available on-line from the HIV/AIDS Treatment Information Service (http://hivatis.org/) and include current and past recommendations for adult/adolescent, pediatric, and perinatal treatment. Once antiretroviral treatment has been initiated, goals of treatment are maximal and durable suppression of viral load, restoration and/or preservation of immunologic function, improvement in the quality of life, and reduction of HIV-related morbidity and mortality.

Two classes of antiretroviral drugs are available for use in the treatment of HIV infection—reverse transcriptase inhibitors (RTIs) consisting of nucleoside RTIs and nonnucleoside RTIs, and protease inhibitors (PIs) (Durham & Lashley, 2000). These drugs act by different mechanisms to inhibit viral replication. By the end of 2000 nine RTIs and six PIs had been approved to treat HIV infection. Many other drugs are in various stages of development and clinical testing. Because of the high costs of these drugs, individuals in the U.S. needing assistance may gain access to HIV-related medications through the AIDS Drug Assistance Program (ADAP) and national pharmaceutical industry patient assistance/expanded access programs.

As exciting as the developments in antiretroviral drug therapy have been, the lack of access to medications worldwide—often because of high cost, the complexity of the regimens and treatment of side effects, and the paucity of practitioners with the necessary expertise and equipment, combine to make the current therapies impractical for much of the world's people; thus the best therapy is prevention of infection. The two major approaches to prevention are behavioral and pharmacological (namely the development of a vaccine). Were behavioral changes to succeed with consensual sexual behaviors, nonconsensual behaviors such as rape would still need to be addressed. Gang rape as an instrument of war and politics creates the conditions for rapid spread of infection. Further, the status of women in many societies, the paucity of occupational options for women, and dependency on men for economic benefits and protection combine to make women vulnerable for HIV transmission (Cohen & Durham, 1993). Such conditions make the development of a vaccine all the more urgent.

Development of a vaccine must address the mutability of the human immunodeficiency virus as well as the variety of its presentation in different clades. Eliciting an antibody response indicative of resistance rather than exposure is another challenge. Lastly, whether to deploy a less than maximally effective vaccine is a major subject of debate. Is it better to protect some people rather than none at all? Will the imperfect protection of today's vaccines preclude later inoculation with a more advanced product? Will vaccination convey the potentially mistaken perception of protection leading to engagement in risk behaviors? If a perfect vaccine is not available, when is a "good" vaccine good enough? The answers to these questions are not the answers to a mystery but to profound scientific, ethical, and philosophical issues. And the answers are not without political consequences.

The infection of large portions of the adult population (30–40% in some African countries) will also have profound political and demographic consequences. The deaths of parents of young children often leave these "AIDS orphans" without food and shelter let alone the money for school fees. Unless these children are educated, their ability to participate in the economic sector will be impaired, potentially leading to political destabilization. The ramifications of this pandemic are profound on every level. While there are numerous scientific mysteries still to be solved, the social and political issues may be the most elusive to solution.

A good mystery ends with the detective having brought the pieces of the puzzle into alignment resulting in a neat conclusion. In this case, while the assailant and modes of attack have been identified, how to prevent further attacks, if not a mystery is still a subject of much debate.

REFERENCES

Ascher, M., Sheppard, H., Winkelstein, W., & Vittinghoff, E. (1993). Does drug use cause AIDS? *Nature, 362*, 103–104.

Barrê-Sinoussi, F., Chermann, J., Rey, F., Nugeyre, M. T., Chamaret, S., Gruest, J., et al. (1983). Isolation of a T-lymphotropic retrovirus from a patient at risk for acquired immune deficiency syndrome (AIDS). *Science, 220*, 868–871.

Carpenter, C. C., Cooper, D. A., Fischel, M. A., Gatell, J. M., Gazzard, B. G., Hammer, S. M., et al. (2000). Antiretroviral therapy in adults: Updated recommendations of the International AIDS Society—USA Panel. *Journal of the American Medical Association, 283*, 381–390.

Centers for Disease Control. (1981a). Kaposi's sarcoma and pneumocytis pneumonia among homosexual men—New York City and California. *Morbidity and Mortality Weekly Report, 30*, 305–308.

Centers for Disease Control. (1981b). Pneumocystis pneumonia—Los Angeles. *Morbidity and Mortality Weekly Report, 30*, 250–252.

Centers for Disease Control. (1982). Possible transfusion-associated acquired immune deficiency syndrome (AIDS)—California. *Morbidity and Mortality Weekly Report, 31*, 652–654.

Centers for Disease Control and Prevention. (2001). *HIV/AIDS Surveillance Supplemental Report*, 7(1) [On-line]. Available: http://www.cdc.gov/hiv/stats/hasrsupp71/commentary.htm

Cohen, F. L., & Durham, J. D. (Eds.). (1993). *Women, children and HIV/AIDS*. New York: Springer Publishing.

Coffin, J., Haase, A., Levy, J. A., Montagnier, L., Oroszlan, S., Teich, N., et al. (1986). What to call the AIDS virus? *Nature, 321*, 10.

Curtis, T. (March 19, 1992). The origin of AIDS. *Rolling Stone*, 54–63.

Delaney, M. (2000). *HIV, AIDS and the distortion of science* [On-line]. Available: http://www/aegis.org/topics/mdelaney.html

Duesberg, P. (1988). HIV is not the cause of AIDS. *Science, 241*, 524, 517.
Duesberg, P. (1989). Human immunodeficiency virus and acquired immunodeficiency syndrome: Correlation but not causation. *Proceedings of the National Academy of Science, United States of America, 86*, 755–764.
Duesberg, P. (1991). AIDS epidemiology: Inconsistencies with human immunodeficiency virus and with infectious disease. *Proceedings of the National Academy of Science, United States of America, 88*, 1575–1579.
Duesberg, P. (1994). Infectious AIDS—stretching the germ theory beyond its limits. *International Archives of Allergy and Immunology, 103*(2), 118–127.
Durham, J. D., & Lashley, F. R. (Eds.). (2000). *The person with HIV/AIDS: Nursing perspectives*. New York: Springer Publishing.
Elswood, B., & Stricker, R. (1994). Polio vaccines and the origin of AIDS. *Medical Hypotheses, 42*, 347–354.
Friedman-Kien, A. (1981). Disseminated Kaposi's sarcoma syndrome in young homosexual men. *Journal of the American Academy of Dermatology, 5*, 468–471.
Gottlieb, M., Schroff, R., Schanker, H., Weisman, J. D., Fan, P. T., Wolf, R. A., et al. (1981). *Pneumocystis carinii* pneumonia and mucosal candidiasis in previously healthy homosexual men: Evidence of a new acquired cellular immunodeficiency. *New England Journal of Medicine, 305*, 1425–1431.
Hahn, B., Shaw, G., De Cock, K., & Sharp, P. (2000). AIDS as a zoonosis: Scientific and public health implications. *Science, 287*, 607–614.
Hillis, D. (2000). Origins of HIV. *Science, 288*, 1757, 1759.
Hooper, E. (1999). *The river: A journey to the source of HIV and AIDS*. New York: Little Brown.
Joint United Nations Programme on HIV/AIDS. (2000a). *AIDS epidemic updates: December 2000* [On-line]. Available: http://www.unaids.org/epidemic_update/report_dec00/index_dec.html#full
Joint United Nations Programme on HIV/AIDS. (2000b). HIV, AIDS and the reappearance of an old myth. *Background Brief* [On-line]. Available: http://www.unaids.org/special/index.html
Korber, B., Muldoon, M., Theiler, J., Gao, F., Gupta, R., Lapedes, A., et al. (2000). Timing the ancestor of the HIV-1 pandemic strains. *Science, 288*, 1789–1796.
Korber, B., Theiler, J., & Wolinsky, S. (1998). Limitations of a molecular clock applied to considerations of the origins of HIV-1. *Science, 280*, 1868–1871.
Kurth, R. (1990). Does HIV cause AIDS? An updated response to Duesberg's theories. *Intervirology, 31*, 301–314.
Levy, J., Hoffman, A., Kramer, S., Landis, J., Shimabukuro, J. M., & Oshiro, L. S. (1984). Isolation of lymphocytopathic retroviruses from San Francisco patients with AIDS. *Science, 225*, 840–842.
Masur, H., Michelis, M. A., Greene, J. B., Onorato, I., Stouwe, R. A., Holzman, R. S., et al. (1981). An outbreak of community-acquired *Pneumocystis carinii* pneumonia: Initial manifestation of cellular immune dysfunction. *New England Journal of Medicine, 305*, 1431–1438.
National Institute of Allergy and Infectious Diseases. (2000a). The evidence that HIV causes AIDS. *Fact Sheet* [On-line]. Available: http//www.niaid.nih.gov/factsheets/evidhiv.htm

National Institute of Allergy and Infectious Diseases. (2000b). *The relationship between the human immunodeficiency virus and the acquired immunodeficiency syndrome* [On-line]. Available: http://www.niaid.nih.gov/publications/hivaids/all.htm

Panel on Clinical Practices for Treatment of HIV Infection (DHHS). (2001). *Guidelines for the use of antiretroviral agents in HIV-infected adults and adolescents* [On-line]. Available: http://www.hivatis.org/guidelines/adult/text/

Poinar, H., Kuch, M., & Pääbo, S. (2001). Molecular analyses of oral polio vaccine samples. *Science, 292,* 743–744.

Popovic, M., Sarngadharan, M., Read, E., & Gallo, R. (1984). Detection, isolation, and continuous production of cytopathic retroviruses (HTLV-III) from patients with AIDS and pre-AIDS. *Science, 224,* 497–500.

Robertson, D. L., Anderson, J. P., Bradac, J. A., Carr, J. K., Foley, B., Funkhouser, R. K., et al. (2000). HIV-1 nomenclature proposal. *Science, 288,* 55–57.

Sarngadharan, M., Popovic, M., Bruch, L., Schupbach, J., & Gallo, R. C. (1984). Antibodies reactive with human T-lymphotropic retroviruses (HTLV-III) in the serum of patients with AIDS. *Science, 224,* 506–508.

Shilts, R. (1987). *And the band played on.* New York: Penguin Books.

13

Legionellosis: Legionnaires' Disease and Pontiac Fever

Alicia M. Fry and
Richard E. Besser

In July 1976, during the annual American Legion convention in Philadelphia, an outbreak of a severe form of pneumonia occurred at the convention hotel. Between July 22 and August 3, 1976, 182 persons were infected, 147 (81%) required hospitalization and 29 (16%) died (Fraser, Tsai, McDade, Shepard, & Brachman, 1977). Scientists at the Centers for Disease Control (CDC) identified a previously unknown pathogen from autopsy lung specimens. The new pathogen was named *Legionella pneumophila*, and the clinical syndrome, Legionnaires' disease (McDade, Shepard, Fraser, Tsai, Redus, & Dowdle, 1977). Subsequently, through stored serum samples, investigators retrospectively identified earlier outbreaks, one from the same hotel in 1974, at a psychiatric hospital in 1965, and at a meat packing plant in 1957 (Breiman & Butler, 1998; Osterholm, Chin, Osborne, Dull, Dean, Fraser, et al., 1983; Terranova, Cohen, & Fraser, 1978; Thacker, Bennett, Tsai, Fraser, McDade, Shepard, et al., 1978). Sporadic cases from 1947 were also found (McDade, Brenner, & Bozeman, 1979).

Legionella, the causative agent of Legionnaires' disease, is a gram-negative, aerobic, unencapsulated bacillus. At least 42 species and 64 serotypes of *Legionella* have been identified, although *L. pneumophila* causes over 90% of the cases of Legionnaires' disease in the United States and Europe (Benson, 1998). Rarely, nonpneumophila *Legionella* species have been associated with Legionnaires' disease in the United

States, including *L. longbeachae*, *L. micdadei*, *L. dumoffii*, and *L. bosemanii* (Butler, Fields, & Breiman, 1997; Knirsch, Jakob, Schoonmaker, Kiehlbauch, Wong, Della-Latta, et al., 2000). In Australia, unlike the United States and Europe, almost half of the cases of Legionnaires' disease are caused by *L. longbeachae*, although *L. pneumophila* still accounts for the majority of cases (Doyle, Steele, McLennan, Parkinson, Manning, & Heusenroeder, 1998; "Legionellosis," 1997).

Two clinically and epidemiologically distinct syndromes are caused by legionellae: Legionnaires' disease and Pontiac fever (Yu, 2000). Legionnaires' disease is a pneumonia that can be severe and which may include systemic symptoms, such as fever, watery diarrhea, and delirium. Other symptoms can include a nonproductive cough, headache, and myalgia. In persons with immune compromising conditions, extrapulmonary involvement and/or dissemination can occur (Yu, 2000). Two to fifteen percent of adult community-acquired pneumonia in the United States is thought to be caused by *L. pneumophila* (Marston, Plouffe, File, Hackman, Salstrom, Lipman, et al., 1997; Yu, 2000). Persons with compromised immune systems and underlying medical conditions, such as the elderly, smokers, persons with chronic cardiovascular or pulmonary conditions, and users of immunosuppressive drugs, are most susceptible. It is rare to diagnose Legionnaires' disease in a healthy, young person. Perhaps it is not surprising, therefore, that the attack rate for Legionnaires' disease in outbreaks is low, less than 5%, and that mortality can be high, ranging from 5%–30% (Hoge & Breiman, 1991). The incubation period for Legionnaires' disease is 2–10 days (Fraser et al., 1977).

In contrast to Legionnaires' disease, Pontiac fever is a self-limited, nonfatal, nonpneumonic illness that presents with flu-like symptoms such as malaise, fever, chills, headache, and myalgia. It has a shorter incubation period than Legionnaires' disease, usually 24–48 hours. Unlike Legionnaires' disease, it generally affects persons without underlying medical conditions and has a high attack rate (up to 95%). The first outbreak of Pontiac fever was described in 1978 in Pontiac, Michigan (Mangione, Remis, Tait, McGee, Gorman, Wentworth, et al., 1985; Yu, 2000). Occasionally, an outbreak of *Legionella* can manifest as both Legionnaires' disease and Pontiac fever (Benin, Arnold, Benson, Fiore, Cook, Williams, et al., 1999).

Why have legionellae only recently been identified as a cause of human disease? The organisms have been isolated from several natural environments including lakes, rivers, thermally polluted ponds, and wet soil (Hoge & Brieman, 1991). Natural freshwater environments, however, have rarely been implicated as a source of human disease; man-made water environments are the principal reservoirs of *Legionella* species that cause human disease because they allow for the growth, amplification, and dissemination of the bacteria.

Legionellae require appropriate conditions to grow and multiply, that is, temperatures of 25°–42° C and environments with appropriate nutritional requirements. These nutritional requirements are met by growth in an intracellular environment, and legionellae survive in the environment as intracellular parasites of free-living protozoa, such as amoebae. Other factors, such as water stagnation and the presence of biofilms and sediment even on materials such as ceramic tile, enhance the amplification of legionellae in water systems, making man-made environments ideal conditions for the growth and amplification of legionellae (Breiman, 1996).

In addition to supporting the growth of legionellae, the man-made water environments must produce aerosols containing fine droplets of water, that can be inhaled and reach the alveoli. Water droplets of 1–5 microliters can reach alveoli in the lung, where they are retained and have the ability to cause disease in susceptible persons (Breiman, 1996). Man-made freshwater environments that have been implicated in the dissemination of *Legionella* include cooling towers, evaporative condensers, whirlpools, and spas, as well as sources that use potable water from plumbing systems, such as showers, cool-mist humidifiers, and supermarket ultrasonic misting machines (Cordes, Wiesenthal, Gorman, Phair, Sommers, Brown, et al., 1981; Garbe, Davis, Weisfeld, Markowitz, Miner, Garrity, et al., 1985; Jernigan, Sanders, Waites, Brookings, Benson, & Pappas, 1994; Keller, Hajjeh, DeMaria, Fields, Pruckler, Benson, 1995; Lepine, Jernigan, Butler, Pruckler, Benson, Kim, et al., 1998; Mahoney, Hoge, Farley, Barbaree, Breiman, Benson, & McFarland, 1992; Politi, Fraser, Mallison, Mohatt, Morris, Patton, et al., 1979; Stout, Yu, & Muraca, 1987; Stout, Yu, Muraca, Joly, Troup, & Tompkins, 1992). In 2000, in Melbourne, Australia, an outbreak of legionellosis, associated with a cooling tower on the aquarium there resulted in 76 cases and 2 deaths (World Health Organization, 2000). If legionellae are present in these water systems, each type of system has the ability to disseminate water droplets containing bacteria to susceptible persons. The largest outbreak of Legionnaires' disease began in June 2001 in Murcia, Spain, and was caused by community-acquired *L. pneumophila* serogroup 1. Approximately 745 persons became ill with suspected disease with more than 310 cases confirmed (Bosch, 2001).

Hospitals are unique environments because highly susceptible persons are concentrated in one location. Numerous outbreaks of nosocomial-acquired legionellosis have been reported. Although the majority have been associated with potable water, cooling towers are another confirmed source of transmission (Campins, Ferrer, Callis, Pelaz, Cortes, Pinart, et al., 2000; Helms, Massanari, Wenzel, Pfaller, Moyer, & Hall, 1988; Johnson, Yu, Wagner, & Best, 1985; Mitchell, O'Mahony, Watson, Lynch, Joseph, Quigley, et al., 1990; Tobin, Bear, Dunnill, Fisher-Hoch, French, Mitchell, et al., 1980).

As advances in technology have improved medical care, persons with underlying medical conditions (see chapter 23) are more likely to be active in their communities and to travel for business and pleasure. Therefore, although legionellae have been in the natural environment for centuries, it is only in the 20th century that technologic advances have provided the ideal setting for multiplication of the bacterium, effective dissemination, and contact with a sizable number of susceptible hosts (Breiman & Butler, 1998).

Four methods are currently available to diagnosis Legionnaires' disease: culture of the organism from respiratory secretions, detection of *Legionella* urinary antigen by either enzyme immunoassay or radioimmunoassay, paired acute- and convalescent-phase serologic testing, and direct fluorescent antibody (DFA). But there are problems with all those currently available (Waterer, Baselki, & Wunderink, 2001). Of the four, culture and *Legionella* urinary antigen detection are most commonly used for the clinical diagnosis of legionellosis; both are highly specific for *L. pneumophila*. Culture of respiratory secretions is 50%–60% sensitive (Breiman, 1996). Legionellae are fastidious and require special media and conditions for growth; techniques for culturing other respiratory pathogens will not detect *Legionella*. Therefore the clinician and laboratory must always consider *Legionella* in the differential diagnosis of pneumonia so that sputum samples can be appropriately evaluated. An advantage of culture as a diagnostic method for Legionnaires' disease is that culture techniques will isolate all *Legionella* species, *pneumophila* and non-*pneumophila*. Also, molecular typing techniques can be used on clinical isolates to determine whether two or more cases are related. Furthermore, an isolate obtained from an environmental source can be compared with a clinical isolate to determine if the water environment is the source of the

Legionella causing disease. Without directly comparing environmental and clinical isolates, it is difficult to definitively implicate a source in a case of Legionnaires' disease.

Urinary antigen tests are simple to perform and give results much sooner than culture of respiratory secretions. Obtaining a urine sample is often easier than obtaining an adequate sputum sample. However, commercially available tests only detect *L. pneumophila* serogroup 1, the cause of more than 70% of cases of Legionnaires' disease in the United States and Europe. Cases due to species and serogroups other than *L. pneumophila* serogroup 1 may go undiagnosed if the evaluation is limited to urinary antigen tests. Also, without a clinical isolate, it is not possible to use molecular techniques to identify an environmental source of a case or outbreak. The other diagnostic methods have limited usefulness in clinical diagnosis and only detect *L. pneumophila* serogroup 1. Serologic testing is useful in epidemiologic studies only.

Because *Legionella* is an intracellular pathogen, those antibiotics that achieve high intracellular concentrations are most effective. The traditional use of erythromycin has largely been replaced by newer agents such as azithromycin, clarithromycin, and other macrolides, and quinolones such as ciprofloxacin, trovofloxacin, and levofloxicin. These can achieve high pulmonary concentrations (Edelstein, 1995; Yu, 2000).

Two surveillance systems at CDC currently collect information about Legionnaires' disease cases in the United States, National Electronic Telecommunications System for Surveillance (NETTS) and the Legionnaires' disease surveillance system. NETTS is most useful as a means to alert state health departments about possible outbreaks; however, it collects limited demographic information about each case. The Legionnaires' disease surveillance system collects demographic and diagnostic information, as well as data on potential risk factors for disease. This system has contributed to knowledge about risk factors for disease, though it is not useful at detecting outbreaks because of the long time before reports are received and analyzed. Underreporting is a problem in both surveillance systems. For example, 8,000–18,000 cases of Legionnaires' disease are estimated to occur yearly, yet NETTS receives fewer than 1,500 reports per year and the Legionnaires' disease surveillance system receives fewer than 400 reports per year (Centers for Disease Control and Prevention, 1999; Marston et al., 1997).

Travelers are exposed to many potential *Legionella* sources, including evaporative coolers and potable water systems in hotels, convention centers, and cruise ships, as well as whirlpools and spas. The first outbreak of Legionnaires' disease described in 1976 was travel related and is an example of how a concentration of susceptible hosts exposed to a single source can result in an outbreak. Because the incubation period is relatively long, onset of illness is often after travelers return home to different locations, and dispersed patients make travel-associated outbreaks difficult to detect. In Europe, surveillance for Legionnaires' disease has focused on detecting travel-associated clusters and outbreaks (see chapter 22). In 1997, 29% of European cases were community-acquired, 16% were nosocomial, and 22% were travel related (World Health Organization, 1998).

Efforts to prevent the transmission of legionellae from the environment to susceptible hosts have focused on either altering aquatic environments so they no longer support the growth of legionellae, or reducing the exposure of susceptible hosts to potentially contaminated aerosols. Several published guidelines are available to reduce transmission of legionellae to susceptible persons and minimize the risk of community- and travel-acquired legionellosis. The American Society of Heating, Refrigerating and Air-conditioning Engineers (ASHRAE) has published guidelines to diminish the risk of legionellosis associated with building water systems (American Society of Heating, 2000). Also, specific guidelines for reducing the transmission of *Legionella* in public spas and hot tubs and for minimizing transmission from whirlpool spas on cruise ships are available from CDC (Centers for Disease Control, 1985; Centers for Disease Control and Prevention, 1997a).

Hospital facilities present a unique situation with a concentration of patients who are highly susceptible to *Legionella* infection. A case of Legionnaires' disease is considered to be a definite nosocomial case if it is laboratory confirmed and occurs in a patient who has been hospitalized continuously for ≥ 10 days before the onset of symptoms. A case is considered a possible case of nosocomial Legionnaires' disease if the infection is laboratory confirmed and occurs 2–9 days after hospital admission. From 1980 through 1989, 23% of cases reported to the CDC Legionaires' disease surveillance system were reported as possibly nosocomial. Thirty-seven percent of the nosocomially-acquired cases were associated with outbreaks, while the majority of non-nosocomial Legionnaires' disease in the community was sporadic; only 3.7% of community-acquired cases were classified as outbreak associated (Marston, Lipman, & Breiman, 1994).

Special guidelines to reduce the transmission of legionellae in hospital environments are available from CDC and other organizations

(Centers for Disease Control and Prevention, 1997b, 1997c; Maryland Scientific Working Group, 2000). In general, routine testing of samples from hospital water systems is not recommended by CDC if legionellosis has not previously been identified in the hospital. The reasons for this recommendation are (a) there is no clear correlation between the results of water sample testing and transmission; (b) *Legionella* can be isolated from water without being associated with known cases; (c) interpretation of results of routine sampling is limited by different sampling and laboratory methods; and (d) risk of disease due to *Legionella* is influenced by multiple factors in addition to the detection of and concentration of legionellae in the water source, including host susceptibility, how well the organism is aerosolized, and strain virulence (Centers for Disease Control and Prevention, 1997c). However, some authorities do recommend routine environmental testing for *Legionella* in hospital facilities (Maryland Scientific Working Group, 2000). Future efforts to evaluate the effectiveness of these different hospital guidelines in decreasing nosocomial cases of Legionnaires' disease will be important. Once one definite or two possible nosocomial cases of Legionnaires' disease have been identified in a hospital facility, a full environmental investigation to identify and subsequently decontaminate sources of *Legionella* in the facility is indicated.

Twentieth century advances in technology have contributed to the emergence of *Legionella* as a human pathogen. Use of appropriate diagnostic tests will help assure optimum treatment. In the future, surveillance for Legionnaires' disease in the United States will be expanded and electronic reporting will be used, improving our ability to detect travel-related and non-travel-related outbreaks especially from various geographic areas.

REFERENCES

American Society of Heating and Air-conditioning Engineers. (2000). *ASHRAE guideline 12-2000—Minimizing the risk of Legionellosis associated with building water systems* (2000). Atlanta, GA: American Society for Heating, Refrigeration, and Air Conditioning Engineers.

Benin, A., Arnold, K., Benson, R., Fiore, A., Cook, P., Williams, K., et al. (1999, November). *An outbreak of Legionnaires' disease and Pontiac fever from a whirlpool spa.* Abstract presented at the Infectious Diseases Society of America, Philadelphia.

Benson, R. F. (1998). Classification of the genus *Legionella*. *Seminars in Respiratory Infections, 13,* 90–99.

Bosch, X. (2001). Legionnaire's outbreak in Spanish town may be the largest ever. *Lancet, 358*, 220.

Breiman, R. F. (1996). Impact of technology on the emergence of infectious diseases. *Epidemiologic Reviews, 18*, 4-9.

Breiman, R. F., & Butler, J. C. (1998). Legionnaires' disease: Clinical, epidemiological, and public health perspectives. *Seminars in Respiratory Infections, 13*, 84–89.

Butler, J., Fields, B. S., & Breiman, R. F. (1997). Prevention and control of legionellosis. *Infectious Diseases in Clinical Practice, 6*, 458–464.

Campins, M., Ferrer, A., Callis, L., Pelaz, C., Cortes, P. J., Pinart, N., et al. (2000). Nosocomial Legionnaires' disease in a children's hospital. *Pediatric Infectious Diseases Journal, 19*, 228–234.

Centers for Disease Control. (1985). *Suggested health and safety guidelines for public spas and hot tubs.* Atlanta: Author.

Centers for Disease Control and Prevention. (1997a). *Final recommendations to minimize transmission of Legionnaires' disease from whirlpool spas on cruise ships.* Atlanta: Author.

Centers for Disease Control and Prevention. (1997b). Transmission of nosocomial Legionnaires' disease. *Journal of the American Medical Association, 277*, 1927–1928.

Centers for Disease Control and Prevention. (1997c). Guidelines for prevention of nosocomial pneumonia. Centers for Disease Control and Prevention. *Morbidity and Mortality Weekly Report, 46*(RR-1), 1–79.

Centers for Disease Control and Prevention. (1999). Summary of notifiable diseases, United States 1998. *Morbidity and Mortality Weekly Report, 47*(53), 1–93.

Cordes, L. G., Wiesenthal, A. M., Gorman, G. W., Phair, J. P., Sommers, H. M., Brown, A., et al. (1981). Isolation of *Legionella pneumophila* from hospital shower heads. *Annals of Internal Medicine, 94*, 195–197.

Doyle, R., Steele, T. W., McLennan, A. M., Parkinson, I. H., Manning, P. A., & Heusenroeder, M. W. (1998). Sequence analysis of the *mip* gene of the soilborne pathogen *Legionella longbeachae. Infections and Immunity, 66*, 1492–1499.

Edelstein, P. H. (1995). Antimicrobial chemotherapy for Legionnaires' disease: A review. *Clinical Infectious Diseases, 21*(Suppl. 3), S265–S276.

Fraser, D. W., Tsai, T., McDade, J. E., Shepard, C. C., & Brachman, P. S. (1977). Legionnaires' disease: Description of an epidemic of pneumonia. *New England Journal of Medicine, 277*, 1189–1198.

Garbe, P. L., Davis, B. J., Weisfeld, J. S., Markowitz, L., Miner, P., Garrity, F., et al. (1985). Nosocomial Legionnaires' disease. Epidemiologic demonstration of cooling towers as a source. *Journal of the American Medical Association, 254*, 521–524.

Helms, C. M., Massanari, R. M., Wenzel, R. P., Pfaller, M. A., Moyer, N. P., & Hall, N. (1988). Legionnaires' disease associated with a hospital water system. A five-year progress report on continuous hyperchlorination. *Journal of the American Medical Association, 259*, 2423–2427.

Hoge, C. W., & Breiman, R. F. (1991). Advances in the epidemiology and control of *Legionella* infections. *Epidemiologic Reviews, 13*, 329–340.

Jernigan, D. B., Sanders, L. I., Waites, K. B., Brookings, E. S., Benson, R. F., & Pappas, P. G. (1994). Pulmonary infection due to *Legionella cincinnatiensis* in renal transplant recipients: Two cases and implications for laboratory diagnosis. *Lancet, 18,* 385–389.

Johnson, J. T., Yu, V. L., Wagner, R. L., & Best, M. G. (1985). Nosocomial *Legionella* pneumonia in a population of head and neck cancer patients. *Laryngoscope, 95,* 1468–1471.

Keller, D., Hajjeh, R., DeMaria, A., Fields, B. S., Pruckler, J. M., Benson, R. S., et al. (1995). Community outbreak of Legionnaires' disease: An investigation confirming the potential for cooling towers to transmit *Legionella* species. *Clinical Infectious Diseases, 22,* 257–261.

Knirsch, C. A., Jakob, K., Schoonmaker, D., Kiehlbauch, J. A., Wong, S. J., Della-Latta, P., et al. (2000). An outbreak of *Legionella micdadei* pneumonia in transplant patients: Evaluation, molecular epidemiology, and control. *American Journal of Medicine, 108,* 290–295.

Legionellosis. (1997). *Communicable Diseases Intelligence, 21,* 137.

Lepine, L. A., Jernigan, D. B., Butler, J. C., Pruckler, J. M., Benson, R. F., Kim, G., et al. (1998). A recurrent outbreak of nosocomial Legionnaires' disease detected by urinary antigen testing: Evidence for long-term colonization of a hospital plumbing system. *Infection Control & Hospital Epidemiology, 19,* 905–910.

Mahoney, F. J., Hoge, C. W., Farley, T. A., Barbaree, J. M., Breiman, R. F., Benson, R. F., & McFarland, L. M. (1992). Communitywide outbreak of Legionnaires' disease associated with a grocery store mist machine. *Journal of Infectious Diseases, 165,* 736–739.

Mangione, E. J., Remis, R. S., Tait, K. A., McGee, H. B., Gorman, G. W., Wentworth, B. B., et al. (1985). An outbreak of Pontiac fever related to whirlpool use, Michigan 1982. *Journal of the American Medical Association, 253,* 535–539.

Marston, B. J., Lipman, H. B., & Breiman, R. F. (1994). Surveillance for Legionnaires' disease. Risk factors for morbidity and mortality. *Archives of Internal Medicine, 154,* 2417–2422.

Marston, B. J., Plouffe, J. F., File, T. M., Hackman, B. A., Salstrom, S. J., Lipman, H. B., et al. (1997). Incidence of community-acquired pneumonia requiring hospitalization—Results of a population-based active surveillance study in Ohio. *Archives of Internal Medicine, 157,* 1709–1718.

Maryland Scientific Working Group. (2000). *Report of the Maryland Scientific Working Group to study Legionella in water systems in healthcare institutions* [On-line]. Available: http://www.dhmh.state.md.us/html/legionella.htm

McDade, J. E., Brenner, D. J., & Bozeman, F. M. (1979). Legionnaires' disease bacterium isolated in 1947. *Annals of Internal Medicine, 90,* 659–661.

McDade, J. E., Shepard, C. C., Fraser, D. W., Tsai, T. R., Redus, M. A., & Dowdle, W. R. (1977). Legionnaires' disease: Isolation of a bacterium and demonstration of its role in other respiratory disease. *New England Journal of Medicine, 297,* 1197–1203.

Mitchell, E., O'Mahony, M., Watson, J. M., Lynch, D., Joseph, C., Quigley, C., et al. (1990). Two outbreaks of Legionnaires' disease in Bolton Health District. *Epidemiology and Infection, 104,* 159–170.

Osterholm, M. T., Chin, T. D., Osborne, D. O., Dull, H. B., Dean, A. G., Fraser, D. W., et al. (1983). A 1957 outbreak of Legionnaires' disease associated with a meat packing plant. *American Journal of Epidemiology, 117,* 60–67.

Politi, B. D., Fraser, D. W., Mallison, G. F., Mohatt, J. V., Morris, G. K., Patton, C. M., et al. (1979). A major focus of Legionnaires' disease in Bloomington, Indiana. *Annals of Internal Medicine, 90,* 587–591.

Stout, J. E., Yu, V. L., & Muraca, P. (1987). Legionnaires' disease acquired within the homes of two patients. Link to the home water supply. *Journal of the American Medical Association, 257,* 1215–1217.

Stout, J. E., Yu, V. L., Muraca, P., Joly, J., Troup, N., & Tompkins, L. S. (1992). Potable water as a cause of sporadic cases of community-acquired legionnaires' disease. *New England Journal of Medicine, 326,* 151–155.

Terranova, W., Cohen, M. L., & Fraser, D. W. (1978). 1974 outbreak of Legionnaires' disease diagnosed in 1977. Clinical and epidemiological features. *Lancet, 2*(8081), 122–124.

Thacker, S. B., Bennett, J. V., Tsai, T. F., Fraser, D. W., McDade, J. E., Shepard, C. C., et al. (1978). An outbreak in 1965 of severe respiratory illness caused by the Legionnaires' disease bacterium. *Journal of Infectious Diseases, 138,* 512–519.

Tobin, J. O., Beare, J., Dunnill, M. S., Fisher-Hoch, S., French, M., Mitchell, R. G., et al. (1980). Legionnaires' disease in a transplant unit: Isolation of the causative agent from shower baths. *Lancet, 2*(8186), 118–121.

Waterer, G. W., Baselski, V. S., & Wunderink, R. G. (2001). *Legionella* and community-acquired pneumonia: A review of current diagnostic tests from a clinician's viewpoint. *American Journal of Medicine, 110,* 41–48.

World Health Organization. (1998). Legionnaires' disease in Europe, 1009. *Weekly Epidemiological Record, 73,* 257–262.

World Health Organization. (2000). Outbreak news. Legionellosis, Australia (update). *Weekly Epidemiological Record, 75,* 173.

Yu, V. (2000). *Legionella pneumophila* (Legionnaires' disease). In G. L. Mandell, J. E. Bennett, & R. E. Dolin (Eds.), *Mandell, Douglas, and Bennett's principles and practice of infectious diseases* (5th ed., pp. 2424–2441). Philadelphia: Churchill Livingstone.

14

Lyme Disease, Ehrlichiosis, and Babesiosis

Felissa R. Lashley

Since the mid-1970s more than 20 tick-borne infectious diseases have been newly identified in humans. Among these emerging diseases are a trio that are clinically important in the United States. Lyme disease, usually caused by *Borrelia burgdorferi*, a spirochete, was first recognized in North America in the 1970s. Ehrlichiosis, which is caused in humans by several members of the bacterial genus *Ehrlichia*, came to attention in 1986. The third, babesiosis, is a parasitic infection caused by *Babesia microti*. All three of these diseases have usual animal reservoirs. Societal and environmental changes such as building suburban and country residential dwellings that increasingly encroach on wooded areas near where deer, large mammals, and certain types of wild rodents usually live facilitate spread. Humans can then come into contact with these microbes through usual maintenance such as gardening and yard work and via pets that may carry ticks into yards and homes. More leisure time in which to pursue outdoor activities such as hiking, fishing, and camping in meadows and wooded areas also afford opportunities for exposure. Changes in weather and climate such as global warming and increased rain can increase reservoir and vector populations. Vector-borne diseases are discussed in general in chapter 3. Lyme disease, ehrlichiosis, and babesiosis are considered here.

LYME DISEASE

The recognition of Lyme disease began with a phone call to the state health department in November 1975 from a mother in Old Lyme,

Connecticut who reported a cluster of 12 cases of a disease that had been diagnosed as juvenile rheumatoid arthritis. Four of these cases lived on the same street (Steere, Malawista, Snydman, & Andiman, 1976; Steere, Malawista, Snydman, Shope, Andiman, Ross, et al., 1977). This report was quickly followed by that of another mother in the same community who told investigators at the Yale Rheumatology Clinic and the state health department about arthritis occurring in herself, her husband, two of their children, and several neighbors (Steere et al., 1977). Researchers began investigating cases of clustering arthritis in Lyme, Old Lyme, and East Haddam, CT, believing that they were not typical juvenile or other type of rheumatoid arthritis. In all, 51 persons, 39 children, and 12 adults comprised the sample investigated at that time with information that some cases began in 1972. They believed that an arbovirus might be responsible and tests were performed for the Ross River, Chikungunya, and O'nyong-nyong viruses. The tests were negative. Thus, investigators referred to this arthritis as a new or previously unrecognized clinical entity, and called it Lyme arthritis (Steere et al., 1976, 1977). As investigations moved forward, an arthropod vector was suspected (Steere et al., 1977). The typical skin lesion known as erythema migrans, a bull's-eye rash, was described in earlier literature in Europe and in a 1970 report in the United States from Connecticut (Parola & Raoult, 2001; Scrimenti, 1970), suggesting earlier times of emergence without recognition of a new agent.

Lyme disease is caused by a gram-negative bacterial spirochete, *Borrelia burgdorferi*, sensu lato that is transmitted to humans by the deer or black-legged tick, specifically *Ixodes scapularis* (also called *I. dammini*), and *I. pacificus* in the West (Centers for Disease Control and Prevention, 2001; Shapiro & Gerber, 2000; Terkeltaub, 2000). It is the most common tick-borne infection in the United States. The life cycle of the tick occurs over a 2-year period and involves the evolution from eggs to the feeding of the larva, particularly on the white-footed mouse, and other small rodents such as chipmunks, where *B. burgdorferi* may be acquired. The life cycle progresses through a nymphal stage the next spring, with feeding again on mice, and progresses to adult stages when the adult ticks feed on and attach to white-tailed deer or other large mammals where they mate, and may fall off (Armstrong & Cohen, 1999; Strickland, 2000). In the Pacific northwest, the life cycle involves woodrats and lizards. Ticks of the *Ixodes* genus can hide in ground litter and leaf litter, and find hosts from the tips of grass and shrubs (Grabenstein, 1999). They prefer shade with high humidity. Humans are incidental hosts (Strickland, 2000). The size of the nymphs that may attach to humans is about that of a poppy seed and thus can be difficult to detect (Centers for Disease Control and Prevention, 2000). While humans may encounter the ticks during recreational activities such as hiking, fishing, and camping in meadows and wooded areas, or when doing activities such as clearing brush, ticks can also be encountered in the backyards of suburban dwellings, as humans have expanded their housing into formerly wooded areas where deer may live. Furthermore, pets such as cats may carry ticks into yards and homes (Strickland, 2000). Therefore, preventing tick bites is an important aspect of prevention of the tick-borne diseases. Preventive measures are shown in Appendix C, Table C.4. It is as yet unclear what human factors are associated with an increased predisposition to acquiring Lyme disease from a tick. One factor does appear to be the length of time the tick is attached to the body. Those to whom it is attached less than 24 hours appear to have a smaller risk of acquiring Lyme disease (Armstrong & Cohen, 1999). Rather recently it has been realized that these ticks may be coinfected with the agents of babesiosis and ehrlichiosis, transmitting multiple infective agents together (Strickland, 2000). These diseases are discussed later in this chapter.

Lyme disease became a nationally notifiable disease in January 1991. Although cases have been reported from 49 of the 50 states, and the District of Columbia, 92% were reported from 8 northeastern and mid-Atlantic states and 2 north-central states. In 1996–1999, the states reporting the highest number of Lyme disease cases in descending order of frequency were New York, Connecticut, Pennsylvania, New Jersey, Wisconsin, Maryland, Rhode Island, Massachusetts, Minnesota, California, Delaware, and Virginia (Centers for Disease Control and Prevention, 2000, 2001). States that reported a Lyme disease incidence per 100,000 population that was greater than the national rate in descending order of frequency were Connecticut, Rhode Island, New York, Pennsylvania, Delaware, New Jersey, Maryland, Massachusetts, and Wisconsin. These states accounted for 92% of reported cases in 1999 (Centers for Disease Control and Prevention, 2001). It is generally agreed that the incidence of Lyme disease is increasing. In 1999, 16,273 cases were reported to CDC as compared with 9,896 reported cases in 1992 (Centers for Disease Control and Prevention, 2000, 2001). Other areas of greater incidence are Missouri, North

Carolina, Vermont, New Hampshire, Kansas, Oklahoma, and Texas (Grabenstein, 1999). Cases have also been reported from Europe, Asia, and Australia as well as other locales (Shapiro & Gerber, 2000). Outside the U.S., different species of *Ixodes* are involved with varying strains and species of *Borrelia* (Parola & Raoult, 2001). A Lyme-like disease, transmitted by the Lone Star tick (*Amblyomma americanum*) that is seen in the southern U.S. appears to result from a spirochete, tentatively called *Borrelia lonestarii* (Terkeltaub, 2000).

Lyme disease can cause acute and chronic manifestations that may be localized and/or disseminated and multisystem with both early and late signs and symptoms (Armstrong & Cohen, 1999; Terkeltaub, 2000). The case definition includes the previously described skin lesion known as either erythema chronicum migrans or erythema migrans that appears in 60%–80% of affected persons at the site of the tick bite within a few days. It appears as a macule/papule that expands over days or weeks to form a large round lesion that measures at least 5 cm to 15 cm with partial central clearing or at least one late manifestation of musculoskeletal, neurologic, or cardiovascular disease with laboratory confirmation of *B. burgdorferi* infection. This case definition is considered limited (Centers for Disease Control and Prevention, 2001). Often the person may not be aware of being bitten. Secondary lesions may occur. Stage 1 consists of early infection with localized erythema migrans. This is followed in days or weeks by stage 2, disseminated infection especially affecting the heart, nervous system and/or joints. Within weeks or months late or persistent infection can occur designated by Steere as stage 3 (Steere, 2001). In the early disseminated phase, other symptoms such as secondary rash, malaise, fatigue, lethargy, headache, chills, fever, backache, anorexia, and intermittent arthralgias and myalgias may occur. Even if untreated, these may remit for a period of time.

The chief later effects are arthritis, and neurological and cardiac manifestations. The arthritis is generally asymmetric and oligoarticular, and the knee is nearly always a site occurring at a median time of 6 months after infection if untreated. Arthritis may become chronic in 10%–20% of untreated persons, and association with specific HLA types may predict arthritic outcome (Armstrong & Cohen, 2000; Lashley, 1998; Steere, 2001). Neurological symptoms may occur early as mild symptoms such as headache and photophobia. In some persons, they progress to meningitis, peripheral or cranial neuropathy, especially Bell's palsy or bilateral facial nerve palsy, or encephalopathy.

Late neurological syndromes, occurring years after infection in the form of sensory peripheral neuropathy, headache, encephalopathy, and cognitive deficits involving concentration, sleep disturbances, and short-term memory may be seen (Armstrong & Cohen, 1999; Steere, 2001; Strickland, 2000). For the latter, a long-term follow-up in children indicated that those treated appropriately did not show long-term cognitive deficits (Adams, Rose, Eppes, & Klein, 1999). Carditis and heart block may occur a few weeks to months after infection (Armstrong & Cohen, 1999; Steere, 2001; Terkeltaub, 2000). Chronic inflammatory eye disease such as keratitis may be seen, and in Europe, chronic atrophic dermatitis may occur at the site of the bite (Steere, 2001; Terkeltaub, 2000). Persistent disease after treatment, also called chronic Lyme disease or post-Lyme syndrome, occurring after antibiotic therapy, has been described but is controversial, and some believe that the original diagnosis in these instances was in error (Strickland, 2000). Diagnosis is by serology, or by direct isolation if needed, and can be difficult (Dumler, 2001). Usually the history of the tick bite and symptoms suffice (Armstrong & Cohen, 1999). Detailed treatment protocols have been developed and disseminated for different situations (Steere, 2001; Wormser, Nadelman, Dattwyler, Dennis, Shapiro, Steere, et al., 2000).

It is important to treat Lyme disease early and completely. In a 10–20-year follow-up study, patients with Lyme disease who developed facial palsy who were not initially treated with antibiotics had more residual deficits even though these were mild (Kalish, Kaplan, Taylor, Jones-Woodward, Workman, & Steere, 2001). Practice guidelines recommend doxycycline, 100 mg twice daily, or amoxicillin, 500 mg three times daily for 14–21 days for early localized or disseminated Lyme disease. Doxycycline has the advantage of also being effective against human granulocytic ehrlichiosis, which is useful since persons may be coinfected (Wormser et al., 2000). Although it has been found that in a study by Nadelman, Nowakowski, Fish, Falco, Freeman, McKenna, et al. (2001), a single dose of doxycycline was 87% effective in preventing Lyme disease within 72 hours after a bite from the *I. scapularis* tick, this prophylaxis is not a universal recommendation (Shapiro, 2001). A vaccine has now been developed against Lyme disease (LYMErix, SmithKline Beecham) and is recommended for those 15–70 years old who live in endemic areas, although those who are at risk due to occupation such as loggers are also candidates. Although it is being widely advertised, the long-term safety is not known ("Lyme disease vaccine," 1999). It appears only cost-effective for those who have a seasonal probability of infection of greater than 1% (Shadick, Liang, Phillips, Fossel, & Kuntz, 2001). Persons who are vaccinated still need to use personal protective measures (Rahn, 2001). Persons with Lyme disease may be coinfected with ehrlichiosis or babesiosis.

EHRLICHIOSIS

In 1986, human ehrlichial infections in North America were first identified in Ft. Chaffee, Arkansas (McQuiston, Paddock, Holman, & Childs, 1999). The agent was subsequently named *Ehrlichia chaffeensis* and was found to cause human monocytic ehrlichosis (HME). In 1992 and 1993, an outbreak of ehrlichiosis in the Midwest was recognized but was realized to be due to an agent distinct from *Ehrlichia chaffeensis.* The agent was closely related to *Ehrlichia phagocytophila* and *Ehrlichia equi* becoming known as the HGE agent. The causative agent in this outbreak resulted in human granulocytic ehrlichiosis (HGE). Human monocytotropic ehrlichiosis (HME) and HGE are similar in many ways. Infection results from the bite of a tick infected with *Ehrlichia,* which it acquires from feeding on infected animal reservoirs (McQuiston et al., 1999; Parola & Raoult, 2001).

Ehrlichia are gram-negative bacteria in the family *Rickettsiaceae.* The species of the genus *Ehrlichia* known to be human rather than animal pathogens are relatively few at this time. These are (a) *E. chaffeensis* causing HME; (b) *E. sennetsu,* which has been known to cause an illness similar to mononucleosis in Japan and Malaysia and that was first reported upon in 1985; (c) *E. canis,* mainly affecting dogs but with reported human asymptomatic infection; (d) the agent causing HGE that is closely related to *Ehrlichia phagocytophila* and *Ehrlichia equi* (referred to subsequently as the HGE agent); and (e) *E. ewingii,* a known pathogen of dogs recently recognized as a human pathogen, that was first reported from Missouri in 1999 (Buller, Arens, Hmiel, Paddock, Sumner, Rikhisa, et al., 1999). The tick vector for *E. chaffeensis* is the Lone Star tick (*Amblyomma americanum*) and the white-tailed deer is the principal wildlife reservoir, although it has been suggested that wild canids such as coyotes and domestic dogs may hold a future potential for cross-species transmission (Kocan, Levesque, Whitworth, Murphy, Ewing, & Barker, 2000). The Lone Star tick also appears to be the vector for the more recently identified *E. ewingii*

(Buller et al., 1999). For the HGE agent, the *Ixodes scapularis* and *Ixodes pacificus* ticks appear to be insect vectors while white-tailed deer, mice and other small mammals are important reservoirs (Bakken & Dumler, 2000). HGE has been most frequently reported from northeastern and upper midwestern states especially Connecticut, Wisconsin, Minnesota, and New York, while HME has been most frequently reported from southeastern and southcentral states including Arkansas, North Carolina, Missouri, and Oklahoma (McQuiston et al., 1999).

HME usually presents after a tick bite. More than 1,500 cases have been diagnosed in the United States. Symptoms at onset include fever, headache, chills, myalgia, and malaise with nausea, anorexia, vomiting, diarrhea, and weight loss developing later. A maculopapular, petechial rash may develop in about 20%–30% of patients (Strickland, 2000). The case fatality rate is estimated as being as high as 5%, and complications can include acute renal failure, prolonged fever, meningoencephalitis, a toxic shock-like syndrome, respiratory insufficiency, and multiorgan failure (Dumler & Walker, 1999; McQuiston et al., 1999).

The clinical course for HGE is very similar to HME with the exception that rash is rarely present. The usual incubation period is 7–10 days after a tick bite. It typically presents as an undifferentiated acute febrile illness after a tick bite with signs and symptoms including headache, fever, myalgia, arthralgia, and malaise. Gastrointestinal symptoms such as nausea, diarrhea, and vomiting; respiratory symptoms such as cough; and central nervous system signs or symptoms such as stiff neck may occur in some patients. Thromobocytopenia, elevation of serum hepatic transaminases, anemia, and elevated creatinine and leukopenia can occur. Most patients recover completely within 2 months. There is a range of illness, however, and some individuals may have asymptomatic infection while others may develop severe illness including shock, seizures, pneumonitis, rhabdomyolysis, acute renal failure, hemorrhage, multiorgan failure, and death. Opportunistic infections may set in and be the cause of mortality (Bakken & Dumler, 2000; Dumler & Walker, 1999; Parola & Raoult, 2001). The case fatality rate may be as high as 10% (McQuiston et al., 1999). There has been less clinical experience with HGE than HME to date.

Both HME and HGE can have a range of severity from asymptomatic or mild illness through life-threatening illness and death. For both

HME and HGE, diagnosis is through serologic methods such as indirect immunofluorescence assays (IFA) and PCR assays for detection of specific rRNA gene targets and DNA. More rapid testing is anticipated in the near future (Comer, Nicholson, Sumner, Olson, & Childs, 1999). Early treatment with doxycyline is important in avoiding severe illness, although sometimes complications develop despite treatment. However, chronic illness similar to that following Lyme disease is not recognized (Bakken & Dumler, 2000; Parola & Raoult, 2001). Persons with ehrlichiosis may be coinfected with Lyme disease and/or babesiosis.

BABESIOSIS

Babesiosis is a zoonotic disease caused by protozoal parasites of the genus, *Babesia.* These organisms are sometimes known as piroplasms because of their pear-like shape (Homer, Aguilar-Delfin, Telford, Krause, & Persing, 2000). There are more than 100 species known. Among those affecting humans, *Babesia microti* is the major species found in the United States, especially in the eastern portion, while a newly recognized strain of *Babesia* called WA-1 was found on the west coast in 1991 and MO-1 was identified in Missouri in 1992 (Herwaldt, 2000; Mylonakis, 2001). In Europe, *Babesia bovis* and *B. divergens* are the species that are recognized to cause human disease (Gelfand & Callahan, 1998). In 1956, the first human case was recognized in a splenectomized man in Yugoslavia, followed by a 1966 report from California and a 1969 report from Nantucket, Massachusetts (Herwaldt, 2000; Skrabolo & Deanovic, 1957). Babesiosis may be an ancient disease. It has been suggested that the plague of Pharaoh's cattle known as murrain, referred to in Exodus 9:3 was actually babesiosis (Gelfand & Callahan, 1998). The most common geographic locations in the U.S. for babesiosis are the northeast—especially on the offshore islands of Connecticut, Rhode Island, Massachusetts—and New York and the upper midwest, especially Wisconsin (Herwaldt, 2000).

Babesiosis is transmitted from its usual animal reservoir to humans via a tick vector. In the eastern U.S., the usual tick vector is *Ixodes scapularis,* also called *I. dammini,* while in Europe, the hard-bodied cattle tick, *I. ricinus,* is the common vector. Human babesiosis has been described in the U.S. outside the range of the usual vector, and thus either the range may be expanding or a similar *Ixodes* tick may also be a vector. In the U.S., common hosts are the white-footed mouse (a major reservoir), the white-tailed deer, and other large and small mammals that include field mice, rats, chipmunks, and occasionally bats, certain birds, and lizards. Babesiosis may also be acquired via blood transfusion (Gelfand & Callahan, 1998; Mylonakis, 2001).

The incubation period for *Babesia* infection that is tick-borne ranges from 1 to several weeks and is shorter for those cases from blood transfusion. In Europe, most of the symptomatic cases have been in asplenic or immunocompromised persons; this is not the case in the U.S. *Babesia* invade the erythrocytes, launching a complicated cycle. Thus, laboratory findings commonly include hemolytic anemia signs. Signs and symptoms include fever, chills, sweating, malaise, weakness, headache, and myalgia, and may appear malaria-like. Also seen may be arthralgia, nausea, vomiting, anorexia, abdominal pain, depression, emotional lability, dark urine, and mild hepatosplenomegaly (Herwaldt, 2000; Homer et al., 2000). Complications can include myocardial infarction, pulmonary edema, adult respiratory distress syndrome, disseminated intravascular coagulation, renal failure, and death (Gelfand, & Callahan, 1998; Herwaldt, 2000). Diagnosis is by examination of blood smears, serology, and PCR analysis. Standard therapy has been a combination of clindamycin and quinine but frequently results in adverse reactions. A combination of atovaquone and azithromycin is being evaluated for effectiveness and appears to have fewer adverse reactions (Krause, Leopore, Sikand, Gadbaw, Burke, Telford, et al., 2000; Mylonakis, 2001). Sometimes exchange transfusion is done. For tick-borne cases, preventive measures to avoid tick bites is recommended as shown in Appendix C, Table C.4. Co-infection with Lyme disease is relatively common, so the practitioner should test for concurrent infection, especially if a rash is present (Herwaldt, 2000).

SUMMARY

These three diseases provide examples of how changes in human activities result in increased opportunities for exposure to emerging infectious disease agents. In a short 25 years, Lyme disease has progressed from a virtually unknown problem to a clinically significant endemic disease in parts of the northeastern United States. Preventive measures to prevent tick bites are considered in Appendix C, Table C.4.

REFERENCES

Adams, W. V., Rose, C. D., Eppes, S. C., & Klein, J. D. (1999). Long-term cognitive effects of Lyme disease in children. *Applied Neuropsychology, 6*, 39–45.

Armstrong, D., & Cohen, J. (Eds.). (1999). *Infectious diseases*. London: Mosby.

Bakken, J. S., & Dumler, J. S. (2000). Human granulocytic ehrlichiosis. *Clinical Infectious Diseases, 31*, 554–560.

Buller, R. S., Arens, M., Hmiel, S. P., Paddock, C. D., Sumner, J. W., Rikhisa, Y., et al. (1999). *Ehrlichia ewingii*, a newly recognized agent of human ehrlichiosis. *New England Journal of Medicine, 341*, 148–155.

Centers for Disease Control and Prevention. (2000). Surveillance for Lyme disease—United States, 1992–1998. *Morbidity and Mortality Weekly Report, 49*(No. SS-3), 1–11.

Centers for Disease Control and Prevention. (2001). Lyme disease—United States, 1999. *Morbidity and Mortality Weekly Report, 50*, 181–185.

Comer, J. A., Nicholson, W. L., Sumner, J. W., Olson, J. G., & Childs, J. E. (1999). Diagnosis of human ehrlichiosis by PCR assay of acute-phase serum. *Journal of Clinical Microbiology, 37*, 31–34.

Dumler, J. S. (2001). Molecular diagnosis of Lyme disease: Review and meta-analysis. *Molecular Diagnostics, 6*, 1–11.

Dumler, J. S., & Walker, D. H. (1999). Ehrlichiosis. In R. L. Guerrant, D. H. Walker, & P. F. Weller (Eds.), *Tropical infectious diseases* (pp. 598–604). Philadelphia: Churchill Livingstone.

Gelfand, J. A., & Callahan, M. V. (1998). Babesiosis. *Current Clinical Topics in Infectious Diseases, 18*, 201–216.

Grabenstein, J. D. (1999). Lyme disease: Geography predicts risk. *Journal of the American Pharmaceutical Association, 39*, 86–91.

Herwaldt, B. (2000). Babesiosis. In G. T. Strickland (Ed.), *Hunter's tropical medicine and emerging infectious diseases* (pp. 688–690). Philadelphia: WB Saunders Co.

Homer, M. J., Aguilar-Delfin, I., Telford, S. R., III, Krause, P. J., & Persing, D. H. (2000). Babesiosis. *Clinical and Microbiological Reviews, 13*, 451–469.

Kalish, R. A., Kaplan, R. F., Taylor, E., Jones-Woodward, L., Workman, K., & Steere, A. C. (2001). Evaluation of study patients with Lyme disease, 10–20-year follow-up. *Journal of Infectious Diseases, 183*, 453–460.

Kocan, A., Levesque, G. C., Whitworth, L. C., Murphy, G. L., Ewing, S. A., & Barker, R. W. (2000). Naturally occurring *Ehrlichia chaffeensis* infection in coyotes from Oklahoma. *Emerging Infectious Diseases, 6*, 477–480.

Krause, P. J., Lepore, J., Sikand, V. K., Gadbaw, J. J., Jr., Burke, G., Telford, S. R., et al. (2000). Atovaquone and azithromycin for the treatment of babesiosis. *New England Journal of Medicine, 343*, 1454–1458.

Lashley, F. R. (1998). *Clinical genetics in nursing practice* (2nd ed.). New York: Springer Publishing Co.

McQuiston, J. H., Paddock, C. D., Holman, R. C., & Childs, J. E. (1999). The human ehrlichioses in the United States. *Emerging Infectious Diseases, 5*, 635–642.

Nadelman, R. B., Nowakowski, J., Fish, D., Falco, R. C., Freeman, K., McKenna, D., et al. (2001). Prophylaxis with single-dose doxycycline for the prevention of Lyme disease after an *Ixodes scapularis* tick bite. *New England Journal of Medicine, 345*, 79–84.

Parola, P., & Raoult, D. (2001). Ticks and tickborne bacterial diseases in humans: An emerging infectious threat. *Clinical Infectious Diseases, 32*, 897–928.

Rahn, D. W. (2001). Lyme vaccine: Issues and controversies. *Infectious Disease Clinics of North America, 15*, 171–187.

Scrimenti, R. J. (1970). Erythema chronicum migrans. *Archives of Dermatology, 102*, 104–105.

Shadick, N. A., Liang, M. H., Phillips, C. B., Fossel, K., & Kuntz, K. M. (2001). The cost-effectiveness of vaccination against Lyme disease. *Archives of Internal Medicine, 161*, 554–561.

Shapiro, E. D. (2001). Doxycycline for tick bites—not for everyone. *New England Journal of Medicine, 345*, 133–134.

Shapiro, E. D., & Gerber, M. A. (2000). Lyme disease. *Clinical Infectious Diseases, 31*, 533–542.

Skrabolo, Z., & Deanovic, Z. (1957). Piroplasmosis in man. *Documenta de Medicina Geographica et Tropica, 9*, 11–16.

Steere, A. C. (2001). Lyme disease. *New England Journal of Medicine, 345*, 115–124.

Steere, A. C., Malawista, S. E., Snydman, D. R., & Andiman, W. A. (1976). A cluster of arthritis in children and adults in Lyme, Connecticut. *Arthritis and Rheumatism, 19*, 824.

Steere, A. C., Malawista, S. E., Snydman, D. R., Shope, R. E., Andiman, W. A., Ross, M. R., et al. (1977). Lyme arthritis: An epidemic of oligoarticular arthritis in children and adults in three Connecticut communities. *Arthritis and Rheumatism, 20*, 7–16.

Strickland, G. T. (Ed.). (2000). *Hunter's tropical medicine and emerging infectious diseases*. Philadelphia: WB Saunders Co.

Terkeltaub, R. A. (2000). Lyme disease 2000. Emerging zoonoses complicate patient work-up and treatment. *Geriatrics, 55*(7), 34–47.

Wormser, G. P., Nadelman, R. B., Dattwyler, R. J., Dennis, D. T., Shapiro, E. D., Steere, A. C., et al. (2000). Practice guidelines for the treatment of Lyme disease. *Clinical Infectious Diseases, 31*(Suppl. 1), S1–S14.

15

Malaria

Roslyn Sykes and Gladys Mabunda

On August 18th, 1999, an 11-year-old boy residing in Suffolk County, New York, was seen by his physician, with a 5-day history of fever, rigors, abdominal pain, arthralgias, and vomiting. Intracellular parasites consistent with *P. vivax* were noted on a complete blood count. The patient was admitted to a local hospital on August 21st with a temperature of 102.0° F (38.9° C), hepatosplenomegaly, and several healing maculopapular bite lesions. Initial laboratory examinations revealed leukopenia (white blood cell count: 2,800/ mm^3 [normal: 4,500–13,500/mm^3]), anemia (hemoglobin: 9.8 g/dL [normal: 11.5–15.5 g/dL]), and severe thrombocytopenia (platelet count: 21,000 mm^3 [normal: 150,000–400,000/mm^3]). Serology was negative for Lyme disease and babesiosis. Serum electrolytes and chest radiograph were normal. Urinalysis demonstrated a slightly elevated urobilinogen. Examination of peripheral thick and thin blood smears at the New York State Department of Health (NYSDH) and CDC confirmed *P. vivax* infection. The patient was treated with chloroquine phosphate, quinine, clindamycin, and primaquine and was discharged from the hospital on August 25th.

The patient's parents reported he had never traveled to a malarious area or had a history of a blood transfusion or organ transplantation. During August 1–7, the patient spent 1 week at a summer camp 20 miles from his hometown. He slept in a tent and went swimming in the camp pond. After his return home on August 7th, the patient attended another camp in Massachusetts for 2 days. This case is an example of locally acquired malaria in the United States (Centers for Disease Control and Prevention, 2000b, p. 495).

Malaria is a serious worldwide health problem with about 300–500 million cases reported per year, and about 2.7 million deaths per year mostly in sub-Saharan African children (Martens & Hall, 2000; Warhurst, 2001). It is endemic in nearly 100 countries with 41% of the world's population considered to be at risk (Martens & Hall, 2000). At one time, malaria was endemic in the United States (U.S.), but it was eradicated by the mid-20th century. The mosquito vectors are still present in the U.S. Today, each year there are about 1,000 cases of malaria reported in the U.S., most of which occur in immigrants, refugees, and travelers. The reemergence of malaria in the U.S. has attracted much attention from the public health community. Many causes contribute to the reemergence such as travel; population growth and movement including immigration; global warming; resistance to insecticides and antimalarial drugs; and disruptions from wars and natural disasters (Martens & Hall, 2000). Immigrants and migrants from malaria-endemic countries provide sources of the malarial parasite for feeding the mosquito vectors. Warm humid weather facilitates completion of the cycle, and the infected *Anopheles* mosquito can transmit the malarial parasite to a previously uninfected human. Thus, local transmission can, and does, occur (Taylor & Strickland, 2000). Airport malaria is discussed in chapter 22.

In the U.S. in the last decade, there have been reported cases of malaria in Georgia, Vermont, and Tennessee (Centers for Disease Control and Prevention, 1997a), Missouri and Pennsylvania (Centers for Disease Control and Prevention, 1999a), New York (McNeeley, Chu, Lowe, & Layton, 1998; Viani & Bromberg, 1999), Houston, Texas (Zucker, 1996), Minnesota (Adair & Nwaneri, 1999; Fritz & Hedemark, 1998), Illinois and Florida (Centers for Disease Control and Prevention, 1999b), and southwestern states (Barat, Barnett, Smolinski, Epsey, Levy, & Zucker, 1999). There are occasional diagnoses in infants with congenital infections (Ahmed, Cerilli, & Sanchez, 1998), in persons exposed to infected blood or blood products (Kachur, Reller, Barber, Barat, Koumans, Parise, et al., 1997), and in persons whose infection was acquired through local mosquito-borne transmission (Centers for Disease Control and Prevention, 2000b). In the U.S., most locally-acquired cases are *Plasmodium vivax*, which is usually milder. For imported cases, the most frequent species seen is *P. vivax*, followed closely by *P. falciparum*. Most imported cases in the U.S. were from Africa followed by India and Central America and the Caribbean. The U.S. states reporting the largest number of cases were

California, New York, Illinois, and Florida (Centers for Disease Control and Prevention, 1999b). A review of malaria in Europe over a 30-year span may be found in Sabatinelli, Ejov, and Joergensen (2001).

Malaria is caused by obligate intracellular protozoan parasites of the genus *Plasmodium*. There are over 100 species of *Plasmodium* known. Four species, *P. falciparum*, *P. vivax*, *P. ovale*, and *P. malariae* infect humans, although rarely some others do so. Their distribution varies. For example, *P. vivax* is rare in Africa because most native Africans do not have a specific receptor—the Fy6 Duffy blood group protein—which is necessary for the parasite to be able to enter the erythrocyte (Lashley, 1998; Rios & Blanco, 2000). *P. falciparum* is the most serious. The other *Plasmodium* species are usually not as life threatening except in the young, the old, and persons with a concurrent disease or immunodeficiency. The usual mode of transmission of the infecting parasite is through the bite of an infected female *Anopheles* mosquito, but in rare instances can result through the transfusion of blood, contaminated needles, or congenitally. The malaria parasite life cycle involves a mosquito and human host. It is usually transmitted between sunset and sunrise by the bite of an infected female *Anopheles* mosquito. In brief, the infective stage is the sporozoite in the mosquito's saliva. A large number of sporozoites enter through the human skin with each mosquito bite. Those that survive the body's initial defenses infect the liver cells (hepatocytes). In the liver they undergo asexual reproduction (exoerythrocytic shizogony/merogony), resulting in hepatic schizonts/meronts. As they mature, they release merozoites into the bloodstream. Merozoites infect red blood cells and undergo a second phase of asexual reproduction (erythrocytic schizogony). The infected red blood cells mature and rupture, releasing still more merozoites into the bloodstream and starting another cycle of asexual development and multiplication. The multiplication of the blood stage parasites is responsible for the clinical features of malaria.

In the blood, some merozoites differentiate into sexual forms called gametocytes. Both male and female gametocytes circulate without causing symptoms and can be ingested by a mosquito at the next blood meal. Sexual reproduction occurs within the mosquito. The gametocytes, after ingestion by an *Anopheles* mosquito during a blood meal, undergo a sporogonic cycle yielding sporozoites. The life cycle starts again when the infective mosquito bites another human. Some variations occur depending on the specific species of *Plasmodium*. *P. vivax* and *P. ovale* can produce a dormant form (hypnozoites) that can stay in the liver for 3 or 4 years, causing periodic relapses. While *P. falciparum* and *P. malariae* do not form hypnozoites, infection can result in residual undetectable levels after resolution of symptoms. This very low-level parasitemia can result in recurrence of clinical disease.

A few individuals will experience a predromal stage consisting of malaise, anorexia, myalgia, fever, and headache 2 to 3 days before an acute paroxysm begins. Manifestations typically include fever, chills, dizziness, malaise, tachycardia, fatigue, backache, and myalgia, often called "total body pain" (Taylor & Strickland, 2000, p. 625). Some have a prominence of gastrointestinal symptoms such as anorexia, nausea, vomiting, abdominal pain, and diarrhea, while others may have dyspnea and a nonproductive cough. The symptoms of malarial illness can be rather nonspecific and the diagnosis can be missed if health providers are not alert to the possibility of the disease. Additional clinical features may include enlarged liver and spleen, anemia, thrombocytopenia, pulmonary or renal dysfunction, jaundice, hyponatremia, and neurologic involvement. Clinical presentation depends on the infecting species, the level of parasitemia, and the immune status of the patient. In primary cases, paroxysms beginning with chills, and then sweating and feelings of warmth with headache, malaise, and myalgia may occur that can last for 9–10 hours and occur with a periodicity dependent on the length of the life cycle of the infecting species. *P. vivax* and *P. falciparum* have a tertian periodicity (every 48 hours) while *P. malariae* has a quartan periodicity associated with schizonts rupturing at 72-hour intervals. These usually begin in the afternoon (Taylor & Strickland, 2000). *P. falciparum* is the most severe species, and if untreated may result in death in up to 25% of the nonimmune adults experiencing a primary attack. Untreated *P. falciparum* can progress to coma, renal failure, pulmonary edema, and death. Asymptomatic parasitemia can occur among persons who have been long-term residents of malarious areas. Persons can be co-infected by more than one *Plasmodium* species. Malaria due to *P. malariae* tends to be the mildest and most chronic. This parasite tends to invade older erythrocytes with lower parasitemia, and less severe anemia. It may recur following a stressful event such as surgery, even 30–50 years after initial infection (Taylor & Strickland, 2000). Pregnant women are particularly vulnerable to malaria and relapses are seen in those who have been previously infected. Epidemic malaria can result in fetal loss and neonatal death, and in endemic areas can result in low birth weight and contribute to the effects of anemia in pregnancy. Falciparum malaria in pregnant women can result in hypoglycemia and renal insufficiency. Susceptibility is greatest in the second and third trimester as well as post-partum (Diagne, Rogier, Sokhna, Tall, Fontenille, Roussilhon, et al., 2000; Taylor & Strickland, 2000). Major complications tend to occur in nonimmune persons with *P. falciparum* infections. These may include cerebral malaria, with altered consciousness; adult respiratory distress syndrome; pulmonary edema; acute renal failure; severe anemia; acidemia; spontaneous bleeding or disseminated intravascular coagulation; convulsions; and/or hypoglycemia. In endemic areas repeated attacks can lead to chronic conditions such as hyperactive malarial splenomegaly and nephrotic syndrome, the latter often due to *P. malariae* (Taylor & Strickland, 2000).

It is important to remember that periodic fever is uncommon in imported malaria (malaria acquired outside a specific area, e.g., the United States). It is also important to always obtain a travel history of persons presenting with a fever. Failure to obtain a travel history may delay diagnosis and treatment. This error results in 40% of deaths due to *P. falciparum* in travelers from the United States. Malaria is the great imitator and should be ruled out in all cases with history of travel or immigration from endemic areas (Viani & Bromberg, 1999).

The first step toward diagnosis of malaria is to consider malaria in the differential diagnosis. Laboratory confirmation of the infection is made by microscopic identification of an active infection. Molecular diagnosis techniques can complement microscopy, especially in species identification. Antibody detection can detect past infections and immunologic/biochemical detection of malaria parasite products are available and under evaluation. Microscopic examinations of the parasite in thick and thin film of peripheral blood (Giemsa-stained smears) are common. It is recommended that both films be used (Centers for Disease Control and Prevention, 2001c). The thin film smears are useful for species identification of parasites already detected in the thick smears and rapid screening while the thick smear is drying. The thick film lyses erythrocytes and is useful for screening for parasites and for detecting mixed infections. New technology for diagnosing malaria is based on an antigen-capture dipstick methodology using a monoclonal antibody to *P. falciparum* histidine-rich protein-2 (van Agtmael, Eggelte, & van Boxtel, 1999). Dipsticks have the potential of enhancing speed and accuracy of the diagnosis (Jelinek, Grobusch, Schwenke, Steidl, von Sonnenburg, Nothdurft, et al., 1999). Other diagnostic tests are available and have varying degrees of application depending on geographic area. These include the Kawamoto technique using fluorescent dyes to detect blood parasites and the polymerase chain reaction test which detects the malarial parasites directly, irrespective of the immunocompetence and previous history of the patient (Iqbal, Sher, Hira, & Al-Owaish, 1999).

Treatment varies according to the infecting species, the geographic area where the infection was acquired (known resistance), drug sensitivity, economic constraints, a patient's level of immunity, side effects, and the severity of the disease. Drug resistance is becoming problematic. Frequently used antimalarial drugs for chloroquine sensitive strains include chloroquine, and sulfadoxine-pyrimethamine (Fansidar). Resistant cases require quinine, doxycycline, mefloquine, primaquine and/or malarone. Artemisinin and proguanil may be used outside the U.S. Because of the increasing problem of drug resistance, it is recommended that the parasitologic response to treatment be followed, to confirm elimination of the parasites. For severe malaria, the drug of choice is quinine used intravenously, supplemented with tetracycline, clindamycin, or Fansidar when the patient recovers. Where there is multidrug resistance, oral quinine may also be combined with an antibiotic (Centers for Disease Control and Prevention, 2000a; Newton & White, 1999). Newer agents for treatment include triclosan (Surolia & Surolia, 2001).

Prevention includes individual and population control methods. Five principles of malaria prevention should receive the attention of people who travel internationally:

- Get adequate pre-travel advice.
- Be aware of the risk in order to be able to recognize main symptoms.
- Avoid being bitten by mosquitoes (see Appendix C, Table C.5).
- Take appropriate chemoprophylaxis and adhere to the recommended doses and schedule of the selected drug for effective protection.
- Get early diagnosis and treatment (Viani & Bromberg, 1999). The recommended chemoprophylaxis is chloroquine in sensitive areas. Mefloquine, doxycycline, or malarone (a combination of atovaquone and proguanil) are the CDC-recommended options for malaria chemoprophylaxis in areas of chloroquine-resistant malaria (Centers for Disease Control and Prevention, 2001a).

Terminal prophylaxis with primaquine may also be used (Viani & Bromberg, 1999; World Health Organization, 2000).

Chemoprophylaxis is usually begun 1 week before travel and discontinued 4 weeks after the last exposure or after returning from travel to areas where *P. vivax* or *P. ovale* is prevalent. Primaquine should be given after exposure to prevent relapses. It is important to note that chemoprophylaxis may not be 100% efficacious. The type of chemoprophylactic regimen prescribed will depend on the itinerary of the travelers, the length of a stay, the risk of exposure, the age of the traveler, whether the traveler is pregnant, any history of allergies or hypersensitivities, and current medications being taken. Doxycycline is the best alternative to mefloquine. It is the drug of choice for those who plan to travel to areas with a high incidence of mefloquine resistance. Doxycycline has a short half-life, so it requires a high degree of compliance. Travelers must understand that even one missed dose may compromise the drug's efficacy. Chloroquine is reserved for those travelers who cannot take mefloquine or doxycycline or for those who travel to regions with no known chloroquine resistance. The antimalarial drug Fansidar should be carried for self-medication if medical care is not immediately available (Bloland, Neafie, & Marty, 1998).

Population-based methods of prevention include measures to prevent or reduce mosquito breeding by eliminating collections of water, by destroying mosquito larvae and adult mosquitoes, vaccine development, public education, and mass prophylactic campaigns (Taylor & Strickland, 2000). Biological control measures are used as well including manipulation of mosquito genomes so they cannot serve as vectors (Phillips, 2001).

The malaria situation is getting worse in many areas of the world, and prevention and treatment of malaria are becoming more difficult because of the increasing resistance of the *P. falciparum* to antimalarial drugs. Small increases in global warming in temperate and subtropical climates can markedly increase the future number of malaria cases (Phillips, 2001). A specific mutation in resistant strains may allow for better surveillance in the future (Djimdé, Doumbo, Cortese, Kayentao, Doumbo, Diourté, et al., 2001). Poor adherence to prophylactic regimens, however, remains the major reason behind travelers acquiring malaria. On a positive note, the World Health Organization initiative,

Roll Back Malaria, is focusing new attention on this significant global health problem (Kombe & Darrow, 2001).

REFERENCES

Adair, R., & Nwaneri, O. (1999). Communicable disease in African immigrants in Minneapolis. *Archives of Internal Medicine, 159*, 83–85.

Ahmed, A., Cerilli, A., & Sanchez, P. (1998). Congenital malaria in a preterm neonate: Case report and review of the literature. *American Journal of Perinatology, 15*(1), 19–22.

Barat, L., Barnett, B., Smolinski, M., Espey, D., Levy, C., & Zucker, J. (1999). Evaluation of malaria surveillance using retrospective, laboratory-based active case detection in four southwestern states. *American Journal of Tropical Medicine & Hygiene, 60*, 910–914.

Bloland, P. B., Neafie, R. C., & Marty, A. M. (1998). Malaria: A reemerging disease. In A. M. Nelson & C. R. Horsburgh, Jr. (Eds.), *Pathology of emerging infections 2* (pp. 283–316). Washington, DC: American Society for Microbiology Press.

Centers for Disease Control and Prevention. (1997a). Malaria in an immigrant and travelers: Georgia, Vermont, and Tennessee, 1996. *Morbidity & Mortality Weekly Report, 46*, 536–539.

Centers for Disease Control and Prevention. (1999a). Transfusion-transmitted malaria—Missouri and Pennsylvania, 1996–1998. *Morbidity and Mortality Weekly Report, 48*, 253–256.

Centers for Disease Control and Prevention. (1999b). Malaria surveillance—United States, 1995. *Morbidity and Mortality Weekly Report, 48*(SS-1), 1–23.

Centers for Disease Control and Prevention. (2000a). Notice to readers: Availability and use of parenteral quinidine gluconate for severe or complicated malaria. *Morbidity and Mortality Weekly Report, 49*, 1138–1140.

Centers for Disease Control and Prevention. (2000b). Probable locally acquired mosquito-transmitted Plasmodium *vivax* infection—Suffolk county, New York, 1999. *Morbidity and Mortality Weekly Report, 49*, 495–498.

Centers for Disease Control and Prevention. (2001a). Malaria deaths following inappropriate malaria chemoprophylaxis—United States, 2001. *Morbidity and Mortality Weekly Report, 50*, 597–599.

Centers for Disease Control and Prevention. (2001b). Malaria surveillance–United States, 1997. *Morbidity and Mortality Weekly Report, 50*, 597–599.

Centers for Disease Control and Prevention. (2001c). Microscopic procedures for diagnosing malaria. *Morbidity and Mortality Weekly Report, 50,(SS-05)*, 19–20.

Diagne, N., Rogier, C., Sokhna, C., Tall, A., Fontenille, D., Roussilhon, C., et al. (2000). Increased susceptibility to malaria during the early postpartum period. *New England Journal of Medicine, 343*, 598–603.

Djimdé, A. D., Doumbo, O. K., Cortese, J. F., Kayentao, K., Doumbo, S., Diourté, Y., et al. (2001). A molecular marker for chloroquine-resistant falciparum malaria. *New England Journal of Medicine, 344*, 257–263.

Fritz, M., & Hedemark, L. (1998). Somali refugee health screening in Hennepin County. *Minnesota Medicine, 81*(4), 43–47.

Iqbal, J., Sher, A., Hira, P. R., & Al-Owaish, R. (1999). Comparison of the OptiMAL test with PCR for diagnosis of malaria in immigrants. *Journal of Clinical Microbiology, 37*, 3644–3646.

Jelinek, T., Grobusch, M. P., Schwenke, S., Steidl, S., von Sonnenburg, F., Nothdurft, H. D., Klein, E., & Loscher, T. (1999). Sensitivity and specificity of dipstick tests for rapid diagnosis of malaria in nonimmune travelers. *Journal of Clinical Microbiology, 37*, 721–723.

Kachur, S., Reller, M., Barber, A., Barat, L., Koumans, E., Parise, M., et al. (1997). Malaria surveillance—United States, 1994. *Morbidity & Mortality Weekly Report, 46*(SS-5), 1–16.

Kombe, G. C., & Darrow, D. M. (2001). Revisiting emerging infectious diseases: The unfinished agenda. *Journal of Community Health, 26*, 113–122.

Lashley, F. R. (1998). *Clinical genetics in nursing practice* (2nd ed.). New York: Springer Publishing Co.

Martens, P., & Hall, L. (2000). Malaria on the move: Human population movement and malaria transmission. *Emerging Infectious Diseases, 6*, 103–109.

McNeeley, D., Chu, A., Lowe, S., & Layton, M. (1998). Malaria surveillance in New York City: 1991–1996. *International Journal of Infectious Diseases, 2*, 132–136.

Newton, P., & White, N. (1999). Malaria: New developments in treatment and prevention. *Annual Review of Medicine, 50*, 179–192.

Phillips, R. S. (2001). Current status of malaria and potential for control. *Clinical Microbiology Reviews, 14*, 208–226.

Rios, M., & Bianco, C. (2000). The role of blood group antigens in infectious diseases. *Seminars in Hematology, 37*, 177–185.

Sabatinelli, G., Ejov, M., & Joergensen, P. (2001). Malaria in the WHO European Region. *Eurosurveillance, 6*, 61–65.

Surolia, N., & Surolia, A. (2001). Triclosan offers protection against blood stages of malaria by inhibiting enoyl-ACP reductase of *Plasmodium falciparum*. *Nature Medicine, 7*, 167–173.

Taylor, T. E., & Strickland, G. T. (2000). Malaria. In G. T. Strickland (Ed.), *Hunter's tropical medicine and emerging infectious diseases* (8th ed., pp. 614–643). Philadelphia: WB Saunders Co.

van Agtmael, M., Eggelte, T., & van Boxtel, C. S. (1999). Artemisinin drugs in the treatment of malaria: From medicinal herb to registered medication. *Trends in Pharmacological Sciences, 20*(5), 199–205.

Viani, R., & Bromberg, K. (1999). Pediatric imported malaria in New York: Delayed diagnosis. *Clinical Pediatrics, 38*, 333–337.

Warhurst, D. C. (2001). A molecular marker for chloroquine-resistant falciparum malaria. *New England Journal of Medicine, 344*, 299–302.

World Health Organization. (2000). *Malaria: Protective measures against malaria* [On-line]. Available: www.who/int/ith/english/protect

Zucker, J. (1996). Changing patterns of autochthonous malaria transmission in the United States: A review of recent outbreaks. *Emerging Infectious Diseases, 2*, 37–43.

16

Multidrug-Resistant Tuberculosis

Neil W. Schluger

M. T., a 45-year-old man, presented to the chest clinic complaining of fever, cough, and a 15-pound weight loss. The patient, a recent immigrant from the former Soviet Union, had a history of tuberculosis (TB), for which he had been treated several years ago. He was unsure of his treatment while in the Soviet Union, but he stated that his medications were changed frequently. After being released he took his medications sporadically, as he could not afford all the drugs that were prescribed for him. Since entering the United States he had had no medical care. On examination the patient was a thin male with rhonchi over the upper left lung field. A chest radiograph showed a cavitary infiltrate in the left upper lobe, and a sputum sample contained numerous acid-fast bacilli. He was started on a regimen of six antituberculous medications, including isoniazid, rifampin, pyrazinamide, ethambutol, streptomycin, and levofloxacin, all of which were administered by directly observed therapy (DOT). A sputum culture was positive for *Mycobacterium tuberculosis* 2 weeks after beginning therapy.

Two months after beginning treatment, the mycobacteriology laboratory reported that the patient's isolate was resistant to rifampin and isoniazid. These drugs were discontinued, and the patient was treated with the remaining drugs. Streptomycin injections were discontinued after 9 months, and the patient received ethambutol, pyrazinamide, and levofloxacin for a total of 18 months. He regained all the weight he had lost, and sputum cultures were negative for the last 15 months of his therapy. He continues to do well. This case illustrates many of the important principles involved in understanding the epidemiology, pathogenesis, diagnosis, and treatment of multidrug-resistant tuberculosis (MDR-TB), to be discussed further below.

Both tuberculous infection and tuberculosis are caused by the tubercle bacilli that include *Mycobacterium tuberculosis, M. africanum, M. bovis,* and *M. microti. M. tuberculosis* is the most common and most important in the United States. *M. tuberculosis* is a nonmotile, non-spore-forming rod-shaped bacillus that has no capsule and does not produce toxin. It is known as acid fast because of its staining characteristics. It can survive for long periods under adverse conditions. Like other microbes, it can mutate, affecting characteristics such as drug sensitivity (Cohen & Durham, 1995), the focus of this chapter. *M. tuberculosis* can cause pulmonary or extrapulmonary TB. Common symptoms of pulmonary TB include cough (usually productive), fatigue or malaise, anorexia, weight loss, low-grade fever, sweating and/or chills at night, and dull, aching chest pain or tightness (Schluger & Rom, 1994). Extrapulmonary TB may include systemic symptoms and those related to the affected organ system (Cohen & Durham, 1995). For detailed treatment regimens see Small and Fujiwara (2001).

Tuberculosis remains the leading cause of death due to infection in the world today among persons older than 5 years of age. The global burden of disease due to *M. tuberculosis* is staggering. The World Health Organization estimates that roughly one third of the world's population, or some 2 billion people, are infected with *M. tuberculosis* (Dye, Scheele, Dolin, Pathania, & Raviglione, 1999). Of these, between 8 and 12 million people will actually develop active disease each year (new, or incident, cases). At any given time there are approximately 16 million total prevalent cases in the world, and 2–3 million people die each year of tuberculosis around the world. The vast majority (95%) of both cases and deaths due to tuberculosis occur in resource-poor countries, with most cases found in sub-Saharan Africa, south and southeast Asia, and parts of South America. In some of these regions, the annual case rate exceeds 300 cases per 100,000 population annually. By contrast, in the United States, the case rate for tuberculosis in 1999 was a historic low of 6.4 cases per 100,000 population (Centers for Disease Control and Prevention, 2000).

Drug-resistant tuberculosis was first noted after the introduction of streptomycin as the first useful antibiotic with activity against *M.*

tuberculosis. When used as a single agent, as was the case in the early clinical trials of the drug, initial exhilaration over treatment success was soon tempered with the realization that most patients taking the single agent soon failed therapy or relapsed with organisms resistant to streptomycin (Fox, Ellard, & Mitchison, 1999). This problem was alleviated by the coadministration of isoniazid and streptomycin together, although soon after the introduction of isoniazid in the early 1950s, resistance to this drug was noted as well.

The truly modern era of chemotherapy for tuberculosis began in the 1970s with the introduction of rifampin, which allowed the shortening of chemotherapy regimens to 9 and eventually 6 months (Schluger, Harkin, & Rom, 1996). The addition of rifampin simplified treatment programs greatly, although resistance to rifampin was noted in a few regions around the world, notably in a report in the mid-1980s from the Philippines. However, since culture and drug susceptibility testing for *M. tuberculosis* was and is not routinely performed in many parts of the world because of the substantial expense involved, true and systematic estimates of the prevalence of MDR-TB (now generally defined as cases of tuberculosis that are resistant to at least both isoniazid and rifampin), was not known.

Renewed attention to and concern about MDR-TB arose again in the early 1990s when a sharp rise in multidrug-resistant tuberculosis cases was noted in New York City and Florida (Centers for Disease Control, 1990, 1991; Centers for Disease Control and Prevention, 1993). This rise accompanied an overall increase in tuberculosis cases that was caused by a dismantling of the city's public health infrastructure; a deterioration in the living conditions among the indigent, with increased use of homeless shelters and a larger percentage of persons incarcerated; and the AIDS epidemic, which facilitated rapid transmission of tuberculosis cases among extremely vulnerable populations. In addition, inadequate infection control procedures in hospitals and prisons, as well as poor prescribing practices of physicians caring for tuberculosis cases contributed greatly to the emergence of MDR-TB as a significant threat to public health in New York City (Frieden, Sterling, Pablos-Méndez, Kilburn, Cauthen, & Dooley, 1993). In 1992, New York City reported a total of 450 cases of MDR-TB out of a overall caseload of 3,811 persons with tuberculosis. In other words, 11.8% of all cases of tuberculosis in New York City in that year were due to MDR-TB. Remarkably, in 1999, the MDR-TB case burden in New York City had fallen to only 30 out of a total of 1,460, or only

2% of the total. The reasons behind this dramatic turnaround have been studied extensively and will be discussed later in this chapter.

Globally, little was known about the prevalence of drug-resistant tuberculosis until the World Health Organization (WHO) conducted the first global survey of 35 countries in 1994, and reported the results a few years later (Pablos-Mêndez, Raviglione, Laszlo, Binkin, Rieder, Bustreo, et al., 1998). The results of this survey sparked great concern in the global public health community. No region was found to be without multidrug-resistant tuberculosis cases, and in some regions the incidence of MDR-TB was astoundingly high. Countries as diverse as the Dominican Republic, India, Latvia, Estonia, Russia, and Côte d'Ivoire had rates of MDR-TB that ranged from 7%–22% of total cases. As these countries have extremely high overall rates of tuberculosis (in the state of Delhi in India the tuberculosis case rate may be as high as 450 cases/100,000 population), the absolute numbers of MDR-TB patients in these nations are quite high. In prisons in parts of the former Soviet Union, the tuberculosis case rate may be as high as 4,000/100,000 population, and some reports indicate that MDR-TB cases constitute at least 20% of this total (Centers for Disease Control and Prevention, 1999; Kimerling, Kluge, Vezhnina, Iacovazzi, Demeulenaere, Portaels, et al., 1999; Viljanen, Vyshnevsky, Otten, Vyshnevskaya, Marjamaki, & Soini, 1998). An international working group has recommended enhanced surveillance including reports of drug susceptibility (World Health Organization, 2001).

An update of the WHO's report of the global burden of MDR-TB completed in 1999 indicated that in several regions of the world, the problem is getting worse, not better (World Health Organization, 2000). In Denmark and Germany, although the absolute numbers are small, MDR cases have increased by 50%. In Estonia, MDR-TB cases now account for 18% of the total tuberculosis burden. Other regions or countries where MDR-TB cases have continued to rise include China (Henan and Zhejiang), India (Tamil Nadu), Iran, Mozambique, Russia (Tomsk), Israel, Italy, and Mexico (Baja California, Oaxaca, and Sinaloa). Because of the ease and frequency with which persons travel around the globe today, it is reasonable to expect that MDR-TB cases will continue to appear in every region of the world in the forseeable future (Schluger, 2000).

Compounding the gravity of the above situation is the fact that no new class of drugs has been developed since the introduction of rifamycins in the late 1960s and early 1970s. This situation is not likely to improve in the near future. From the perspective of pharmaceutical manufacturers, tuberculosis drug development is economically unattractive, as most of the cases occur in countries with little money available to buy new agents (Pecoul, Chirac, Trouiller, & Pinel, 1999). This acts as a powerful disincentive to development of new antibiotics for tuberculosis. This disincentive is reflected in the fact that at present there is no new class of antituberculosis drugs in a phase III trial anywhere in the world. If fundamentally new drugs are introduced, it will probably be at least 10 years hence.

Resistance to antimycobacterial drugs occurs naturally in any population of mycobacteria, although at different frequencies for different drugs. Resistance to isoniazid is found in approximately 1 in 10^6 organisms, which is the same frequency at which resistance to ethambutol occurs. On the other hand, resistance to rifampin is quite a bit less common, occurring spontaneously at a rate of about 1 in 10^8 organisms. These naturally occurring rates of resistance provide the basis for understanding the need for multidrug therapy of TB. If only a single drug were used (say, isoniazid) eventually, the 1 in 10^6 organisms with naturally occurring resistance would be selected for and would lead to a treatment failure or relapse due to isoniazid-resistant tuberculosis. On the other hand, if two drugs are used initially (say, isoniazid and rifampin), naturally occurring resistance to both would be present in only 1 in 10^{14} organisms, and the likelihood of selecting for one of these would be very, very low. Not only does the natural occurrence of drug resistance explain the need for multidrug chemotherapy at the outset of treatment, but it also underlies the most important rule for treating cases of suspected drug resistance, namely, never add a single drug to a failing regimen. Successful treatment of drug-susceptible TB is part of the prevention of MDR-TB (Espinal, Laszlo, Simonsen, Boulahbal, Kim, Reniero, et al., 2001).

In recent years, there has been substantial progress in the molecular understanding of the basis of antibiotic resistance in mycobacteria (Riska, Jacobs, & Alland, 2000). Resistance to isoniazid occurs as a result of mutations in genes that encode enzymes that normally convert INH to its active form (catalase), or genes that produce proteins that normally bind INH to form a complex that prevents cell wall synthesis (inhA). Rifampin normally works by binding to the b subunit of RNA polymerase, thus interfering with RNA synthesis. Mutations in the *rpoB* gene prevent the rifampin from binding, and RNA synthesis continues uninterrupted. Streptomycin interferes with ribosomal protein synthesis, and mutations in the ribosomal protein gene *rrs* prevent this from occurring. The fluoroquinolones work by inhibiting a group of enzymes called DNA gyrases. Although the elucidation of the molecular basis of mycobacterial drug resistance may target drug development and may lead to rapid molecular-based diagnostic techniques, at present the clinical application of this information is somewhat limited (Drobniewski, Watterson, Wilson, & Harris, 2000; McNerney, Kiepiela, Bishop, Nye, & Stoker, 2000; Piatek, Telenti, Murray, El-Hajj, Jacobs, Kramer, et al., 2000).

In practice, a patient develops MDR-TB in one of two ways. The patient is either infected initially with a drug-resistant strain of *M. tuberculosis* (so-called primary drug resistance), or he or she is initially infected with a drug-susceptible strain and only later does this strain become resistant (so-called secondary drug resistance). A high prevalence of primary drug-resistant cases may indicate failure of an infection control program or treatment program or both, so that vulnerable patients are exposed to infectious cases on an ongoing basis. On the other hand, a high prevalence of secondary drug resistance indicates a serious problem with either the prescribing practices of treating physicians (the wrong drugs are being used in an improper fashion) or in the adherence of patients to the medical regimen (patients take their medicine sporadically and erratically). Unfortunately, none of the circumstances leading to the development of secondary drug resistance are rare. Difficulties in adherence to tuberculosis treatment have been well-chronicled (Cohen, 1997), and a study from a leading referral center found that in the typical case of MDR-TB, treating physicians had made an average of nearly four management errors per patient (Mahmoudi & Iseman, 1993).

There is nothing in the clinical presentation of the patient that leads one to initially suspect MDR-TB. Signs, symptoms, and radiographic findings are all indistinguishable from drug-susceptible tuberculosis. Rather, the major clinical clue to the presence of drug resistance is in the patient's history (Telzak, Chirgwin, Nelson, Matts, Sepkowitz, Benson, et al., 1999). Drug resistance should be suspected in any patient with active tuberculosis who has a history of previously treated tuberculosis. In such cases, every effort must be made to obtain all the details of the patient's prior treatment. This includes not only all previous culture and drug susceptibility reports, but also records of the previous drug treatment regimen and the record of the patient's adherence to it. If a patient has relapsed after excellent adherence to a proper regimen, then in fact the development of drug resistance is extremely uncommon, and empiric therapy for drug resistance is not generally indicated. If on the other hand a patient develops relapse or treatment failure in the setting of poor adherence to the prescribed regimen, or the regimen turns out not to have been adequate based on the known drug susceptibility pattern, MDR-TB should be suspected. Other reasons to suspect MDR-TB are community rates for isoniazid resistance above 4%, patient is from a country with a high rate, a positive HIV status, and a high likelihood of exposure to nosocomial, prison, or community sources of MDR-TB (Telenti & Iseman, 2000).

When MDR-TB is suspected on clinical grounds, every effort should be made to obtain a relevant clinical specimen for culture and drug susceptibility testing. There will be a significant delay in treatment, however, if drugs are held until drug susceptibility results are obtained, so empiric therapy must be instituted. When beginning treatment for MDR-TB on clinical grounds, there is one rule that must always be obeyed: *never add a single agent to a failing (or failed) regimen.* One must assume that the patient is resistant to all previous drugs used, so that the regimen to be used should contain at least two, and preferably at least three, drugs that the patient has not received before.

The selection of drugs used in the treatment of MDR-TB depends obviously on the pattern of drug resistance present. Although it is clear that the outcome of treatment for MDR-TB is not as good as it is for drug-susceptible TB (which is essentially always curable), studies demonstrate that aggressive therapy is associated with a very high likelihood of cure (Goble, Iseman, Madsen, Waite, Ackerson, & Horsburgh, 1993; Park, Davis, Schluger, Cohen, & Rom, 1996; Salomon, Perlman, Friedmann, Buchstein, Kreiswirth, & Mildvan, 1995; Telenti & Iseman, 2000; Turett, Telzak, Torian, Blum, Alland, Weisfuse, et al., 1995). Specific treatment regimens for MDR-TB are beyond the scope of this chapter (see Horsburgh, Feldman, and Ridzon, 2000; Small & Fujiwara, 2001). As a general rule treatment of drug-resistant TB should only be attempted by persons with expertise in the field. In addition, treatment for MDR-TB can best be accomplished in the setting of a program of directly observed therapy (DOT), so that adherence to the therapeutic regimen can be assured (Horsburgh, 2000). Globally, WHO has established a Working Group for a DOTS-plus approach (Gupta, Kim, Espinal, Caudron, Pecoul, Farmer, et al., 2001).

The key drug in the treatment of tuberculosis is rifampin. If a patient has tuberculosis that is resistant to isoniazid and streptomycin, a regimen of rifampin, pyrazinamide, and ethambutol can be used for 6–9 months, and excellent results can generally be expected. In the relatively unusual setting of rifampin-monoresistant tuberculosis, seen primarily, for poorly understood reasons, in persons with HIV disease (Sandman, Schluger, Davidow, & Bonk, 1999), a 9-month regimen of isoniazid, streptomycin, and pyrazinamide has been reported (in the pre-AIDS era) to be associated with a relapse rate of 5%–6% (British Medical Research Council 1975, 1977). On the other hand, if neither rifampin nor isoniazid can be used, treatment regimens will always need to be prolonged to 18–24 months (Telenti & Iseman, 2000). In the case of isoniazid- and rifampin-resistant tuberculosis, the combination of an aminoglycoside such as streptomycin with a fluoroquinolone forms the cornerstone of the regimen. If these drugs can be used, particularly in combination with pyrazinamide, a good outcome can be expected. Patients in this circumstance will typically be treated with the aminoglycoside for the first 6–9 months of therapy, and the remaining drugs will be continued for a total of 18–24 months, depending on the extent of disease and response to treatment. If, on the other hand, the patient is resistant to isoniazid, rifampin, and all of the aminoglycosides (or the related drug capreomycin), the potential for a medical cure becomes less certain, and consideration of early surgical intervention to resect lung tissue at the site of disease should be given. Obviously, this can only be done if the disease is localized (Iseman, 1993; Telenti & Iseman, 2000).

MDR-TB represents one of the most worrisome infectious diseases to emerge in the last several years because of the magnitude of the problem, the potential for significant morbidity and mortality, and the lack of new drugs at present or on the horizon with which to treat these infections (Farmer, Bayona, Becerra, Furin, Henry, Hiatt, et al., 1998; Gupta et al., 2001). At present, careful prescribing and assurances of adherence to therapy are the best tools clinicians have to prevent the emergence and spread of MDR-TB.

REFERENCES

British Medical Research Council. (1975). Controlled trial of 6- and 9-month regimens of daily and intermittent streptomycin plus isoniazid plus pyrazinamide for pulmonary tuberculosis in Hong Kong. *Tubercle, 56,* 81–96.

British Medical Research Council. (1977). Controlled trial of 6-month and 9-month regimens of daily and intermittent streptomycin plus isoniazid plus pyrazinamide for pulmonary tuberculosis in Hong Kong. The results up to 30 months. *American Review of Respiratory Disease, 115*, 727–735.

Centers for Disease Control. (1990). Nosocomial transmission of multidrug-resistant tuberculosis to health-care workers and HIV-infected patients in an urban hospital—Florida. *Morbidity and Mortality Weekly Report, 39*, 718–722.

Centers for Disease Control. (1991). Nosocomial transmission of multidrug-resistant tuberculosis among HIV-infected persons—Florida and New York, 1998–1991. *Morbidity and Mortality Weekly Report, 40*, 585–591.

Centers for Disease Control and Prevention. (1993). Outbreak of multidrug-resistant tuberculosis at a hospital—New York City, 1991. *Morbidity and Mortality Weekly Report, 42*, 427–434.

Centers for Disease Control and Prevention. (1999). Primary multidrug-resistant tuberculosis—Ivanovo Oblast, Russia, 1999. *Morbidity and Mortality Weekly Report, 48*, 661–664.

Centers for Disease Control and Prevention. (2000). *Reported tuberculosis cases in the United States, 1999*. Atlanta: Centers for Disease Control and Prevention.

Cohen, F. L. (1997). Adherence to therapy in tuberculosis. In J. J. Fitzpatrick (Ed.), *Annual review of nursing research* (Vol. 15, pp. 153–184). New York: Springer Publishing Co.

Cohen, F. L., & Durham, J. D. (Eds.). (1995). *Tuberculosis: A sourcebook for nursing practice*. New York: Springer Publishing Co.

Drobniewski, F. A., Watterson, S. A., Wilson, S. M., & Harris, G. S. (2000). A clinical, microbiological and economic analysis of a national service for the rapid molecular diagnosis of tuberculosis and rifampicin resistance in *Mycobacterium tuberculosis*. *Journal of Medical Microbiology, 49*, 271–278.

Dye, C., Scheele, S., Dolin, P., Pathania, V., & Raviglione, M. C. (1999). Consensus statement. Global burden of tuberculosis: Estimated incidence, prevalence, and mortality by country. WHO Global Surveillance and Monitoring Project. *Journal of the American Medical Association, 282*, 677–686.

Espinal, M. A., Laszlo, A., Simonsen, L., Boulahbal, F., Kim, S. J., Reniero, A., et al. (2001). Global trends in resistance to antituberculosis drugs. *New England Journal of Medicine, 344*, 1294–1303.

Farmer, P., Bayona, J., Becerra, M., Furin, J., Henry, C., Hiatt, H., et al. (1998). The dilemma of MDR-TB in the global era. *International Journal of Tuberculosis and Lung Diseases, 2*, 869–876.

Fox, W., Ellard, G. A., & Mitchison, D. A. (1999). Studies on the treatment of tuberculosis undertaken by the British Medical Research Council tuberculosis units, 1946–1986, with relevant subsequent publications. *International Journal of Tuberculosis and Lung Diseases*, 3(10 Suppl. 2), S231–S279.

Frieden, T. R., Sterling, T., Pablos-Mêndez, A., Kilburn, J. O., Cauthen, G. M., & Dooley, S. W. (1993). The emergence of drug-resistant tuberculosis in New York City. *New England Journal of Medicine, 328*, 521–526.

Goble, M., Iseman, M. D., Madsen, L. A., Waite, D., Ackerson, L., & Horsburgh, C. R., Jr. (1993). Treatment of 171 patients with pulmonary tuberculosis resistant to isoniazid and rifampin. *New England Journal of Medicine, 328*, 527–532.

Gupta, R., Kim, J. Y., Espinal, M. A., Caudron, J-M, Pecoul, B., Farmer, P. E., et al. (2001). Responding to market failures in tuberculosis control. *Science, 293*, 1049–1051.

Horsburgh, C. R., Jr. (2000). The global problem of multidrug-resistant tuberculosis: The genie is out of the bottle. *Journal of the American Medical Association, 283*, 2575–2576.

Horsburgh, C. R., Jr., Feldman, S., & Ridzon, R. (2000). Practice guidelines for the treatment of tuberculosis. *Clinical Infectious Diseases, 31*, 633–639.

Iseman, M. D. (1993). Treatment of multidrug-resistant tuberculosis. *New England Journal of Medicine, 329*, 784–791.

Kimerling, M. E., Kluge, H., Vezhnina, N., Iacovazzi, T., Demeulenaere, T., Portaels, F., & Matthys, F. (1999). Inadequacy of the current WHO re-treatment regimen in a central Siberian prison: Treatment failure and MDR-TB. *International Journal of Tuberculosis and Lung Diseases, 3*, 451–453.

Mahmoudi, A., & Iseman, M. D. (1993). Pitfalls in the care of patients with tuberculosis. Common errors and their association with the acquisition of drug resistance. *Journal of the American Medical Association, 270*, 65–68.

McNerney, R., Kiepiela, P., Bishop, K. S., Nye, P. M., & Stoker, N. G. (2000). Rapid screening of *Mycobacterium tuberculosis* for susceptibility to rifampicin and streptomycin. *International Journal of Tuberculosis and Lung Diseases, 4*, 69–75.

Pablos-Mêndez, A., Raviglione, M. C., Laszlo, A., Binkin, N., Rieder, H. L., Bustreo, F., et al. (1998). Global surveillance for antituberculosis-drug resistance, 1994–1997. World Health Organization-International Union against Tuberculosis and Lung Disease Working Group on Anti-Tuberculosis Drug Resistance Surveillance. *New England Journal of Medicine, 338*, 1641–1649.

Park, M. M., Davis, A. L., Schluger, N. W., Cohen, H., & Rom, W. N. (1996). Outcome of MDR-TB patients, 1983–1993. Prolonged survival with appropriate therapy. *American Journal of Respiratory and Critical Care Medicine, 153*, 317–324.

Pecoul, B., Chirac, P., Trouiller, P., & Pinel, J. (1999). Access to essential drugs in poor countries: A lost battle? *Journal of the American Medical Association, 281*, 361–367.

Piatek, A. S., Telenti, A., Murray, M. R., El-Hajj, H., Jacobs, W. R., Jr., Kramer, F. R., et al. (2000). Genotypic analysis of *Mycobacterium tuberculosis* in two distinct populations using molecular beacons: Implications for rapid susceptibility testing. *Antimicrobial Agents and Chemotherapy, 44*, 103–110.

Riska, P. F., Jacobs, W. R., Jr., & Alland, D. (2000). Molecular determinants of drug resistance in tuberculosis. *International Journal of Tuberculosis and Lung Diseases, 4*(2 Suppl. 1), S4–S10.

Salomon, N., Perlman, D. C., Friedmann, P., Buchstein, S., Kreiswirth, B. N., & Mildvan, D. (1995). Predictors and outcome of multidrug-resistant tuberculosis. *Clinical Infectious Diseases, 21*, 1245–1252.

Sandman, L., Schluger, N. W., Davidow, A. L., & Bonk, S. (1999). Risk factors for rifampin-monoresistant tuberculosis: A case-control study. *American Journal of Respiratory and Critical Care Medicine, 159*, 468–472.

Schluger, N., Harkin, T., & Rom, W. (1996). Principles of therapy of tuberculosis. In W. N. Rom & S. Garay (Eds.), *Tuberculosis* (pp. 751–761). Boston: Little Brown.

Schluger, N. W., & Rom, W. N. (1994). Current approaches to the diagnosis of active pulmonary tuberculosis. *American Journal of Respiratory and Critical Care Medicine, 149*, 264–267.

Schluger, N. W. (2000). The impact of drug resistance on the global tuberculosis epidemic. *International Journal of Tuberculosis and Lung Diseases, 4*(2 Suppl. 1), S71–S75.

Small, P. M., & Fujiwara, K. I. (2001). Management of tuberculosis in the United States. *New England Journal of Medicine, 345*, 189–200.

Telenti, A., & Iseman, M. (2000). Drug-resistant tuberculosis: What do we do now? *Drugs, 59*, 171–179.

Telzak, E. E., Chirgwin, K. D., Nelson, E. T., Matts, J. P., Sepkowitz, K. A., Benson, C. A., et al. (1999). Predictors for multidrug-resistant tuberculosis among HIV-infected patients and response to specific drug regimens. Terry Beirn Community Programs for Clinical Research on AIDS (CPCRA) and the AIDS Clinical Trials Group (ACTG), National Institutes for Health. *International Journal of Tuberculosis and Lung Diseases, 3*, 337–343.

Turett, G. S., Telzak, E. E., Torian, L. V., Blum, S., Alland, D., Weisfuse, I., et al. (1995). Improved outcomes for patients with multidrug-resistant tuberculosis. *Clinical Infectious Diseases, 21*, 1238–1244.

Viljanen, M. K., Vyshnevsky, B. I., Otten, T. F., Vyshnevskaya, E., Marjamaki, M., Soini, H., et al. (1998). Survey of drug-resistant tuberculosis in northwestern Russia from 1984 through 1994. *European Journal of Clinical Microbiology and Infectious Disease, 17*, 177–183.

World Health Organization. (2000). *Global tuberculosis report 2000*. Geneva: World Health Organization.

World Health Organization. (2001). European recommendations on surveillance of antituberculosis drug resistance. *Weekly Epidemiological Record, 76*, 2–5.

17

Prion Diseases: Creutzfeldt-Jakob Disease and Other Transmissible Spongiform Encephalopathies

Noreen J. Mocsny and Felissa R. Lashley

Stephen, a 19-year-old English man, became the first officially acknowledged victim of what was then known popularly as "mad cow disease" or more technically, bovine spongiform encephalopathy (BSE). Like most people, Stephen ate beef, and he had visited his aunt's farm every year for 8 years, coming into contact with cows as well as drinking unpasteurized milk. However, no cases of mad cow disease had been reported in his aunt's herd. The first hints of illness came in 1994 when Stephen's college grades were worse than expected. He became depressed and dizzy, and his parents watched him deteriorate into a living nightmare of madness and hallucinations. As his condition grew worse, he lost coordination and balance until he could no longer walk, swallow, talk, or move, until finally dying in May of 1995 (Rampton & Stauber, 1997).

In March of 1996, the British government announced that 10 young Britons, whose average age was 27 years, were dead or dying of what looked like Creutzfeldt-Jakob disease (CJD), a fatal neurodegenerative disorder that usually affects older persons. Thus, the condition was named new variant CJD, now usually called variant CJD (vCJD). A link was made between eating beef from cows with BSE and developing vCJD. Altered prions were believed to be the agent responsible (Brown, Will, Bradley, Asher, & Detwiler, 2001).

PRIONS AND TRANSMISSIBLE SPONGIFORM ENCEPHALOPATHIES

Prions are usually defined as normally occurring proteins that are widely expressed in the body and are components of the neuronal cell membrane. They are transported along neurons (Lueck, McIlwaine, & Zeidler, 2000). Prusiner (2001) defines prions as infectious proteins. The prion protein gene, *PRNP*, has been located on chromosome 20 (Painter, 2000). The normal prion protein is known as PrP^{C} (C for cellular). When this particle is converted into an abnormal form or isoform, it is known as PrP^{SC} (SC for scrapie) or PrP^{Res} (Res for resistant) or PrP^{CJD} (for Creutzfeldt-Jakob disease) (Hope, 2000; Painter, 2000; Pruisner, 2001). In its abnormal form, it is resistant to proteinase K, an enzyme (Dormont, 1999), and PrP accumulates in neurons, eventually causing cell damage or death.The prion is highly resistant to disinfection and sterilization processes but strong chemicals such as sodium hydroxide or bleach render it biologically inactive. The recognition of prions, which are believed to be devoid of nucleic acids, caused considerable discussion and controversy in the scientific community but resulted ultimately in a Nobel prize in 1997 for Stanley B. Prusiner. He coined the term "prion"—which he originally referred to as the scrapie agent, discovered a new biological principle of infection, and published detailed work about the properties of prions beginning in 1977 (Prusiner, 1982). Polymorphisms or variations are noted in the human prion protein gene. Persons who are homozygous for either methionine or valine at codon 129 of the gene may be predisposed to developing sporadic or iatrogenic CJD while heterozygosity at that locus seems to have a protective effect, but this picture is still evolving. Other specific mutant allele patterns appear to be related to the clinical picture (Belay, 1999).

When the abnormal form of the prion comes into contact with the normal form, the previously normal form changes shape and becomes abnormal. How this change occurs is not yet known. Prion diseases then result from the accumulation of PrP^{SC}, which can have a variety of conformations, and according to Prusiner (2001), each conformation is associated with a specific disease. Prion diseases may be infectious (including iatrogenic), genetic or sporadic (Prusiner, 2001). There are still unknowns regarding transmission as well. Prions are considered to be the etiologic agents of a group of fatal neurodegenerative diseases known as the transmissible spongiform encephalopathies (TSEs), also called the prion diseases (Alter, 2000). These have in common brain changes resembling a "swiss cheese" look. Prion diseases or TSEs occur in both animals and humans. Scrapie in sheep, a TSE, had long been known and described and was believed for many years to be caused by a slow-acting virus before it was realized that abnormal prions were the etiologic agent. TSEs occur in many animal species. Besides the ones in nature, they have been identified in pets, and in captive animals of at least 17 species in zoos and in animal laboratories in the United Kingdom and in France (Blakeslee, 1999, March 30; Brown, Will, et al., 2001; Daszak, Cunningham, & Hyatt, 2000). The known animal and human prion diseases are shown in Tables 17.1 and 17.2, and selected ones are discussed in detail below.

Scrapie

Scrapie can be transmitted from ewe to lamb. Its name comes from affected animals trying to scrape or rub their fleece off their sides. Affected animals become wasted and ataxic. The incubation period for scrapie is about 3 years. Some scientists believe that the agent that causes scrapie crossed the species barrier to cows as BSE (Brown, 2001). In the United States, scrapie was identified in Vermont sheep, and two flocks were quarantined and then euthanized under a declaration of extraordinary emergency ("USDA removes quarantined," 2001).

Bovine Spongiform Encephalopathy

Bovine spongiform encephalopathy (BSE), commonly known as mad cow disease, was first formally identified in cattle in the United Kingdom (UK) in 1986 (Wells, Scott, Johnson, Gunning, Hancock, & Jeffrey, 1987). It resembled scrapie, a transmissible spongiform encephalopathy (TSE), affecting sheep in England for more than 200

TABLE 17.1 Human Transmissible Spongiform Encephalopathies

Creutzfeldt-Jakob disease: iatrogenic/ infectious, inherited, variant, sporadic	See text.
Fatal familial insomnia	Genetically determined. Inherited in an autosomal dominant manner. Associated with a mutation on codon 178 of the prion protein gene (*PRNP*) but requires the normal methionine codon at position 129 for expression. Appears between ages 40 to 60 years often between 45 and 51 years. Signs and symptoms include restlessness; marked reduction in sleep time; specific polysomnographic changes; alteration of autonomic functions such as hyperthermia, tachycardia, hypertension, ataxia, myoclonus, dysarthria, and endocrine disturbances. May also see decreased attention, hallucinations, confusion, and memory impairment. Progresses rapidly with death occurring at a mean of 13 months after presentation.
Gerstmann-Sträussler-Scheinker syndrome	First described in 1936. Genetically determined. Most have autosomal dominant inheritance. Much heterogeneity. Very rare—only about 2 dozen families known. Certain specific gene mutations appear associated with certain clinical features. Symptoms include progressive cerebellum degeneration with ataxia, dementia.
Sporadic fatal insomnia	Recently identified. Have normal *PRNP* but same symptoms as familial form.

Sources: Gambetti & Parchi (1999); Mastrianni, Nixon, Layzer, Telling, Han, DeArmond, et al. (1999); Tyler (1999).

TABLE 17.2 Transmissible Spongiform Encephalopathies in Animals

TSE	Hosts	Comments
Bovine spongiform encephalopathy	Cattle	See text. Signs and symptoms include kicking, abnormal gait, nervousness, and pelvic limb ataxia.
Chronic wasting disease of deer and elk	Wild deer, elk	Endemic in northeast Colorado and Wyoming. Estimated to affect 6%–15% of deer and 17% of elk in this area. Humans are warned to avoid contacting brain, spinal cord, eyes, spleen, or lymph nodes of any deer or elk they kill and use rubber gloves in cutting up carcasses. Found/reported in mid-1960s at Wildlife Research Station in Ft. Collins, Colorado, and in the wild in 1981. Present in game farms in South Dakota, Nebraska, Oklahoma, and Saskatchewan. Symptoms include excessive drooling, staggering, and weight loss.
Feline spongiform encephalopathy	Domestic cats, cheetahs, pumas, ocelots, tigers	Found to date in captive animals, beginning in 1990 with the domestic cat.
Scrapie	Sheep, goats	First prion strain to be identified. Enzootic in the United Kingdom. Recognized as a distinct disorder in 1738. Affected animals develop ataxia and scrape fleece off sides of body. Can be transmitted from ewe to lamb. The placenta can contaminate the environment. Many strains of agent known. Worldwide distribution. Relatively common.
Transmissible mink encephalopathy	Mink	Very rare. Occurs in mink farms in U.S.
Unnamed spongiform encephalopathy	A variety of ruminants such as eland, greater kudu, Arabian oryx, bison	So far only identified in captive populations beginning in 1986.

Sources: Blakeslee (1999, February 23); Blakeslee (2000); Enserink (2001); Ironside (1997); Lueck, McIlwain, & Zeidler (2000); Patterson & Painter (1999).

years. Until 1988, cattle, other ruminants, and other animals were fed a meat and bonemeal product as a supplement that was made from the rendered carcasses of livestock including sheep. Around 1980, the rendering process was changed in a way that may have allowed the etiologic agent to survive, contaminate the supplement, and thus infect cattle. Cattle carcasses were also recycled through the rendering plants, eventually causing a large-scale BSE epidemic in the UK. This accounting of BSE originating from scrapie in this way is not universally accepted, and another theory is that it arose from unrecognized endemic BSE (Brown, Will, et al., 2001). In experiments, brain homogenates from BSE-infected cattle were fed to goats who developed BSE, demonstrating that transmission from ingestion could occur (Foster, Hope, & Fraser, 1993). Beef might also be contaminated by contact with nervous system tissue during processing (Brown, Will, et al., 2001). Although other countries used rendering processes similar to the UK's around the same time, it is theorized that the proportion of sheep and the proportion of scrapie in the carcasses used in rendering in the UK was higher than in other countries or that a pathogenic mutation occurred in cattle (Brown, Will, et al., 2001). Imported cases in other countries have resulted from importation of either live animals or of food supplements. Nonimported cases of BSE have been described in Ireland, Portugal, Switzerland, France, Belgium, the Netherlands, Germany, Liechtenstein, Denmark, Luxembourg, and Japan (Brown, Will, et al., 2001).

In 1988, the UK took action that included making BSE a notifiable disease, conducting BSE surveillance with brain histologic examination, banning ruminant protein in ruminant feed, banning the export of UK cattle born before the July, 1988 feed ban, the compulsory slaughter of nearly 200,000 BSE infected cattle, and the destruction of milk from affected cattle. Countries in the European Union as well as the U.S. also took action in 1989 and 1990 by banning UK cattle importation. Other measures to prevent the spread of BSE are found in Brown, Will, and colleagues (2001). An economic impact not only on British beef but on related industries such as gelatin, and tallow for candles, was also felt with the various bans on export and import. Within weeks after the identification of BSE in the UK, concern was raised about the possibility of human infection, and in May 1990, a CJD Surveillance Unit was established in Scotland. Its activities were later extended to other countries in Europe (Brown, Will, et al., 2001). Ironically, at the same time, the British agriculture minister claimed that beef was "completely safe" and was on TV encouraging his 4-year-old daughter to bite into a hamburger ("Timeline: How the crisis unfolded," 2000). Consumer reaction has been intense, at times bordering on panic (Cowley, 2001; Daley, 2000). Various other recommendations related to trade and animal health have been developed through WHO and other worldwide agencies (World Health Organization, June 14, 2001).

Kuru

Among the Fore women of New Guinea (and rarely, men), ritualistic cannibalism was formerly practiced in what was described by Rhodes (1997) as "a mortuary feast of love." In this cultural tradition, when kin died, a ceremony was held that involved the cooking and eating of virtually the entire body during which women would share the feast with their children. Often those who were dying assigned certain body parts in advance of their death to specific relatives to eat after they died. By the early 1950s, kuru, a progressive, fatal, neurological disorder, came to Western attention. It is thought, but not known, that kuru may have originated as a sporadic case of CJD, and that cannibalism of an infected person facilitated its spread. None of the Fores born since the government mandated cessation of cannibalism have acquired the disease, but observation has indicated that the incubation period could be 25–30 years (Alter, 2000; Tyler, 1999). The Fore described kuru in three stages, translated to "walk-about yet" (still ambulatory), "sit down finish" (no longer able to walk), and "sleep finish" (stupor), the final phase (Rhodes, 1997). It occurred mainly in women and children, and was investigated by a team led by D. Carleton Gajdusek (Gajdusek & Zigas, 1957) who ultimately received a Nobel prize in 1976 for his work demonstrating that kuru was infectious. Persons with the *PRNP* methionine/methionine genotype are preferentially infected (Lee, Brown, Cervenáková, Garruto, Alpers, Gajdusek, et al., 2001).

Creutzfeldt-Jakob Disease

The so-called classical form of Creutzfeldt-Jakob disease (CJD) was first described in the 1920s independently by two German neurologists, Creutzfeldt and Jakob. The overall incidence is about 1 in 1 million per year. The mean age of onset is between 55 and 65 years, but has occurred in persons as young as 14 years and in a person 92 years of age (Lueck et al., 2000). CJD may occur sporadically, in a familial or inherited form, or through infectious/iatrogenic transmission (Prusiner, 2001). Approximately 85% of classic CJD cases are sporadic (Brandel, 1999). The World Health Organization (WHO) developed a revised subtype definition for CJD that is shown in Table 17.3. In sporadic CJD, neurodegeneration is rapidly progressive and signs and symptoms include dementia, behavioral changes, myoclonus, cerebellar ataxia, visual symptoms, delusions, speech abnormalities, and other signs. No cure is known. Pathology may include neuronal cell death with spongiform changes and vacuolation in the central nervous system, reactive astrocytosis and in some cases, amyloid plaques. Onset may be sudden or be insidious over weeks. Other forms and variations may occur, and it is postulated that the clinical picture might ultimately be related to varying prion strains or to varying prion gene mutations (Belay, 1999; Brandel, 1999; Murphy, 1999; Prusiner, 2001). In the familial form, onset is typically earlier with a longer duration, and there are at least 11 known mutations in the *PRNP* gene (Parker & Snyder, 1999).

Iatrogenic CJD is believed to account for only about 5% of all CJD cases. The implications of these cases, however, are frightening. Iatrogenic CJD cases have been documented to follow dura mater graft transplants in neurosurgery such as for aneurysm repair (over 80 reports, many from a single manufacturer, LYODURA), corneal transplants, liver transplants, the use of contaminated neurosurgical instruments or stereotactic depth electroencephalographic electrodes during surgery, and the administration of cadaveric human pituitary hormones. In the latter case, inadvertent CJD transmission occurred in some patients who received intramuscular injections of human growth hormone for treating short stature, and a few cases occurred in women treated for infertility using human pituitary gonadotrophin. There are over 100 reports of CJD via human pituitary hormone transmission (Lueck et al., 2000). The use of recombinant pituitary hormone therapy instead of pooled human tissue has largely eliminated this source of infection. Of great concern has been the possible transmission of CJD through blood or blood product transfusion. To date, no documented cases of CJD in humans acquired via transfusion of blood or blood products have been reported. CJD has been transmitted from humans to animals via blood, however, and blood can transmit scrapie between

TABLE 17.3 Revised WHO Definition of CJD Subtypes

Sporadic CJD

Definite

Diagnosed by standard neuropathological techniques *and/or* immunocytochemically and/or Western blot confirmed protease resistant PrP *and/or* presence of scrapie-associated fibrils

Probable

Progressive dementia and at least two out of the following four clinical features:

- myoclonus
- visual or cerebellar disturbance
- pyramidal/extrapyramidal dysfunction
- akinetic mutism

and

- A typical EEG during an illness of any duration *and/or* a positive 14-3-3 CSF assay and a clinical duration to death less than 2 years
- Routine investigations should not suggest an alternative diagnosis

Possible

Progressive dementia and at least two out of the following four clinical features:

- myoclonus
- visual or cerebellar disturbance
- pyramidal/extrapyramidal dysfunction
- akinetic mutism

and

- No EEG or atypical EEG and a duration less than 2 years

Iatrogenic CJD

Progressive cerebellar syndrome in a recipient of human cadaveric-derived pituitary hormone or sporadic CJD with a recognized exposure risk, e.g., antecedent neurosurgery with dura mater graft

Familial CJD

Definite or probable CJD plus definite or probable CJD in a first degree relative *and/or* neuropsychiatric disorder plus disease-specific PrP gene mutation

Source: World Health Organization (1998).

animals (Lueck et al., 2000). Prion diseases can be transmitted via stainless steel surgical instruments and infective prions have shown resistance to the usual sterilization procedures (Frosh, Joyce, & Johnson, 2001; Zobeley, Flechsig, Corrizio, Enari, & Weissman, 1999). Other reusable instruments such as angioplasty catheters have been scrutinized as potential vehicles for CJD transmission as have certain procedures involving lymphoid tissue such as appendectomy and tonsillectomy, and procedures such as electromyography (Barbeau, 1999). In Great Britain, by the end of 2001, disposable instruments will be used in all adenotonsillectomy procedures (Frosh et al., 2001).

Variant Creutzfeldt-Jakob Disease

In 1995, the CJD Surveillance Unit received notification about three cases of CJD. These patients were young (16, 19, and 29 years of age), and had amyloid plaques that were usually found in only 5%–10% of sporadic cases of CJD (Bateman, Hilton, Love, Zeidler, Beck, & Collinge, 1995; Britton, Al-Sarraj, Shaw, Campbell, & Collinge, 1995; Brown, Will, et al., 2001). By December, 1995, the unit had been informed of 10 suspected cases of CJD in persons under 50 years of age, some of whom were ultimately found to have sporadic or familial CJD. By early 1996, a distinct clinical syndrome was identified in 10 cases and led to the conclusion that a previously unrecognized variant of CJD was "probably due to exposure to BSE." This was named new variant and then variant CJD (vCJD) (Brown, Will, et al., 2001; Will, Ironside, Zeidler, Cousens, Estibeiro, Alperovitch, et al., 1996). Neurologists in the UK were contacted in an effort to try to identify additional cases. More cases continue to be reported. The connection with BSE is considered probable but not proven completely, however, evidence increasingly implicates the BSE agent in causation (Lasmézas, Fournier, Nouvel, Boe, Marcé, Lamoury, et al., 2001). For a review see Coulthart and Cashman (2001).

At the end of June 2001, 105 cases of vCJD had been reported worldwide, 101 from the UK, 3 from France, and 1 from Ireland (World Health Organization, June, 2001). In contrast to sporadic CJD, vCJD cases had an earlier age of onset, usually below 50 years of age, and tended to present with behavioral changes or psychiatric symptoms such as agitation, aggression, anxiety, depression, and poor concentration. The median duration of illness is about 14 months.

TABLE 17.4 New WHO vCJD Case Definition (17 May 2001)

I	A	Progressive neuropsychiatric disorder
	B	Duration of illness > 6 months
	C	Routine investigations do not suggest an alternative diagnosis
	D	No history of potential iatrogenic exposure
	E	No evidence of a familial form of TSE
II	A	Early psychiatric symptoms[a]
	B	Persistent painful sensory symptoms[b]
	C	Ataxia
	D	Myoclonus or chorea or dystonia
	E	Dementia
III	A	EEG does not show the typical appearance of sporadic CJD[c] (or no EEG performed)
	B	Bilateral pulvinar high signal on MRI
IV	A	Positive tonsil biopsy[d]

Definite vCJD:	I A and neuropathological confirmation of vCJD[e]
Probable vCJD:	I and 4/5 of II and III A and III B or I and IV A[d]
Possible vCJD:	I and 4/5 of II and III A

[a]Depression, anxiety, apathy, withdrawal, delusions.
[b]This includes both frank pain and/or dysaesthesia.
[c]Generalized triphasic periodic complexes at approximately one per second.
[d]Tonsil biopsy is not recommended routinely, nor in cases with EEG appearances typical of sporadic CJD, but may be useful in suspect cases in which the clinical features are compatible with vCJD and MRI does not show bilateral pulvinar high signal.
[e]Spongiform change and extensive PrP deposition with florid plaques, throughout the cerebrum and cerebellum.
TSE: Transmissible Spongiform Encephalopathies; EEG: Electroencephalogram; MRI: Magnetic Resonance Imaging.
Source: World Health Organization Communicable Disease Surveillance and Response (2001).

Overt neurological signs, usually appearing about 6 months after the onset of illness signal rapid progression, and cerebellar ataxia often appears first. This may be followed by cognitive impairment, involuntary movements, and incontinence of urine progressing to mutism, progressive immobility, and unresponsiveness. Delusions may accompany the neurologic signs (Belay, 1999; Brandel, 1999). A revised case definition for vCJD was released on May 17, 2001 by the World Health Organization and is found in Table 17.4. Neuropathologically, extensive "florid" amyloid plaques are seen in the brain with surrounding spongiform changes (Brown, Will, et al., 2001; Prusiner, 2001).

IMPLICATIONS

The outbreak of vCJD raises many questions and issues. Major concerns include what the magnitude of the outbreak will ultimately be—in other words, how many people will be affected; what the geographic distribution will be since as of 2001, about 99% of known cases are in the UK; and what will be the length of the incubation period. The knowledge that persons may be infected with abnormal prions and be clinically asymptomatic for long periods of time leads to questions about the potential transmission of vCJD by blood or blood product transfusion, or during medical/surgical procedures on such individuals who would not be recognized as bearers. These procedures would include endoscopies, vascular catheterizations, as well as surgical operations and blood and organ donation (Bonn, 2000; Brown, Will, et al., 2001). The question of direct person-to-person transmission appears unlikely but has not been resolved. Mathematical models using various assumptions regarding such parameters as the incubation period and infecting dose predict varying numbers of total cases in the outbreak ranging from 100 to hundreds of thousands (Brown, Will, et al., 2001). Since prions may concentrate in lymphoid tissue, prevalence studies of tonsils and appendices are underway in the UK, and these organs are proving useful in developing diagnostic tests by biopsy (Ironside, Hilton, Ghani, Johnston, Conyers, McCardle, et al., 2000). Screening tests are in development (Brown, Cervenáková, & Diringer, 2001; MacGregor, 2001). Various countries have issued recommendations excluding donors with certain characteristics and risks from donating blood. For example, initially in the U.S., potential donors who spent 6 months or more in the UK since 1980 were excluded from being donors (Gottlieb, 1999). In 2001, the FDA proposed more stringent blood-donation restrictions. The following would be indefinitely barred from donating blood. Donors who: (a) spent 3 or more months in the U.K. from 1980 through 1996; (b) spent 5 years in France from 1980–present; (c) were diagnosed with any form of CJD; (d) were at risk for CJD because of being a blood relative of someone with CJD or someone who used pituitary growth hormone, or had a dura mater graft; (e) were U.S. military personnel or civilian military employees and their dependents who resided at U.S. military bases in Northern Europe for 6 months or more from 1980 through 1990 or elsewhere in Europe from 1980 through 1996; (f) received whole blood from a person who lived cumulatively for 5 years or more in Europe from 1980 through present; (g) received a transfusion of blood or blood components in the U.K. between 1980 and the present; or (h) injected bovine insulin since 1980 unless the product was not manufactured after 1980 from cattle in the U.K. (Food and Drug Administration, 2001). The Pentagon originally proposed implementation of these restrictions for military personnel effective September 14, 2001. However, the terrorist attacks in New York City, Washington, DC, and Pennsylvania caused a delay to October 29th (U.S. Department of Defense, 2001). In the UK, all blood from UK donors is filtered to eliminate leukocytes since they have been implicated as carriers of infectivity. Prevention also extends to appropriate disinfection and sterilization processes, to revision of guidelines for transfusion of blood, and for modifications to surgical procedures such as appendectomies to minimize risk of transmission. In early 2001, it came to light that more than 1,500 Spaniards had apparently been treated with a drug made from the blood of multiple donors, one of whom died of vCJD, setting off anger at Britain over its "failure to control" BSE ("Exposure to CJD," 2001). Protection of health care workers and morticians from inadvertent infection has also been raised as an issue, and groups such as WHO have published guidelines available on the Internet (World Health Organization, 2000 [on-line: Available: http://www.who.int/emc/diseases/bse/index.html]).

Breaches in infection control in hospitals have come to light and posed ethical dilemmas. In one instance, in the UK, a baby was born to a mother by cesarean section. The mother had vCJD. The instruments were used on other such births with sterilization procedures that would not have killed prions, and there was a delay in notification of those families. The baby in the original case was found to have vCJD in February, 2000. In another instance, a Melbourne, Australia hospital notified nine neurosurgical patients that they might have been exposed to CJD. Surgical equipment used on an elderly person with CJD was used again with routine sterilization not adequate to destroy abnormal prions if present (Zinn, 2000).

SUMMARY

Many uncertainties exist about the most worrisome human prion disease—vCJD. The concept of a conformationally altered protein causing transmissible disease is a relatively recent one. Attention brought to the BSE epidemic and the connection to the development of vCJD in humans has been intense. Social, economic, and political consequences and consumer reactions, sometimes bordering on hysteria, have occurred as detailed previously and reviewed recently in the popular press by Cowley (2001). Because the incubation period is long, a test for detection of infection with abnormal prions before symptoms appear would be very desirable. Preliminary results of a technique called protein misfolding cyclic amplification might lead for a test for early diagnosis (Orellana, 2001). To date, definitive diagnosis of vCJD is usually made through pathological examination of the brain, although altered prions can now be detected through pathological study of lymphoid tissue such as the tonsils. Rational policies for preventing infection by blood transfusion and other means are being developed. A rapid diagnostic test and successful treatment approaches are needed. While in the U.S., officials state that no one has contracted vCJD from eating U.S. beef, concern is escalating (Cowley, 2001). As of November 2001, the number of CJD cases in the UK was 111 (Department of Health, 2001), with a few reported outside. The true prevalence of this disorder remains unknown at this time as does certainty about how the altered prions are transmitted to humans. Further information about CJD statistics can be found on-line at http://www.cjd.ed.ac.uk, the website for the UK CJD Surveillance Unit. Other informational Web sites are in Appendix D.

REFERENCES

Alter, M. (2000). How is Creutzfeldt-Jakob disease acquired? *Neuroepidemiology, 19*, 55–61.

Barbeau, G. R. (1999). Reuse of coronary catheters: Old questions, new environment. *American Heart Journal, 137*, 1010–1011.

Bateman, D., Hilton, D., Love, S., Zeidler, M., Beck, J., & Collinge, J. (1995). Sporadic Creutzfeldt-Jakob disease in an 18-year-old in the UK. *Lancet, 346*, 1155–1156.

Belay, E. D. (1999). Transmissible spongiform encephalopathies in humans. *Annual Review of Microbiology, 53*, 283–314.

Blakeslee, S. (1999, February 23). Weighing 'mad cow' risks in American deer and elk. *New York Times* [On-line]. Available: http://www.nytimes.com/library/national/science/022399sci-mad-elk.html

Blakeslee, S. (1999, March 30). 'Mad cow disease' seen in French zoos. *New York Times* [On-line]. Available: http://www.nytimes.com.science/033099sci-lemur-madcow.html

Blakeslee, S. (October 31, 2000). Biologists say hunters should beware of brain disease. *New York Times* [On-line]. Available: http://www.nytimes.com/2000/10/31/science/31HUNT.html

Bonn, D. (2000). Healthy carriers could increase vCJD risk, scientists say. *Lancet, 356,* 833.

Brandel, J. P. (1999). Clinical aspects of human spongiform encephalopathies, with the exception of iatrogenic forms. *Biomedicine & Pharmacotherapy, 53,* 14–18.

Britton, T. C., Al-Sarraj, S., Shaw, C., Campbell, T., & Collinge, J. (1995). Sporadic Creutzfeldt-Jakob disease in a 16-year-old in the UK. *Lancet, 346,* 1155.

Brown, P. (2001). Bovine spongiform encephalopathy and variant Creutzfeldt-Jakob disease. *British Medical Journal, 322,* 841–844.

Brown, P., Cervenáková, L., & Diringer, H. (2001). Blood infectivity and the prospects for a diagnostic screening test in Creutzfeldt-Jakob disease. *Journal of Laboratory and Clinical Medicine, 137,* 5–13.

Brown, P., Will, R. G., Bradley, R., Asher, D. M., & Detwiler, L. (2001). Bovine spongiform encephalopathy and variant Creutzfeldt-Jakob disease: Background, evolution, and current concerns. *Emerging Infectious Diseases, 7,* 6–16.

Coulthart, M. B., & Cashman, N. R. (2001). Variant Creutzfeldt-Jakob disease: Summary of current scientific knowledge in relation to public health. *Canadian Medical Association Journal, 165,* 51–58.

Cowley, G. (2001, 12 March). Cannibals to cows: The path of a deadly disease. *Newsweek,* 52–61.

Daley, S. (2000, December 1). As mad cow disease spreads in Europe, consumers panic. *New York Times* [On-line]. Available: http://www.nytimes.com/2000/12/01/world/01COW.html

Daszak, P., Cunningham, A. A., & Hyatt, A. D. (2000). Emerging infectious diseases of wildlife—threats to biodiversity and human health. *Science, 287,* 443–449.

Department of Health. (2001, Nov. 5). *Monthly Creutzfeldt-Jakob disease statistics* [On-line]. Available: http://www.doh.gov.uk/cjd/stats/nov01.htm

Dormont, D. (1999). Agents that cause transmissible subacute spongiform encephalopathies. *Biomedical Pharmacotherapy, 53*(1), 3–8.

Exposure to CJD from blood product? (2001). *ProMED Digest, 2001*(029), unpaginated.

Food and Drug Administration. (2001). *Guidance for industry. Revised preventive measures to reduce the possible risk of transmission of Creutzfeldt-Jakob disease (CJD) and variant Creutzfeldt-Jakob disease (vCJD) by blood and blood products. Draft guidance.* [Online]. Available: http://www.fda.gov/cber/guidelines.htm

Foster, J. D., Hope, J., & Fraser, H. (1993). Transmission of bovine spongiform encephalopathy to sheep and goats. *Veterinary Record, 128,* 119–203.

Frosh, A., Joyce, R., & Johnson, A. (2001). Iatrogenic vCJD from surgical instruments. *British Medical Journal, 322,* 1558–1559.

Gajdusek, D. C., & Zigas, V. (1957). Degenerative disease of the central nervous system in New Guinea: The endemic occurrence of 'kuru' in the native population. *New England Journal of Medicine, 257,* 974–981.

Gambetti, P., & Parchi, P. (1999). Insomnia in prion diseases: Sporadic and familial. *The New England Journal of Medicine, 340*, 1675–1677.

Gottlieb, S. (1999). FDA bans blood donation by people who have lived in UK. *British Medical Journal 319*, 535.

Hope, J. (2000). Prions and neurodegenerative diseases. *Current Opinion in Genetics and Development, 10*, 568–574.

Ironside, J. W., Hilton, D. A., Ghani, A., Johnston, N. J., Conyers, L., McCardle, L. M., et al. (2000). Retrospective study of prion-protein accumulation in tonsil and appendix tissues. *Lancet, 355*, 1693–1694.

Lasmézas, C. I., Fournier, J-G., Nouvel, V., Boe, H., Marcé, D., Lamoury, F., et al. (2001). Adaptation of the bovine spongiform encephalopathy agent to primates and comparison with Creutzfeldt-Jakob disease: Implications for human health. *Proceedings of the National Academy of Sciences of the United States of America, 98*, 4142–4147.

Lee, H-S, Brown, P., Cervenáková, L., Garruto, R. M., Alpers, M. P., Gajdusek, D. C., et al. (2001). Increased susceptibility to kuru of carriers of the *PRNP* 129 methionine/methionine genotype. *Journal of Infectious Diseases, 183*, 192–196.

Lueck, C. J., McIlwaine, G. G., & Zeidler, M. (2000). Creutzfeldt-Jakob disease and the eye. *Eye, 14*, 263–290.

Mastrianni, J. A., Nixon, R., Layzer, R., Telling, G. C., Han, D., DeArmond, S. J., et al. (1999). Prion protein conformation in a patient with sporadic fatal insomnia. *New England Journal of Medicine, 340*, 1630–1638.

Murphy, M. F. (1999). New variant Creutzfeldt-Jakob disease (nvCJD): The risk of transmission by blood transfusion and the potential benefit of leukocyte-reduction of blood components. *Transfusion Medicine Reviews, 13*, 75–83.

Orellana, C. (2001). Test for early detection of BSE, vCJD on horizon? *Canadian Medical Association Journal, 165*, 199.

Painter, M. J. (2000). Variant Creutzfeldt-Jakob disease. *Journal of Infection, 41*, 117–124.

Parker, J. C., Jr., & Snyder, J. W. (1999). Prion infections in Creutzfeldt-Jakob disease and its variants. *Annals of Clinical Laboratory Science, 29*(2), 112–117.

Patterson, W. J., & Painter, M. J. (1999). Bovine spongiform encephalopathy and new variant Creutzfeldt-Jakob disease: An overview. *Communicable Disease and Public Health, 2*(1), 5–13.

Prusiner, S. B. (1982). Novel proteinaceous infectious particles cause scrapie. *Science, 216*, 136–144.

Prusiner, S. B. (2001). Shattuck lecture—neurodegerative diseases and prions. *New England Journal of Medicine, 344*, 1516–1524.

Rampton, S., & Stauber, J. (1997). *Mad cow USA: Could the nightmare happen here?* Monroe, Maine: Common Courage Press.

Rhodes, R. (1997). *Deadly feasts.* New York: Simon and Schuster.

Timeline: How the crisis unfolded. (2000, October 25). *CNN.com* [On-line]. Available: wysiwyg://26/http://europe.cnn.com

Tyler, K. L. (1999). Prions and prion diseases of the central nervous system. *Current Clinical Topics in Infectious Diseases, 19*, 226–251.

USDA removes quarantined sheep from second Vermont farm (2001, 23 March). *USDA News Release* (No. 0053.01), unpaginated.

U.S. Department of Defense. (September 14, 2001). New blood donation policy delayed. Press Advisory, No. 189-P. Unpaginated.

Wells, G. H., Scott, A. C., Johnson C. I., Gunning, R. F., Hancock, R. D., & Jeffrey, M. (1987). A novel progressive spongiform encephalopathy in cattle. *Veterinary Record, 121*, 419–420.

Will, R. G., Ironside, J. W., Zeidler, M., Cousens, S. N., Estibeiro, K., Alperovitch, A., et al. (1996). A new variant of Creutzfeldt-Jakob disease in the U.K. *Lancet, 347*, 921–925.

World Health Organization. (1998). Human transmissible spongiform encephalopathies. *Weekly Epidemiological Record, 73*, 361–366.

World Health Organization. (June 14, 2001). Joint WHO/FAO/OIE technical consultation on BSE: Public health, animal health and trade. Press release WHO/28, unpaginated. [online]. Available: http://www.who.int/inf-pr-2001/en/pr2001-28.html

World Health Organization. (June, 2001). Variant Creutzfeldt-Jakob disease (vCJD). Fact Sheet No. 180. Unpaginated.

World Health Organization. (May 17, 2001). New case definition for variant Creutzfeldt-Jakob disease (vCJD). *Communicable Disease Surveillance and Response (CSR)*. Online Available: http://www.who.int/emc/diseases/bse/index.html

World Health Organization. (2000). WHO infection control guidelines for transmissible spongiform encephalopathies. Report of a WHO consultation, Geneva, Switzerland, 23-26 March 1999. WHO/CDS/CSR/APH/2000.3. Online Available: http://www.who.int/emc/diseases/bse/index.html

Zinn, C. (2000). Nine hospital patients may have been exposed to CJD. *British Medical Journal, 320*, 1296.

Zobeley, E., Flechsig, E., Corrizio, A., Enari, M., & Weissman, C. (1999). Infectivity of scrapie prions bound to a stainless steel surface. *Molecular Medicine, 5*, 240–243.

18

Drug-Resistant *Streptococcus pneumoniae*

Victoria L. Anderson

Streptococcus pneumoniae, sometimes called pneumococcus, is the most frequent cause of otitis media, pneumonia, meningitis, and sinusitis in the United States, and can cause other conditions such as septicemia, peritonitis, arthritis, and endocarditis (Musher, 2000). Pneumococcal disease in the United States accounts for 3,000 cases of meningitis, 50,000 case of bacteremia, 500,000 cases of pneumonia, and 7 million cases of otitis media each year. It causes or contributes to an estimated 40,000 deaths in the United States alone each year (Centers for Disease Control and Prevention, 1997). Despite effective antibiotic treatment, about 20% mortality is seen for bacteremia in the elderly, and in the past about 80% of those hospitalized for pneumococcal infections died. Thus, the appearance of multidrug-resistant strains of *S. pneumoniae* in the early 1990s has become a matter of major concern (Whitney, Farley, Hadler, Harrison, Lexau, Reingold, et al., 2000).

First identified in the late 1800s as *Microbe septicemique du salve* and *Micrococcus pasteur* by Sternberg and Pasteur, respectively, the organism's name evolved to *Pneumococcus* in 1886, *Diplococcus pneumoniae* in 1920, and finally came to be *Streptococcus pneumoniae* in 1974 (Musher, 2000). *Streptococcus pneumoniae* is a catalase negative, gram-positive, lancet shaped bacteria. *S. pneumoniae* replicates in pairs or chains and is usually encapsulated. The organism is a facultative anaerobe and metabolizes through lactic acid fermentation. There are

90 different serotypes of *S. pneumoniae*. The serotypes are differentiated by the type or types of presenting antigens on the polysaccharide capsule (Musher, 2000).

Early investigators of *S. pneumoniae* learned that this organism incorporates DNA from other bacteria in a process called transformation (Musher, 2000). This ability of the organism to transform means that it can change capsules and thus become a different serotype. This is especially significant, in that *S. pneumoniae* can develop antibiotic resistance when it replicates, using DNA of other pneumococci or bacteria whose genetic information defines such resistance (Jacobs, 1999). *S. pneumoniae* virulence is not from production of toxins but in its ability to "replicate in host tissues and to generate an inflammatory response" (Musher, 2000, p. 2131). The organism's capsule defends against host phagocytosis by means of inhibiting the function of macrophages and neutrophils. Musher (2000) has pointed out that in a naïve person, *S. pneumoniae* is not readily killed by phagocytes, given their lack of receptors to the organism. *S. pneumoniae* can also escape death by electrostatically repelling phagocytes and degrading specific cytokines needed for chemical attraction of the phagocytes (Musher, 2000). Genomics has revealed new understanding of virulence factors (Hollingshead & Briles, 2001).

As discussed previously, *S. pneumoniae* is a common bacterial pathogen in infections of the upper and lower respiratory tract and in meningitis (Musher, 2000). In addition, it is commonly carried in the nasopharynx of about 40% of healthy adults, and a greater percentage of children, and reports indicate that nearly all infants are colonized with *S. pneumoniae* at some time in the first 2 years of life (Gray, Converse, & Dillon, 1980). *S. pneumoniae* is usually acquired in a community setting. Epidemiological surveillance of *S. pneumoniae* is, therefore, quite difficult, and the scope of the problem always remains somewhat unknown (Jacobs, 1999). The CDC convened a working group to look at the impact of drug-resistant *S. pneumoniae*, and develop an action plan (Centers for Disease Control and Prevention, 1997).

Those at highest risk for invasive infection with *S. pneumoniae* include the following: persons who are immunosuppressed due to primary or secondary defective antibody formation such as congenital agammaglobulinemia and lymphomas respectively; those with defective complement, diminished numbers of polymorphonuclear leukocytes such as from aplastic anemia; those with poorly functioning polymorphonuclear leukocytes such as from alcoholism, renal insufficiency, or glucocorticoid therapy; those who cannot clear pneumococcal bacteremia effectively; and those with prior respiratory infections or inflammatory respiratory conditions such as asthma, or cigarette smoking. Others at risk are infants, the elderly, persons who are malnourished, persons who have cirrhosis of the liver, diabetes mellitus, renal insufficiency, other chronic illnesses, or who are under stress or fatigued. Those who live in, or spend substantial time in, contained or crowded living conditions such as day care centers, prisons, homeless shelters, long-term living facilities, or military training camps are also at increased risk (Bonomo, 2000; Musher, 2000).

The incidence of infection with pneumococcus in children under 2 years of age in the U.S. is 160 cases per 100,000, while in adults over 65 years, this incidence is 50–83 cases per 100,000 (Centers for Disease Control and Prevention, 1997). Invasive pneumococcal infection is often the defining illness of previously undiagnosed HIV-infected children (Centers for Disease Control and Prevention, 1997). Poland (1999) reports that in underdeveloped nations, pneumococcal-related illnesses are estimated to account for the deaths of 1.2 million children, surpassing death related to diarrheal illnesses. In hospitalized cases of community-acquired pneumonia, *S. pneumoniae* is the causative agent in 25%–35% of cases (Centers for Disease Control and Prevention, 1997). Although the causative agent in otitis media is rarely sought after, in those cases in which an organism has been cultured, *S. pneumoniae* accounts for 30%–50% (Centers for Disease Control and Prevention, 1997). Deaths related to *S. pneumoniae* are primarily related to bacteremia and meningitis in elderly, immunocompromised, and asplenic patients.

ANTIBIOTIC-RESISTANT *S. PNEUMONIAE*

The identification of antibiotic resistance in *S. pneumoniae* was first seen in the 1940s during experiments in which mice infected with the organism received multiple low dose penicillin injections. The first clinical case of drug-resistant *S. pneumoniae* (DRSP) was first reported in 1964 (Ball, 1999). The emergence of antibiotic-resistant strains of *S. pneumoniae* began to be reported more widely in the 1960s and 1970s (Jacobs, 1999). Penicillin-resistant strains of *S. pneumoniae* are occurring worldwide. In the 1990s, strains resistant to multiple antibiotics began to be seen, and now more than 20 different strains of *S. pneumoniae* showing penicillin-resistant isolates have been identified (Jacobs, 1999). In 1998, about one third of *S. pneumoniae* isolates were resistant to penicillin in the United States, although some believe this is the lower end of the range (Jacobs, 1999; Whitney et al., 2000). Worldwide, the resistance rate of DRSP is 40%–70% (Jacobs, 1999). To date, there are reports of *S. pneumoniae* with resistance to all antibiotics except vancomycin (Musher, 2000).

Individuals especially at risk for developing antibiotic-resistant *S. pnuemoniae* include adults older than 65 years, children under 2 years, children who attend day care centers, those with a history of prior administration of antibiotics, and individuals with HIV infection (Ball, 1999). While there was no noted increase between 1995 and 1998 in the number of penicillin-susceptible isolates that were resistant to other antimicrobial agents, the proportion of penicillin-resistant strains that were resistant to other antimicrobial agents including cefotaxime, meropenem, erythromycin, trimethoprim-sulfamethoxazole, ofloxacin, and rifampin increased. The proportion of isolates that were resistant to three or more classes of antimicrobial agents also increased between 1995 and 1998 from 9% to 14%. This emerging multidrug resistance is of "major concern," and treatment failures due to drug resistance have been reported for various *S. pneumoniae* infections (Whitney et al., 2000). Concern is heightened because while otitis media is relatively benign when treated promptly and appropriately, resistant strains complicate treatment and may lead to long-term sequelae such as hearing loss (Cohen & Tartasky, 1997). Conditions such as pneumonia and meningitis are serious, and while treatment is usually effective in those with drug-susceptible infection, the spectre of multidrug resistance is frightening in its potential consequences.

A contributing factor to DRSP is inappropriate antibiotic usage. Pressures exerted on prescribing clinicians by their patients in an era of increased consumer knowledge of antibiotic choices has led to inappropriate prescribing of antibiotics for viral syndromes. The problem is complex and is likely a result of poor diagnostic skills of primary care providers, an increase of children in day care situations, and better access to health care (Bauchner & Phillips, 1998). The pressure to prescribe antibiotics is most likely based on the practitioners intentions to please their patients or their patients' parents. Bauchner and Philipps (1998) report that in a study of 400 parents, greater than 50% agreed that antibiotics were needed in cough and fever. Furthermore, the authors suggested that parents greatly influence the specific kind of antibiotic prescribed (Bauchner & Phillips, 1998). Inappropriate antibiotic use involves complex issues that are not within the scope of this chapter. It is important to note, however, that educating the public about the appropriateness of antibiotics should be as important as educating them about conditions for which they seek treatment. Discussion of approaches to patient, provider, and public education and practices regarding antibiotics is considered in detail in Cohen and Tartasky (1997).

SINUSITUS AND OTITIS MEDIA

Infection of the middle ear accounts for millions of visits to health care providers each year in the United States (Centers for Disease Control and Prevention, 1997). Patient presentation is with fever and ear pain and on examination one observes a bulging erythematous, tympanic membrane, often with an air-fluid level. Presentation of infection in the sinuses includes facial pressure, dental pain, headache, fever, purulent rhinorrhea, post-nasal discharge, and cough. Diagnosis can be confirmed from the history and presentation of symptoms. Often radiological evaluation with standard X-rays and CT scan is helpful in confirming the diagnosis. The Drug Resistance Streptococcus Therapeutic Working Group convened by the CDC recommends management of otitis media with amoxicillin at doses of 80–90 mg/kg/day. If there is no response in 3 days, amoxicillin should be replaced with amoxicillin-clavulinic acid, intramuscular ceftriaxone, or cefuroxime axetil (Dowell et al., 1999). The approach to sinusitis is similar, except in adults the use of quinilones is available. The time frame for antibiotic coverage for otitis media remains 10 days and for an acute sinusitus 14 days.

PNEUMONIA

S. pneumoniae is the most common cause of community-acquired pneumonia (CAP). Patients with *S. pneumoniae* pneumonia are more likely to undergo hospitalization than those with other organisms (Marrie, 1998). *S. pneumoniae* causes pneumonia through its replication process and the significant amount of inflammation it produces via pneumolysin and autolysin. This process is especially noted in the elderly where unchecked inflammation leads to clinically worse disease and the known increased level of morbidity and mortality in this age group (Bruunsgaard, Skinhoj, Qvist, & Pederson, 1999). A patient with *S. pneumoniae* pneumonia usually presents with high fever up to 104° F, productive cough, chest pain, tachypnea, and dyspnea. The sputum is typically rust colored and may be copious. The physical exam will most likely reveal adventitious breath sounds including rales, bronchial or tubular breath sounds (in consolidation), egophony, decreased breath sounds, and possibly wheezing. Children often present with associated symptoms of nausea, vomiting, diarrhea, and poor feeding. In the elderly, fever may be blunted and mental confusion may be more prominent. In younger individuals the absence of fever or hypothermia is ominous and may be indicative of sepsis.

Treatment of *S. pneumoniae* pneumonia in the outpatient setting for adults and children who appear stable includes oral amoxicillin, a β lactamase inhibitor (Augmentin), or an oral cephalosporin (cefuroxime axetil) (Jacobs, 1999). Quinilones can also be used in adults. Patients who require hospitalization can be treated with continuous penicillin G infusions, ceftraixone or cefotaxime (Jacobs, 1999).

MENINGITIS

The incidence of meningitis in the United States is reported to be 3 per 100, 000 (Eskola & Anttila, 1999). Despite the availability of appropriate antimicrobial therapy the mortality rate from meningitis is still about 25%, and about 10% have a persistent neurological deficit (Aronin & Quagliarello, 2001). Infection of the meninges with *S. pneumoniae* is likely to arise from an infection in the upper respiratory tract followed by hematogenous seeding of the choroid plexus (Musher, 2000). The triad of fever, nuchal ridgity, and mental status changes remains the hallmark diagnostic criteria for meningitis (Eskola & Anttila, 1999). A lumbar puncture provides further diagnostic information. Treatment of known *S. pneumoniae* meningitis should include intravenous administration of a beta lactamase inhibiting antibiotic (e.g., ceftriaxone), along with vancomycin until laboratory studies confirm that the organism is penicillin sensitive.

BACTEREMIA

Septicemia caused by *S. pneumoniae* usually occurs in the setting of a known pneumonia or meningitis. Asplenic patients are at high-risk for *S. pneumoniae* bacteremia. Other high-risk patients are those at risk for *S. pneumoniae* as discussed earlier. The overall annual incidence of bacteremia in the U.S. is estimated to be 15–50 cases per 100,000 people. In adults 60%–80% of bacteremia cases are associated with pneumonia (Centers for Disease Control and Prevention, 1997). The elderly and children under 2 years of age account for the majority of these cases. Individuals with bacteremia usually present with body temperature abnormalities (fever or hypothermia), tachycardia, tachypnea, hypotension, and may be confused. Blood counts usually reveal an elevated white blood cell count with a shift to immature cells (bands or segmented neutrophils). Management includes immediate support of vital signs and infusion of appropriate broad spectrum antibiotics until blood cultures can identify the pathogen.

PREVENTION AND PROPHYLAXIS

Preventing the occurrence of *S. pneumoniae* infection would be the primary way of preventing problems from antibiotic-resistant strains. Development of the first vaccine for *S. pneumoniae* occurred in the 1940s and was removed from the market because of the development of adequate antimicrobial therapy (Fedson, Musher, & Eskola, 1999; Hollingshead & Briles, 2001). The current adult pneumococcal vaccine covers 23 serotypes and is marketed as Pneumovax, Pnu-Immune, and Pneumo-23 around the world (Fedson et al., 1999). The pneumococcal vaccine induces serotype-specific antibodies that enhance recognition, attachment, and killing of *S. pneumoniae* by leukocytes and phagocytic cells (Butler, Shapiro, & Carlone, 1999).

Identifying those individuals at high risk for infection and ensuring appropriate antibiotic prophylaxis and vaccine immunization is the key to preventing serious illness from *S. pneumoniae*. The vaccine is highly recommended for the following individuals:

- persons older than 65 years;
- sufferers of chronic illness such as diabetes mellitus, congestive heart failure, chronic obstructive pulmonary disease (COPD), chronic renal or hepatic dysfunction;
- persons with congenital or acquired asplenia from surgery, sickle cell disease (vaccinate patients if possible 2 weeks before planned splenectomy);
- persons with HIV infection;
- persons with hematological neoplasms;

- persons planning to undergo bone marrow or solid organ transplant (immunization 2 weeks prior to and following procedure); and
- institutionalized individuals.

It is important to note that in immunocompromised individuals the current pneumococcal vaccine does not confer the same level of effectiveness as observed in the immunocompetent recipient and therefore vaccination may need to occur more frequently (Centers for Disease Control and Prevention, 1997).

The vaccine is contraindicated only in individuals with a known allergic reaction to previous doses (Fedson et al., 1999). Current recommendations are for repeat vaccination at 5-year intervals for the unconjugated vaccine, in individuals over 65 years and those over 2 years at high risk for invasive pneumococcal disease (Nguyen-Van Tam & Neal, 1999). Butler and associates (1999) report that postlicensure epidemiologic studies have documented the vaccine's efficacy at 75% for elderly (less than 65 years) immunocompetent individuals, and that this efficacy decreases with advancing age. Cost-benefit analysis still supports the use of the pneumococcal vaccine, however (1998).

A pneumococcal conjugate vaccine that corrects for the problem of antibody and memory response was licensed in February 2000, and should confer a high level of protection to young children who represent the highest number of cases of infection with *S. pnemoniae*. The new vaccine is T-cell dependent and induces higher antibody concentrations and primed B cells (Butler et al., 1999). The major drawback of the conjugated vaccine is that it covers fewer (i.e., 7) *S. pneumoniae* serotypes, suggesting that children will need vaccination with multiple conjugated vaccines to cover the majority of serotypes (Jacobs, 1999). The new vaccine reduces nasopharyngeal carriage of *S. pnemoniae* by inducing mucosal immunity, a quality missing from the current vaccines (Eskola & Anttila, 1999). To date there have been no reported severe adverse effects of the vaccine (Eskola & Anttila, 1999). It is marketed as Prevnar®. The schedule for immunization in children is 2, 4, 6, and 15 to 18 months (American Academy of Pediatrics, 2000). Special recommendations may be found in Dennehy (2001).

S. pneumoniae poses a real threat to all age groups in causing significant disease. Because *S. pneumoniae* shows strong resistance patterns, the need for enthusiastic support of immunization programs is necessary. Research suggests that the reason for low pneumococcal immunization rates is due to providers' failure to recommend such therapy (Ehresmann, Ramesh, Como-Sabetti, Peterson, Whitney, & Moore, 2001; Rhew, Glassman, & Goetz, 1999). Reminder systems and the better use of nurses and other health workers are all potential means to improve immunization rates. The appearance of the new conjugated pneumococcal vaccines for children under 2 years are especially hopeful in reducing carriage and disease in this population and appear cost-effective (Lieu, Ray, Black, Klein, Breiman, Miller, et al., 2001). The vaccine has been recommended by various groups including CDC, the American Academy of Pediatrics, and the American Academy of Family Physicians (Centers for Disease Control and Prevention, 2001; Zimmerman, 2001).

REFERENCES

American Academy of Pediatrics. Committee on Infectious Diseases. (2000). Policy statement: Recommendations for the prevention of pneumococcal infections, including the use of pneumococcal conjugate vaccine (Prevnar), pneumococcal polysaccharide vaccine, and antibiotic prophylaxis. *Pediatrics, 106*(2 Pt. 1), 363–366.

Aronin, S. I., & Quagliarello, V. J. (2001). New perspectives on pneumococcal meningitis. *Hospital Practice, 36*(2), 43–51.

Ball, P. Therapy for pneumococcal infection at the millennium: doubts and certainties. *American Journal of Medicine, 107*(1A), 77S–85S.

Bauchner, H., & Phillips, B. (1998). Commentaries: Reducing inappropriate oral antibiotic use: A prescription for change. *Pediatrics, 107*, 142–145.

Bonomo, R. A. (2000). Multiple antibiotic-resistant bacteria in long-term-care facilities: An emerging problem in the practice of infectious diseases. *Clinical Infectious Diseases, 31*, 1414–1422.

Bruunsgard, H., Skinhoj, P., Qvist, J., & Pederson, B. K. (1999). Elderly humans show prolonged in-vivo inflammatory activity during pneumococcal infections. *Journal of Infectious Diseases, 180*, 551–554.

Butler, J. C., Shapiro, E. D., & Carlone, G. M. (1999). Pneumococcal vaccines: History, current status and future directions. *American Journal of Medicine, 107*, 69S–76S.

Centers for Disease Control and Prevention. (1997). Prevention of pneumococcal disease: Recommendations of the advisory committee on immunization practices. *Morbidity and Mortality Weekly Report, 46*(RR-08), 1–24.

Centers for Disease Control and Prevention. (2001). Recommended childhood immunization schedule—United States, 2001. *Morbidity and Mortality Weekly Report, 50*, 7–10, 19.

Cohen, F. L., & Tartasky, D. (1997). Microbial resistance to drug therapy: A review. *American Journal of Infection Control, 25*, 51–64.

Dennehy, P. H. (2001). Active immunization in the United States: Developments over the past decade. *Clinical Microbiology Reviews, 14,* 872–908.

Dowell, S. F., Butler, J. C., Giebink, G. S., Jacobs, M. R., Jernigan, D., Musher, D. M., et al. (1999). Acute otitis media: Management and surveillance in an era of pneumococcal resistance—A report from the Drug-resistant *Streptococcus pneumoniae* Therapeutic Working Group. *Pediatric Infectious Disease Journal, 18,* 1–9.

Ehresmann, K. R., Ramesh, A., Como-Sabetti, K., Peterson, D. C., Whitney, C. G., & Moore, K. A. (2001). Factors associated with self-reported pneumococcal immunization among adults 65 years of age or older in the Minneapolis-St. Paul metropolitan area. *Preventive Medicine, 32,* 409–415.

Eskola, J., & Anttila, M. (1999). Pneumococcal conjugate vaccines. *Pediatric Infectious Diseases Journal, 18,* 543–551.

Fedson, D. S., Musher, D. M., & Eskola, J. (1999). Pneumococcal vaccine. In S. Plotkin & W. Orebstein (Eds.), *Vaccines* (3rd ed., pp. 553–607). Philadelphia: WB Saunders Co.

Gray, B. M., Converse, G. M., III, & Dillon, H. C., Jr. (1980). Epidemiologic studies of *Streptococcus pneumoniae* in infants: Acquisition, carriage, and infection during the first 24 months of life. *Journal of Infectious Diseases, 142,* 923–933.

Hollingshead, S. K., & Briles, D. E. (2001). *Streptococcus pneumoniae*: New tools for an old pathogen. *Current Opinion in Microbiology, 4,* 71–77.

Jacobs, M. (1999). Drug resistant *Streptococcus pneumoniae*: Rational antibiotic choices. *American Journal of Medicine, 106*(5A), 19S–25S.

Lieu, T., Ray, G., Black, S., Klein, J., Breiman, R., Miller, M., & Shinefeld, H. (2000). Projected cost-effectiveness of pneumococcal conjugate vaccination of healthy infants and children. *Journal of the American Medical Association, 283,* 1460–1468.

Marrie, T. J. (1998). Community-acquired pneumonia: Epidemiology, etiology and treatment. *Infectious Disease Clinics of North America, 12,* 723–739.

Musher, D. (2000). *Streptococcus pneumoniae.* In G. Mandell, J. Bennett, & R. Dolin (Eds.), *Principles and practices of infectious diseases* (5th ed., pp. 2128–2147). Philadelphia: Churchill Livingstone.

Nguyen-Van Tam, J. S., & Neal, K. R. (1999). Clinical effectiveness, policies and practices for influenza and pneumococcal vaccines. *Seminars in Respiratory Infections, 14,* 184–195.

Poland, G. A. (1999). The burden of pneumococcal disease: The role of conjugate vaccines. *Vaccine, 17,* 1674–1679.

Rhew, D. C., Glassman, P. A., & Goetz, M. B. (1999). Improving pneumococcal vaccine rates: Nurse protocols versus clinical reminders. *Journal of General Internal Medicine, 14,* 351–356.

Whitney, C. G., Farley, M. M., Hadler, J., Harrison, L. H., Lexau, C., Reingold, A., et al. (2000). Increasing prevalence of multidrug-resistant *Streptococcus pneumoniae* in the United States. *New England Journal of Medicine, 343,* 1917–1924.

Zimmerman, R. K. (2001). Pneumococcal conjugate vaccine for young children. *American Family Physician, 63,* 1919, 1923.

19

Vancomycin-Resistant Enterococci

Nancy Khardori

A 42-year-old male with multiple medical problems, including end-stage renal disease, hepatitis B, hepatitis C, recurrent pancreatitis, and peptic ulcer disease, was admitted for a cadaveric kidney transplant. The patient received perioperative antibiotic therapy and was in the intensive care unit postoperatively. Two weeks after the transplant, blood and perinephric fluid cultures grew *Serratia marcescens*. The patient had multiple invasive devices including central venous catheters, abdominal (perinephric) drainage tube, and a chest tube. He was treated with imipenem and switched to oral ciprofloxacin on the third day. The central venous catheter tip grew vancomycin-resistant *Enterococcus faecium* (VRE). Ten days later blood cultures also grew VRE. The patient was started on synercid 7.5 mg/kg every 8 hours intravenously. Repeat blood cultures continued to grow VRE. On the eleventh day, rifampin was added. After more than 3 weeks of therapy, synercid was discontinued. The patient was started on doxycycline and amikacin, based on in vitro susceptibility to both of these agents. Blood cultures remained positive for VRE after 1 week of therapy. The patient's clinical status deteriorated and he died 7 weeks after the first isolation of VRE.

Organisms in the genus *Enterococcus* are facultatively anaerobic gram-positive cocci that are widely distributed in the environment and among animals. Enterococci are normal inhabitants of the intestinal tract of humans and animals. In humans, enterococci can colonize the oral cavity, vagina, and hepatobiliary tract. There are at least 17 species in the genus, the most common being *Enterococcus faecalis*, followed by *Enterococcus faecium* (Sahm, 1994). The isolation of enterococci from clinical specimens should be interpreted with caution due to their ubiquitous nature. Nonetheless, their role in a variety of infections, some life-threatening, is well established.

Enterococci are frequent causes of nosocomial surgical site infection, as well as other infections such as endocarditis (Cetinkaya, Falk, & Mayhall, 2000). They are considered emerging because they have developed resistance to both ampicillin and vancomycin (Rice, 2001). For example, the percent of VRE recovered from surgical site infections were 0.3% in 1989 and more than 20% in 1997 (Fleenor-Ford, Hayden, & Weinstein, 1999), and in hemodialysis centers, the percent reporting one or more patients colonized or infected with VRE rose from 11% in 1995 to 21% in 1996 (D'Agata, Green, Schulman, Li, Tang, & Schaffner, 2001). Microbial resistance in general is discussed in chapter 2.

VRE have been recovered from patients in many areas of the world including the United Kingdom, France, Australia, Belgium, Canada, Denmark, Germany, Italy, Malaysia, the Netherlands, Spain, Sweden, and the United States (Boyce, 1997). Studies of genotypes in various geographic areas suggest that the same resistance determinants have spread worldwide.

Contaminated food products and colonized animals may serve as a reservoir from which nonhospitalized individuals acquire VRE. VRE has been recovered from processed chickens in England, Denmark, and Germany, from minced pork meat in Germany, and from chicken carcasses delivered to a hospital kitchen in Germany (Klare, Heier, Claus, Reissbrodt, & Witte, 1995). The occurrence of VRE in animals could be related to the fact that avoparcin (a glycopeptide) has been available as a feed additive for more than 18 years in the United Kingdom and Europe. Animals fed avoparcin are more likely to yield VRE than animals raised on farms where this agent is not fed to animals. The possibility of a community reservoir of VRE is further supported by the presence of VRE in fecal samples of a community-based patient sample in Oxford, England, and recovery of VRE from nonhospitalized patients in rural Germany (Witte & Klare, 1995). VRE isolates recovered from farm animals and humans in one study had similar genotypes (Bates, Jordens, & Griffiths, 1994). In the U.S., avoparcin has not been licensed as a feed additive for animals and limited surveys have failed to show VRE in chickens. Hospitalized patients with gastrointestinal carriage of VRE appear to be the major reservoir for the organism in the United States because asymptomatic colonization is common (Murray, 2000). This reservoir can only be revealed by surveillance cultures. Environmental surfaces and medical items in patients' rooms frequently become contaminated with VRE and may also serve as reservoirs. Because of resistance to desiccation and extreme temperatures, VRE on such items may remain viable for days or weeks (Boyce, Mermel, Zervos, Rice, Potter-Bynoe, Giorgio, et al., 1995). For example, they have been cultured from seat cushions in hospital rooms (Noskin, Bednarz, Suriano, Reiner, & Peterson, 2000). The reported colonization rates of residents of long-term care facilities by VRE range from 5%–47%. Most of these VREs are *E. faecium* and colonized residents in long-term care facilities may also serve as a reservoir for VRE. The epidemiologic significance of gastrointestinal colonization of health care workers is not clear.

The most common vehicle for nosocomial transmission of VRE is the transiently contaminated hands of health care workers. Much less important is the transmission by contaminated medical equipment. There is no conclusive proof that VRE are spread by contaminated clothing. There is no evidence of airborne transmission of enterococci. Foodborne transmission may occur in certain geographic areas (Witte & Klare, 1995).

Enterococci rank second or third in frequency as causes of nosocomial infections in the United States (Moellering, 2000). Early studies revealed that most patients with VRE in the United States were in the intensive care unit. Infections due to VRE are now being seen with increasing frequency among patents with chronic renal failure and malignancies, transplant recipients, and other patients requiring prolonged hospitalization. Risk factors for enterococcal colonization or infection in these patients include prior antibiotic therapy (especially with vancomycin, cephalosporins, or aminoglycosides), the presence of urinary or vascular catheters, exposure to contaminated medical equipment such as electronic thermometers, and proximity to a known case of VRE. Risk factors for VRE infections such as bacteremia include malignancy (especially hematologic malignancy), neutropenia, poor acute physiology and chronic health evaluation score, and preceding therapy with antimicrobial agents with activity against anaerobes (Boyce, 1997).

Most patients from whom VRE are recovered are colonized, rather than infected, with the organism. In hospitals in which perirectal or rectal swab specimens from high-risk patients are used for screening, the ratio of colonized to infected patients may reach as high as 10:1. The morbidity and mortality associated with VRE is difficult to determine because of co-morbid conditions and the presence of other potential pathogens in the cultures. Crude mortality rates of 17%–73% have been reported with VRE bacteremia. In some reports, the mortality rate was higher in patients with VRE bacteremia than in those with bacteremia due to vancomycin-susceptible enterococci.

Urinary tract infections are the most common infection caused by enterococci. Other common infections caused by enterococci include bacteremia and endocarditis (1 out of 50 cases of enterococcal bacteremia results in endocarditis), intra-abdominal and pelvic infections, and skin and soft tissue infections. In the latter two infections, enterococci are seen as part of mixed aerobic and anaerobic flora. Enterococci have been documented to cause neonatal sepsis. Several nosocomial outbreaks of bacteremia or meningitis or both have been described in premature or low birth weight neonates with nasogastric tubes and intravascular device (Moellering, 2000). Enterococci rarely cause meningitis in normal adults, and respiratory tract infections due to enterococci are very uncommon.

The percentage of VRE reported to the National Nosocomial Infection Surveillance System increased 20-fold between 1989 and 1993 (Centers for Disease Control and Prevention, 1993). Vancomycin-resistant *E. faecium* commonly are resistant to ampicillin and high levels of aminoglycosides, resulting in a strain that until recently was untreatable with currently available antimicrobial agents. Numerous reports have documented the serious infections and mortality associated with these strains, especially among immunosuppressed patients and patients with underlying illnesses (Morris, Shay, Hebden, McCarter, Perdue, Jarvis, et al., 1995). A significantly higher proportion of the most immunocompromised patients had more persistent VRE bloodstream infections and were more likely to die on the day of the bloodstream infection, suggesting a greater pathogenicity of VRE in this population (Montecalvo, Shay, Patel, Tacsa, Maloney, Jarvis, et al., 1996).

For the detection of VRE carriage, stools or rectal swabs are optimal specimens because enterococci are a normal component of the gut flora (Tenover, 1998). Recovery of VRE from these samples is best achieved by direct inoculation onto selective media such as bile esculin azide agar, triphenyl-tetrazolium chloride azide agar, or an equivalent medium supplemented with 6 μg/ml of vancomycin. Many *Van*B-VRE with minimum inhibitory concentrations (MICs) to vancomycin of less than 30 μg/ml may not be detected even if vancomycin concentrations higher than 6 μg/ml are used in the selective agar.

Because of the increasing significance of enterococci as nosocomial pathogens, emergence of resistance in *E. faecalis* and *E. faecium* to multiple antimicrobial agents, different intrinsic susceptibility profiles of *E. faecalis* and *E. faecium*, and intrinsic glycopeptide resistance of species other than *E. faecalis* and *E. faecium*, the identification of enterococci to the species level and their in vitro susceptibility testing have clinical significance (Willey, Jones, McGeer, Witte, French, Roberts, et al., 1999). The vancomycin-resistant *Enterococcus faecium* also needs to be differentiated from other intrinsically vancomycin-resistant gram-positive bacteria such as lactobacilli, pediococci, and leuconostocs. These genera and *E. casseliflavus* and *E. gallinarum* with inherent low-level vancomycin resistance are rarely associated with clinical infections, secondary transmission, or transferable glycopeptide resistance.

Enterococci have relatively low virulence compared to other gram-positive organisms. The increasing prevalence and significance of infections caused by enterococci are related to the host factors (including serious underlying illnesses, invasive devices, long hospital stays, prolonged antibiotic therapy) and to the fact that enterococci are intrinsically resistant to many commonly used antibiotics and have a profound propensity to acquire resistance to other agents.

Enterococci are inherently more resistant to antimicrobial agents than other clinically important gram-positive bacteria (French, 1998). Antibiotics to which enterococci are virtually always resistant or should be considered so for therapeutic purposes include β-lactams (all cephalosporins, anti-staphylococcal penicillins, and aztreonam); trimethroprim/sulfamethoxazole; clindamycin; and aminoglycosides (gentamicin, tobramycin, amikacin, and streptomycin). The intrinsic resistance of enterococci to cephalosporins along with their widespread use is believed to be a major contributing factor to the emergence of enterococci as predominant nosocomial pathogens.

Enterococci are more resistant to penicillin than the streptococci because of the lower affinity of their penicillin-binding proteins (PBPs) for penicillin. The minimum inhibitory concentrations (MICs) of ampicillin against enterococci are about one dilution lower than that of penicillin. The minimum bactericidal concentrations (MBCs) to both, however, are usually much higher than MICs and therefore bactericidal activity is not achieved by penicillins alone.

This intrinsic resistance of enterococci limits the choices for antimicrobial therapy and makes antimicrobial combinations the primary mode of treating invasive infections. This is particularly important in patients with impaired host defenses. The two primary components of the therapeutic combination include an agent that acts on bacterial cell wall synthesis (i.e., penicillins or vancomycin) and another agent that causes inhibition of protein synthesis (i.e., an aminoglycoside). The use of a cell wall active agent helps by overcoming the barrier to uptake of aminoglycosides leading to inhibition of protein synthesis and eventually resulting in cell death by synergistic activity. This approach has provided an effective strategy for management of serious infections like enterococcal endocarditis.

The acquisition of genes that mediate resistance to the various components of combination therapy has seriously compromised the management of enterococcal infections. The evolution of this resistance abrogates the contribution of individual antimicrobials to synergistic bactericidal activity resulting in suboptimal single agent therapy. When resistance occurs to both components, a multiply drug-resistant strain evolves, including strains resistant to aminoglycosides and penicillin.

In 1988, two strains of *E. faecalis* with inducible high-level resistance to glycopeptides, vancomycin, and teicoplanin, were reported (Leclercq, Derlot, Duval, & Courvalin, 1988). Since the first reports of VRE from France and the United Kingdom in 1988, and the U.S. 1 year later, VRE have been isolated in small community hospitals as well as in large tertiary-care hospitals (Spera & Farber, 1992). Seen most frequently with *E. faecium*, vancomycin resistance has also been described with *E. faecalis*, *E. gallinarum* and *E. durans*. The mechanism of vancomycin resistance involves a cluster of seven acquired genes (Arthur & Courvalin, 1993). The *Van*A and *Van*B phenotypic expressions predominate among *E. faecium* and *E. faecalis*, the most commonly encountered species. Concomitant high-level resistance to penicillins, aminoglycosides, and glycopeptides was first reported in 1991 (Wade, Rolando, & Casewell, 1991).

Being under the selection pressure of antimicrobial agents and the natural ability of enterococci to accept, share, and distribute resistance genes have allowed these organisms to thrive. In addition, vancomycin-dependent *E. faecalis* and *E. faecium* have been reported from clinical infections (Fraimow, Jungkind, Lander, Delso, & Dean, 1994; Green, Shlaes, Barbador, & Shlaes, 1995). These strains grow in vitro only in the presence of vancomycin. Vancomycin-dependent enterococci should be considered potential pathogens when clinical and microbiological data are consistent with infection due to a fastidious or nutritionally deficient organism in a geographic area where resistance to vancomycin is present. The other agents to which enterococci have acquired resistance include fluoroquinolones, clindamycin (high level), macrolides, rifampin, and tetracyclines. Enterococci can be tested using either disk diffusion on Mueller-Hinton agar or broth microdilution trays following the procedures described by the National Committee on Clinical Laboratory Standards (Jones, Ballow, Biedenbach, Deinhart, & Schentag, 1998). Presumptive VRE from surveillance specimens and enterococci from all clinical specimens must be screened for vancomycin resistance following the guidelines described by the National Committee for Clinical Laboratory Standards (2001).

Serious infections caused by enterococci (e.g., bacteremia, endocarditis) require treatment with a bactericidal combination that should include a penicillin (e.g., ampicillin, penicillin G, or vancomycin) and an aminoglycoside (e.g., gentamicin, streptomycin). For the combination to be synergistic and bactericidal, the enterococcus should be susceptible to penicillin or vancomycin and not exhibit high-level resistance to aminoglycosides. The resistance to penicillin either due to alteration of the target penicillin binding proteins or β-lactamase production, high-level resistance to aminoglycosides, and vancomycin resistance can be present in any given isolate, either singly or as any combination of the three. Vancomycin-resistant *E. faecium* often is resistant to penicillin and has high-level resistance to aminoglycosides. Quinupristin-dalfopristin (a streptogramin combination) and linezolid have recently been approved by the FDA for treatment of vancomycin-resistant *Enterococcus faecium*. The therapeutic options for various types and combinations of resistance are beyond the scope of this chapter.

Acquired absolute resistance to antimicrobial agents represents the most serious and difficult type of resistance and renders a previously effective antibiotic inactive, independent of the dose. The critical care areas in the hospital are the areas where resistance is most likely to be encountered because of the intensity of antibiotic use (Cunha, 1998). Multiple antibiotics with high rates of resistance potential are often used in these areas for prolonged periods. In critically ill patients, antibiotics are often used for fever and leukocytosis due to noninfectious causes and for covering resistant colonizing organisms. Therefore, effective antibiotic usage policies are needed to minimize the potential for emergence of resistant strains.

All antibiotics are not equal in terms of their resistance potential. Resistance is not directly related to any one factor (e.g., structure, antibiotic class, mechanism of action, volume of use, or duration of use). Antibiotic selection and use policies must take into consideration all of these factors. For example, if an antibiotic within a class associated with the development of resistance is used in high volume for a prolonged period of time, the emergence of resistance will be accelerated and exacerbated. Antibiotic resistance is a hospital-wide concern even though the intensity is different in different areas. The keys to minimizing antibiotic resistance are as follows:

- Use agents known to have low resistance potential, all other factors being equal.
- Use these agents only for clinically and or microbiologically documented infections.
- Use at full doses for the shortest possible duration that will eradicate the infection.
- Avoid using antibiotics for colonization.
- Combine antibiotics to increase spectrum or achieve synergy. Antipseudomonal penicillins plus an aminoglycoside and TMP/SMX are the only two combinations that have been shown to decrease the emergence of resistant strains.
- Institute formulary restrictions for high resistance potential antibiotics.
- Control the established antibiotic resistance problems by modifications and substitutions in antibiotic use. Recommendations of the Hospital Infection Control Practices Advisory Committee (HICPAC) for preventing the spread of vancomycin resistance include prudent vancomycin use (Centers for Disease Control and Prevention, 1995). The guidelines list the situations in which the use of vancomycin is appropriate or acceptable, situations in which the use of vancomycin should be discouraged, and recommendations about enhancing compliance.

The elements of an effective strategy to control spread of VRE are

- identification, speciation, antimicrobial susceptibility testing and reporting by the microbiology laboratory, and

- infection control practices including screening procedures for VRE; education; and guidelines for patient placement and the use of barrier precautions, isolation precautions, posthospitalization and readmission procedures, and reporting to the local and state health departments.

Control of VRE requires a multidisciplinary institution-wide effort and should be part of the hospital's quality improvement program. The guidelines at any institution should be made with participation from the hospital's pharmacy and therapeutics committee, hospital epidemiologist, infection control, infectious diseases departments, and the nursing, medical, and surgical staffs (Centers for Disease Control and Prevention, 1995).

REFERENCES

Arthur, M., & Courvalin, P. (1993). Genetics and mechanisms of glycopeptide-resistance in enterococci. *Antimicrobial Agents and Chemotherapy, 37*, 1563–1571.

Bates, J., Jordens, J. Z., & Griffiths, D. T. (1994). Farm animals as a putative reservoir for vancomycin-resistant enterococcal infection in man. *Journal of Antimicrobial Agents and Chemotherapy, 34*, 507.

Boyce, J. M. (1997). Vancomycin-resistant enterococcus—detection, epidemiology, and control measures. *Infectious Disease Clinics of North America, 11*, 367–384.

Boyce, J. M., Mermel, L. A., Zervos, M. J., Rice, L. B., Potter-Bynoe, G., Giorgio, C., et al. (1995). Controlling vancomycin-resistant enterococci. *Infection Control and Hospital Epidemiology, 16*, 634–637.

Centers for Disease Control and Prevention. (1993). Nosocomial enterococci resistant to vancomycin—United States 1989–1993. *Morbidity and Mortality Weekly Report, 42*, 597–599.

Centers for Disease Control and Prevention. (1995). Recommendations for preventing the spread of vancomycin resistance. Recommendations of the Hospital Infection Control Practices Advisory Committee (HICPAC). *Morbidity and Mortality Weekly Report, 44*(RR–12), 1–13.

Cetinkaya, Y., Falk, P., & Mayhall, C. G. (2000). Vancomycin-resistant enterococci. *Clinical Microbiology Reviews, 13*, 686–707.

Cunha, B. A. (1998). Antibiotic resistance—control strategies. *Critical Care Clinics, 14*, 309–327.

D'Agata, E. M. C., Green, W. K., Schulman, G., Li, H., Tang, Y-W., & Schaffner, W. (2001). Vancomycin-resistant enterococci among chronic hemodialysis patients: A prospective study of acquisition. *Clinical Infectious Diseases, 32*, 23–29.

Fleenor-Ford, A., Hayden, M. K., & Weinstein, R. A. (1999). Vancomycin-resistant enterococci: Implications for surgeons. *Surgery, 125*, 121–125.

Fraimow, H. S., Jungkind, D. L., Lander, D. W., Delso, D. R., & Dean, J. L. (1994). Urinary tract infection with an *Enterococcus faecalis* isolate that requires vancomycin for growth. *Annals of Internal Medicine, 121*, 22–26.

French, G. L. (1998). Enterococci and vancomycin resistance. *Clinical Infectious Diseases, 27*(Suppl. 1), S75–S83.

Green, M., Shlaes, J. H., Barbador, K., & Shlaes, D. M. (1995). Bacteremia due to vancomycin-dependent *Enterococcus faecium*. *Clinical Infectious Diseases, 20*, 712–714.

Jones, R. N., Ballow, C. H., Biedenbach, D. J., Deinhart, J. A., & Schentag, J. J. (1998). Antimicrobial activity of quinupristin-dalfopristin (RP 59500, Synercid7) tested against over 28,000 recent clinical isolates from 200 medical centers in the United States and Canada. *Diagnostic Microbiology and Infectious Disease, 31*, 437–451.

Klare, I., Heier, H., Claus, H. J., Reissbrodt, R., & Witte, W. (1995). *van*A-mediated high-level glycopeptide resistance in *Enterococcus faecium* from animal husbandry. *FEMS Microbiology Letter, 125*, 165.

Leclercq, R., Derlot, E., Duval, J., & Courvalin, P. (1988). Plasmid-mediated resistance to vancomycin and teicoplanin in *Enterococcus faecium*. *New England Journal of Medicine, 319*, 157–161.

Moellering, R. C., Jr. (2000). *Enterococcus* species, *Streptococcus bovis*, and *Leuconostoc* species. In G. L. Mandell, J. E. Bennett, R. G. Douglas, & R. Dolin (Eds.), *Mandell, Douglas, and Bennett's principles and practice of infectious diseases* (5th ed., pp. 2147–2156). New York: Churchill Livingstone.

Montecalvo, M. A., Shay, D. K., Patel, P., Tacsa, L., Maloney, S. A., Jarvis, W. R., et al. (1996). Bloodstream infections with vancomycin-resistant enterococci. *Archives of Internal Medicine, 156*, 1458–1462.

Morris, J. G., Shay, D. K., Hebden, J. N., McCarter, R. J., Jr., Perdue, B. E., Jarvis, W., et al. (1995). Enterococci resistant to multiple antimicrobial agents, including vancomycin. *Annals of Internal Medicine, 123*, 250–259.

Murray, B. E. (2000). Vancomycin-resistant enterococcal infections. *New England Journal of Medicine, 342*, 710–721.

National Committee for Clinical Laboratory Studies. (2001). *Performance standards for antimicrobial susceptibility testing*. Document M100-S11, NCCLS. Wayne, PA: Author.

Noskin, G. A., Bednarz, P., Suriano, T., Reiner, S., & Peterson, L. R. (2000). Persistent contamination of fabric-covered furniture by vancomycin-resistant enterococci: Implications for upholstery selection in hospitals. *American Journal of Infection Control, 28*, 311–313.

Rice, L. B. (2001). Emergence of vancomycin-resistant enterococci. *Emerging Infectious Diseases, 7*, 183–187.

Sahm, D. (1994). Multidrug-resistant enterococci. *Mediguide to Infectious Diseases, 14*(5), 1–8.

Spera, R. V., & Farber, B. G. (1992). Multiply-resistant *Enterococcus faecium*. *Journal of the American Medical Association, 268*, 2563–2567.

Tenover, F. C. (1998). Laboratory methods for surveillance of vancomycin-resistant enterococci. *Clinical Microbiology Newsletter, 20,* 1–5.

Wade, J., Rolando, N., & Casewell, M. (1991). Resistance of *Enterococcus faecium* to vancomycin and teicoplanin. *Lancet, 337,* 1616.

Willey, B. M., Jones, R. N., McGeer, A., Witte, W., French, G., Roberts, R. B., et al. (1999). Practical approach to the identification of clinically relevant *Enterococcus* species. *Diagnostic Microbiology and Infectious Disease, 34,* 165–171.

Witte, W., & Klare, I. (1995). Glycopeptide-resistant *Enterococcus faecium* outside hospitals: A commentary. *Microbiology and Drug Resistance, 1,* 259–263.

20

West Nile Virus

Felissa R. Lashley

On August 23rd, 1999, a physician from Queens, a borough of New York City, reported two cases of unusual encephalitis to the New York City Department of Health. Investigators identified a cluster of six patients with encephalitis, four of whom required respiratory support. Initial antibody testing was positive for St. Louis encephalitis virus. The first group of cases resided in a 2-mile square area in Queens. Active surveillance was initiated on September 3rd, 1999, and a clinical case was defined as "a presumptive diagnosis of viral encephalitis with or without muscle weakness or acute flaccid paralysis, Guillain-Barré syndrome, aseptic meningitis, or presence of the clinical syndrome characterizing the initial cluster of cases in a patient presenting after August 1st" (Centers for Disease Control and Prevention, 1999a, p. 845). At the same time, local health officers had noted an increase in fatalities among New York City birds, especially crows, and the Bronx zoo reported deaths in several exotic birds—including Chilean flamingos, an Asian pheasant, and a cormorant. Testing of autopsy specimens from the birds revealed meningoencephalitis and myocarditis as well as the presence of a West Nile-like virus sequence found by genomic analysis. Further testing on the human tissue revealed West Nile-like viral presence as well (Centers for Disease Control and Prevention, 1999a, 1999b). Thus, the first identification of West Nile virus in humans in North America was made. Some responses bordered on panic. Airlines, such as one from Brazil, sprayed flights arriving from New York with insecticide before landing to kill any possible infected mosquitoes on board ("West Nile virus—USA," 1999), and there was even speculation that the outbreak represented a bioterrorist attack (Preston, 1999).

West Nile virus is an arbovirus of the *Flaviviridiae* family. It is a member of the Japanese encephalitis serocomplex, which also includes Japanese encephalitis virus, Murray Valley (in Australia), encephalitis virus, St. Louis encephalitis virus, and the Kunjin virus, which appears to be a subtype of West Nile virus (Petersen & Roehrig, 2001). Various strains of the virus exist. West Nile virus was first isolated from a woman in the West Nile province of Uganda in 1937 (Chowers, Lang, Nassar, Ben-David, Giladi, Rubinshtein, et al., 2001; Smithburn, Hughes, Burke, & Paul, 1940).

Endemic disease exists in many countries, predominately in Africa (e.g., South Africa, Uganda, Nigeria, and Botswana), the Middle East, and Eurasia, including Israel, Azerbaijan, Egypt, the Ukraine, Portugal, Pakistan, India and other countries (Hubâlek & Halouzka, 1999). Antibody seroprevalence varies across geography and age groups and can be difficult to detect because of nonspecificity and cross-reactivity with other flaviviruses and because the antibodies can wane over time. The New York outbreak was the first detected in the Western hemisphere (Platonov, Shipulin, Shipulina, Tyutyunnik, Frolochkina, Lanciotti, et al., 2001).

The principal vectors of West Nile virus are mosquitoes, usually those species that feed on birds such as *Culex* (especially *C. pipiens*), but also others such as *Aedes* and *Anopheles*, and occasionally ticks. Birds are the principal host but lemurs, and frogs and especially horses can also harbor the virus at moderate to high levels. High levels of the virus in birds may persist for long periods of time (20–100 days); thus migratory birds are implicated in the introduction of West Nile virus. There is usually a bird-mosquito cycle, although bird-tick cycles or frog-mosquito cycles occur (Centers for Disease Control and Prevention, 1999a; Hubâlek & Halouzka, 1999). In the New York outbreak described above, the principal birds affected were crows, but deaths in many species occurred, and a large number of bird species are now known to harbor the virus including bluejays, bald eagles, American robins, sandhill cranes, yellow-billed cuckoos, house sparrows, owls, mallards, and red-tailed and broad winged hawks (Centers for Disease Control and Prevention, 1999b). A wide variety of animals may be infected with West Nile virus including raccoons, chipmunks, horses, cats, squirrels, bats, and rabbits ("West Nile virus surveillance . . . ," 2000).

The majority of infections with the West Nile virus are asymptomatic and self-limiting. Symptoms, when they occur, are those of a febrile, flu-like illness, including sudden onset of moderate to high fever, anorexia, malaise, nausea, vomiting, headache, lymphadenopathy, myalgia, eye pain, sore throat, and conjunctivitis. A maculopapular or roseolar rash may be present on the trunk, extremities, and head in about half of the cases, particularly in children. In less than 15% of cases, the central nervous system is involved with aseptic meningitis, or encephalitis occurring with nuchal rigidity (stiff neck), somnolence, confusion, dysarthria, convulsions, alterations in consciousness, weakness, and coma. Hepatosplenomegaly, hepatitis, pancreatitis, myocarditis, and anterior myelitis are sometimes seen, more often in tropical countries (Hubâlek & Halouzka, 1999; Platonov, Shipulin, Shipulina, Tyutyunnik, Frolochkina, Lanciotti, et al., 2001). The fatality rate is highest for those who develop acute encephalitis, which is more likely in those over 60 years of age. Symptoms typically develop 2–6 days after exposure. Depression, myalgias, weakness, and lassitude frequently accompany a long convalescence but permanent sequelae have not been reported. Because there is no specific treatment available, care is supportive (Fisher-Hoch & McCormick, 2000; Hubâlek & Halouzka, 1999). The elderly, and those who are immunosuppressed, such as those with HIV, are especially vulnerable to severe illness (Szilak & Minamoto, 2000).

In 1996, a major outbreak of West Nile fever occurred in Bucharest and the lower Danube valley of Romania. With about 500 clinical cases of illness (393 confirmed), thousands of antibody conversions, and a case fatality rate of nearly 10%, this outbreak was the largest arboviral illness in Europe since the epidemics caused by the Sindbis virus in the 1980s (Hubâlek & Halouzka, 1999; Petersen & Roehrig, 2001). Investigators from the National Center for Infectious Diseases were called in to further investigate the Romanian outbreak. Through case control studies, investigators concluded that meningoencephalitic illness was associated with age over 70 years, residence in a house as opposed to an apartment, seeing mosquitoes in the home, the person recalling being bitten by a mosquito five or more times a day, and spending more time outdoors (Han, Popovici, Alexander, Laurentia, Tengelsen, Cernescu, et al., 1999; "NCID investigates West Nile," 1997). Important aspects of this outbreak were the emergence of West Nile fever in epidemic form in a temperate climate as well as its emergence in an urban area in addition to the surrounding rural one.

Investigators have speculated about various factors that may contribute to West Nile fever outbreaks, including heavy rain, flooding, irrigation, and higher than usual temperatures, possibly related to global warming. Also at question is whether and how an arbovirus could overwinter in an adverse climate (Hubálek, Halouzka, & Juricová, 1999). Various possibilities include persistence in hibernating female mosquitos or chronically infected birds or frogs, or reintroduction by chronically infected birds from tropical or subtropical climates who migrated into the area (Hubálek & Halouzka, 1999). In the case of the Romanian outbreak, phylogenetic studies indicated that the virus might have been introduced from birds migrating from sub-Saharan Africa to north Africa to southern Europe (Savage, Ceianu, Nicolescu, Karabatsos, Lanciotti, Vladimiresch, et al., 1999). In 1997, a central European outbreak occurred in the Czech republic (Hubálek, Halouzka, & Juricová, 1999). In 1997 and 1998, sporadic infections continued in Romania, and in two cases the original diagnosis was measles (Cernescu, Nedelcu, Tardei, Ruta, & Tsai, 2000). An outbreak also occurred in the Volograd region of Russia from July through September, 1999, with a varying reported number of suspected cases (826 in one report and 942 in another), of which 84 developed meningoencephalitis and 40 were fatal (Petersen & Roehrig, 2001; Platonov et al., 2001).

In the 1999 New York outbreak, 62 human cases were identified, with 7 deaths. Most occurred in New York City but cases were detected in counties surrounding New York City and in one Canadian citizen who visited New York City in late August and who developed encephalitis on September 5th that was ultimately fatal (Centers for Disease Control and Prevention, 1999b; Enserink, 2000). The wane in reported cases by the end of October was attributed to both cooler weather and the mosquito control programs undertaken. New York City conducted intensive programs of aerial and ground spraying to control mosquitos, and did door-to-door surveys to look for antibody seroprevalence and find those who did not become ill in order to better understand components of infection. Hotlines were set up and mosquito repellents distributed through local firehouses. Public education about avoiding mosquito exposure and about remaining inside during pesticide spraying took place through the media including the Internet (Centers for Disease Control and Prevention, 1999b).

As with the Romanian outbreak, questions were raised about how West Nile virus emerged in an urban, temperate area such as New

York City. Ideas included those mentioned earlier as well as the illegal importation of one or more exotic infected birds, entry to the U.S. through hurricane winds of infected tropical bird(s), entry of an infected traveler from Africa or another endemic area, transportation of an infected mosquito by jet from an endemic area, or even a bioterrorist attack. Of course, even within New York City, green areas and pooled water abide, providing a friendlier environment for vectors. Concern that with the fall migration birds could bring the virus with them to the southern states or to other countries was voiced. Studies indicated the West Nile virus in the New York outbreak was closely related to that detected in a goose from Israel (Giladi et al., 2001; Lanciotti et al., 1999). At the end of October 1999, dead crows and other birds elsewhere on the Atlantic coast (e.g., in Baltimore) were found to harbor West Nile virus. Scientists concluded that either the virus had spread south with migrating birds or the virus had been in the area for a period of time and had just been recognized ("West Nile virus—Migrating . . . ," 1999). There was also concern that the virus might overwinter in vectors living in subway tunnels or basements (Cowley & Kalb, 1999). By February 2000, New York was proactively preparing for the possibility of another outbreak and hiring additional health department staff who had expertise in arboviral infections. And another outbreak did come. At the end of 2000, there were 21 confirmed cases from Connecticut, New York, and New Jersey and 5 deaths (Centers for Disease Control and Prevention, 2001b; "West Nile virus, human cases—USA," 1999). In the U.S., the West Nile virus has been found in birds as far north as Vermont and New Hampshire and also in Canada. It has been found as far south as the Florida Keys and Louisiana (Cornell University Center for the Environment, 2001). In Israel, a human outbreak occurred in 1999 affecting 2 persons and in 2000 affecting 415 persons, of which 33 died (Chowers, Lang, Nassar, Ben-David, Giladi, Rubenshtein, et al., 2001; Giladi, Metzkor-Cotter, Martin, Siegman, Igra, Korczyn, Rosso, et al., 2001). Also in 2000, France experienced an epizootic outbreak in horses, goats, camels, and other animals leading to some import restrictions on these animals from other countries ("West Nile virus, horses," 2001). Economic consequences follow both human and animal outbreaks. In France, the 2000 outbreak in horses resulted in the cancellation of many equestrian events resulting in job layoffs and other loss of income (Murgue, Murri, Zientara, Durand, Durand, & Zeller, 2001). Other West Nile virus epidemics/epizootics than those mentioned in this chapter have included Israel (1951-1954, 1957, human; 1997, 1998, 1999, geese); South Africa (1974, human); Morocco (1996, horses), Tunisia (1997, humans); Italy (1998, horses); Russia (1999, humans, birds); and the U.S. (1999, 2000, horses). By late November 2001, 48 U.S. human West Nile virus encephalitis cases had been reported: New York (12), Florida (10), New Jersey (7), Connecticut (6), Maryland (6), Pennsylvania (3), Massachusetts (2), Georgia (1), and Louisiana (1) (Centers for Disease Control and Prevention, 2001c). Alabama had one possible case. Thus, the geographic range of West Nile fever had widened.

The 1999 New York outbreak called into question how prepared the U.S. was to handle a large vector-borne disease outbreak. The Centers for Disease Control and Prevention and the U.S. Department of Agriculture convened a meeting in November 1999 to establish guidelines to monitor and prevent future outbreaks. The recommendations included

- active mosquito and bird surveillance for West Nile virus, especially for crows, in areas from Massachusetts to Texas along the Atlantic and Gulf coasts;
- veterinary surveillance for reporting neurological illnesses in animals, especially horses;
- enhanced human surveillance to report viral encephalitis and aseptic meningitis in humans;
- prevention through mosquito control programs;
- public education about prevention of vector-borne diseases, including information about modes of transmission;
- recommendations regarding health department resources needed, rapid data exchange mechanisms, and needed research;
- making funds available for surveillance activities to see if the West Nile virus survived the winter, and if it did to ascertain the distribution along the Atlantic and Gulf coasts.
  (Centers for Disease Control and Prevention, 2000).

Detailed information about surveillance and control can be found in the document by CDC (2001a).

SUMMARY

The emergence of West Nile virus as an epidemic illness in temperate and urban climates is an example of how circumstances can broaden the scope and impact of an endemic disease when new territory is affected. Its emergence constituted a major U.S. public health endeavor, particularly in the northeastern states. West Nile virus appears to have established itself as an enzootic disease on the eastern seaboard. Large avian dieoffs may forecast human epidemics. Thus, health care professionals in that area need to be alert for febrile patients who might be infected with West Nile virus. However, for every obvious infection, there may be 120 to 160 inapparent infections since the majority of West Nile virus infections are asymptomatic (Craven & Roehrig, 2001). Because no specific treatment is available, although ribavirin has been used in a small number of persons, the development of an efficacious, safe vaccine especially for use in immunosuppressed persons might be useful. Surveillance needs to be continued along with appropriate mosquito control measures (see Appendix C, Table 5), and public education. A detailed review of many aspects of West Nile virus may be found in the July–August 2001 volume of *Emerging Infectious Diseases*, which is online at http://www.cdc.gov/eid.

REFERENCES

Centers for Disease Control and Prevention. (1999a). Outbreak of West Nile-like viral encephalitis—New York, 1999. *Morbidity and Mortality Weekly Report, 48*, 845–849.

Centers for Disease Control and Prevention. (1999b). Update: West Nile virus encephalitis—New York, 1999. *Morbidity and Mortality Weekly Report, 48*, 944–946, 955.

Centers for Disease Control and Prevention. (2000). Guidelines for surveillance, prevention, and control of West Nile virus infection—United States. *Morbidity and Mortality Weekly Report, 49*, 25–28.

Centers for Disease Control and Prevention. (2001a). *Epidemic/epizootic West Nile virus in the United States: Revised guidelines for surveillance, prevention, and control.* [Online]. Available: http://www.cdc.gov/ncidod/dobid/westnile/resources

Centers for Disease Control and Prevention. (2001b). Serosurveys for West Nile virus infection—New York and Connecticut counties, 2000. *Morbidity and Mortality Weekly Report, 50*, 37–39.

Centers for Disease Control and Prevention. (2001c). Weekly update: West Nile Virus activity—United States, November 14–20, 2001. *Morbidity and Mortality Weekly Report, 50*, 1061–1062.

Cernescu, C., Nedelcu, N. I., Tardei, G., Ruta, S., & Tsai, T. F. (2000). Continued transmission of West Nile Virus to humans in southeastern. Romania, 1997–1998. *Journal of Infectious Diseases, 181*, 710–712.

Chowers, M. Y., Lang, R., Nassar, F., Ben-David, D., Giladi, M., Rubinshtein, E., et al. (2001). Clinical characteristics of the West Nile fever outbreak, Israel, 2000. *Emerging Infectious Diseases, 7,* 675–678.

Cowley, G., & Kalb, C. (1999, October 11). Anatomy of an outbreak. *Newsweek,* 76–78.

Craven, R. B., & Roehrig, J. T. (2001). West Nile virus. *Journal of the American Medical Association, 286,* 651–653.

Enserink, M. (2000). The enigma of West Nile. *Science, 290,* 1482–1484.

Fisher-Hoch, S. P., & McCormick, J. B. (2000). West Nile fever. In G. T. Strickland (Ed.), *Hunter's tropical medicine and emerging infectious diseases* (8th ed., pp. 245–246). Philadelphia: WB Saunders.

Giladi, M., Matzkor-Cotter, E., Martin, D. A., Siegman-Igra, Y., Korczyn, A. D., Rosso, R., et al. (2001). West Nile encephalitis in Israel, 1999: The New York connection. *Emerging Infectious Diseases, 7,* 659–661.

Han, L. L., Popovici, F., Alexander, J. P., Jr., Laurentia, V., Tengelsen, L. A., Cernescu, C., et al. (1999). Risk factors for West Nile virus infection and meningoencephalitis, Romania, 1996. *Journal of Infectious Diseases, 179,* 230–233.

Hubâlek, Z., & Halouzka, J. (1999). West Nile fever—a reemerging mosquito-borne viral disease in Europe. *Emerging Infectious Diseases,* 5, 643–650.

Hubâlek, Z., Halouzka, J., & Juricovâ, Z. (1999). West Nile fever in Czechland. *Emerging Infectious Diseases,* 5, 594–595.

Lanciotti, R. S., Roehrig, J. T., Deubel, V., Smith, J., Parker, M., Steele, K., et al. (1999). Origin of the West Nile virus responsible for an outbreak of encephalitis in the northeastern United States. *Science, 286,* 2333–2337.

Murgue, B., Murri, S., Zientara, S., Durand, B., Durand, J-P., & Zeller, H. (2001). West Nile outbreak in horses in southern France, 2000: The return after 35 years.*Emerging Infectious Diseases, 7,* 692–696.

NCID investigates West Nile fever outbreak in Romania. (1997). *NCID Focus, 6*(1), unpaginated.

Petersen, L. R., & Roehrig, J. T. (2001). West Nile virus: A reemerging global pathogen. *Emerging Infectious Diseases, 7,* 611–614.

Platonov, A. E., Shipulin, G. A., Shipulina, O. Y., Tyutyunnik, E. N., Frolochkina, T., Lanciotti, R. S., et al. (2001). Outbreak of West Nile virus infection, Volgograd region, Russia, 1999. *Emerging Infectious Diseases, 7,* 128–132.

Preston, R. (1999, October 18 and 25). West Nile mystery. *The New Yorker,* 90–95.

Savage, H. M., Ceianu, C., Nicolescu, G., Karabatsos, N., Lanciotti, R., Vladimiresch, A., et al. (1999). Entomologic and avian investigations of an epidemic of West Nile fever in Romania in 1996, with serologic and molecular characterization of a virus isolate from mosquitoes. *American Journal of Tropical Medicine and Hygiene, 61,* 600–611.

Smithburn, K. C., Hughes, T. P., Burke, A. W., & Paul, J. H. (1940). A neurotropic virus isolated from the blood of a native of Uganda. *American Journal of Tropical Medicine, 20,* 471–492.

Szilak, I., & Minamoto, G. Y. (2000). West Nile viral encephalitis in an HIV-positive woman in New York. *New England Journal of Medicine, 342,* 59–60.

West Nile virus, horses—France. (2001, January 13). *ProMED Digest,* unpaginated.

West Nile virus: Migrating birds: Request for information. (1999). *ProMED Digest 99*(241), unpaginated.

West Nile virus—USA. (1999). *ProMED Digest 99*(272), unpaginated.

Part III

Special Considerations

21

The Role of Infection in Some Cancers and Chronic Diseases

Felissa R. Lashley

It is relatively recently that the association has been made between infection with a microbial agent and the development of a cancer or chronic disease, particularly one for which no cause had been established. For some of these conditions, the causative involvement of microbes has been established, for others the association is very strong, and for the rest evidence is suggestive but definitive association is lacking. Difficulties in establishing microbial etiology include the following: the disease is *not* in fact due to an infectious agent, the disease condition is rare, technologies for detection are not advanced enough to detect the microbe, characteristics of the microbe make it difficult to detect, there is failure to consider an infectious etiology for a specific disease, technology is not being appropriately applied, an organism may trigger a host immune response that continues even when the viable organism is no longer present or persists at low levels that are difficult to detect (Fredricks & Relman, 1998), or it may produce a toxin that in turn causes the chronic condition. Clinical, epidemiological, and pathological characteristics may suggest a microbial etiology for certain cancers and chronic diseases. These include seasonality, occurrence in case clusters or epidemic curve, diseases associated with high fever or leukemoid reaction, pathological changes suggestive of an infectious process, response to antimicrobial therapy

(Fredricks & Relman, 1998), and similarities with animal diseases known to be caused by an infectious agent. Some of the microbes associated with a given cancer or chronic disease have recently been identified and are therefore considered emerging; others have been known for a long period of time. The best rationale for seeking to demonstrate a microbial etiology is the potential for successful prevention and treatment.

LINKING SPECIFIC MICROBIAL ORGANISMS WITH CANCERS AND CHRONIC DISEASES

Table 21.1 lists some cancers and chronic diseases for which a microbial etiology is established or strongly suspected. Worldwide, it is estimated that infection may be responsible overall for 15% of malignancies—7% in the developed world and 22% in the developing world. This may be accomplished through the following mechanisms: persistence of the microbe causing chronic inflammation, direct transformation of cells, or immunosuppression (Kuper, Adami, & Trichopoulos, 2000). Human T-lymphotropic virus type I, *Helicobacter pylori*, human herpesvirus 8, and *Chlamydia pneumoniae* are discussed below as examples of specific known associations between emerging microbes and disease. Prion diseases such as Creutzfeldt-Jakob disease, a neurological condition, are discussed in chapter 17. Other associations are under investigation. For example, retroviruses have been suggested as having a role in the etiology or pathogenesis of schizophrenia but this is not established (Karlsson, Bachmann, Schröder, McArthur, Torrey, & Yolken, 2001).

Human T-Lymphotropic Virus, Type I (HTLV-I)

HTLV-I is a complex human oncogenic retrovirus first described in 1980 (Mandell, Bennett, & Dolin, 2000; Poiesz, Ruscetti, Gazdar, Bunn, Minna, & Gallo, 1980). It causes adult T-cell leukemia/lymphoma (ATL) and a HTLV-I-associated myelopathy/tropical spastic paraparesis (HAM/TSP), and in adults has also been linked with uveitis, HTLV-associated arthritis, polymyositis, Sjögren syndrome, and invasive cervical cancer (Danella & Blattner, 2000; Edlich, Arnette, & Williams, 2000). The cumulative lifetime risk in HTLV-I infected people

TABLE 21.1 Selected Chronic Diseases for Which Microbial Etiology Is Known or Suggested

Disease(s)	Putative or Established Microbial Agent(s)	Comments
Adult T-cell leukemia/lymphoma	Human T-lymphotropic virus type I	Discussed in text.
Bladder cancer	*Schistosoma haematobium*	Schistosomiasis from a trematode parasite leads to urinary tract lesions that may result in bladder carcinoma (squamous cell), probably from prolonged irritation leading to hyperplasia and malignancy. Prevalent in Africa.
Burkitt's lymphoma Hodgkin's disease Leiomyosarcoma Nasopharyngeal carcinoma	Human herpesvirus 4 (Epstein-Barr virus) (EBV)	EBV has been linked to a variety of human cancers and is considered a group 1 carcinogen. Other genetic or environmental conditions, however, may play cofactor roles. It also causes infectious mononucleosis.
Castleman's disease (multicentric)	Human herpesvirus 8 (HHV-8)	Discussed in text.
Cervical carcinoma and less strong association for vulvar intraepithelial neoplasia vaginal intraepithelial neoplasia penile intraepithelial neoplasia anal carcinomas	Human papilloma viruses (HPVs)	HPVs include more than 70 types, each with a particular tissue preference. HPV types 16, 18, 31, and 33 are associated with anogenital malignancy. HPVs have been implicated in progression from premalignancy for penile, vulvar, and anal carcinomas. Molecular techniques indicate an association between oral cancer and HPV16.

(continued)

TABLE 21.1 *(continued)*

Disease(s)	Putative or Established Microbial Agent(s)	Comments
Cholangiocarcinoma	*Opisthorchis viverrini*	A parasitic liver fluke. Endemic in Thailand and Laos. Chronic infection is usually asymptomatic unless heavy infestation is present.
Cholangiocarcinoma	*Clonorchis sinensis*	A parasitic liver fluke. Endemic in China, Japan, Korea, Taiwan, and Vietnam. Known as a class 2 carcinogen.
Coronary artery disease	*Chlamydia pneumoniae*	Discussed in text.
Creutzfeldt-Jakob disease	Altered prions	Several slowly progressive fatal neurodegenerative diseases with long incubation periods are due to altered prions. See chapter 17 for discussion.
Crohn's disease	Unknown	Chronic inflammatory enteritis (pathologically similar to mycobacterial enteritis) causing abdominal pain, fever, and diarrhea. Extraintestinal manifestations include uveitis and arthritis.
Guillain-Barrê syndrome	*Campylobacter*	May follow *Campylobacter* enteritis. Establishing causal relationship difficult due to rarity of GBS.
Hepatocellular carcinoma (HCC)	Chronic hepatitis B virus infection Chronic hepatitis C virus infection (See chapter 11)	HCC is the result of cirrhosis often secondary to chronic hepatitis B and C viral infections. About two thirds of HCC occurs in Asia. Prevention by hepatitis B vaccine is possible but is not available for hepatitis C. Treatment of chronic hepatitis such as by alpha interferon may decrease long-term risk.

TABLE 21.1 *(continued)*

Disease(s)	Putative or Established Microbial Agent(s)	Comments
Kaposi's sarcoma	Human herpesvirus 8 (HHV-8)	Discussed in text.
Multiple sclerosis (MS)	Human herpesvirus 6 (HHV-6) implicated	Neurotropic virus. MS is a progressive CNS demyelination disease. HHV-6 DNA sequences and antigens have been found associated with MS lesions, but association is speculative.
Peptic ulcer Gastric lymphoma Gastric adenocarcinoma	*Helicobacter pylori*	Discussed in text.
Rheumatoid arthritis	Unknown for most types. See comments.	Joint neutrophilia and reports of some response to antibiotic agents has suggested microbial etiology. Viral, bacterial, fungal, and parasitic agents have all been associated with specific types of arthritis. For example, the Ross River virus can cause polyarthritis as part of its manifestations. *Borrelia burgdorferi*, the agent of Lyme disease, can cause chronic arthritis. *Bartonella henselae* has been suggested as a cause of juvenile rheumatoid arthritis. A type of arthritis also follows parvovirus B19 infection.
Sarcoidosis	Unknown *Mycobacterium*	A multisystem inflammatory disorder. Higher incidence in winter and spring. Can be acute or chronic. Apparent transmission by organ transplantation possible.

(continued)

TABLE 21.1 *(continued)*

Disease(s)	Putative or Established Microbial Agent(s)	Comments
Tropical sprue	Unknown bacteria	Chronic diarrhea, malabsorption, weight loss, fever, fatigue. Endemic and epidemic in tropical countries.
Wegener's granulomatosis	Unknown bacteria	Granulomatous, necrotizing vasculitis involving kidneys and respiratory tract.
Whipple's disease	*Tropheryma whippelii*	A systemic disease featuring abnormal fat deposits in intestinal tissue and lymph nodes. Findings include lymphadenopathy, polyarthritis, weight loss, diarrhea, and malabsorption. Extraintestinal disease can involve the heart and central nervous system. The causative organism is difficult to cultivate. There are many unknowns about the source and route of infection, pathogenesis, host susceptibility, full clinical spectrum, and therapy.

Sources: Brown (2000); Campadelli-Fiume, Mirandola, & Menotti (1999); Centers for Disease Control and Prevention (1998); Connor, Johnson, & Soave (2001); Del Mistro & Chieco Bianchi (2001); Enborn (2001); Fredricks & Relman (1998); Guerrant, Walker, & Weller (1999); Heyll et al. (1994); Lauer & Walker (2001); Maiwald & Relman (2001); Mandell, Bennett, & Dolin (2000); Nachamkin & Blaser (2000); Newman, Rose, & Maier (1997); Pagano (1999); Parkin & Ziegler (2000); Schafer & Sorrell (1999); Siegel et al. (2001); Strickland (2000); Tomsone, Logina, Millers, Chapenko, Kozireva, & Murovska, 2001; Tsukahara, Tsuneoka, Tateishi, Fujita, & Uchida (2001); Uemura et al. (2001); Yuki (2001).

for developing ATL or HAM/TSP is about 5% (Edlich et al., 2000). Infection with *Strongyloides stercoralis* with therapeutic failure in apparently healthy persons may be a marker of HTLV-I infection (Gotuzzo, Arango, deQueiroz-Campos, & Istúriz, 2000).

HTLV-I was the first human retrovirus to be associated with a malignancy, and it is still believed that the entire disease spectrum of HTLV-I is not yet known (Manns, Hisada, & La Grenade, 1999). Retroviruses preferentially infect vertebrates, and in the early part of the 20th century before their structure and function were known, they were described as filterable agents that caused transmissible tumors in chickens (Gallo & Thomson, 1996). Other recently identified important retroviruses that cause human disease include HTLV-II, which causes hairy cell leukemia, and human immunodeficiency virus (HIV)-1, and HIV-2, which cause the immunodeficiency leading to the spectrum of conditions comprising acquired immunodeficiency syndrome (AIDS). Retroviruses are enveloped RNA viruses that have an enzyme known as reverse transcriptase that allows them to make a DNA copy that is integrated into the host's DNA (Armstrong & Cohen, 1999; Edlich et al., 2000). There are three major strains of HTLV-I: Cosmopolitan (with subtypes A–E), Melanesian, and Congo (Danella & Blattner, 2000).

HTLV-I has a worldwide distribution and is considered endemic in southern Japan, the Caribbean basin, the South Pacific, several Latin American countries, and parts of Africa. The prevalence is also high in the southeastern United States and in central Brooklyn where there is a large Caribbean population. Between 10 and 20 million people worldwide are believed to be infected. In endemic areas such as Okinawa, the prevalence rate is as high as 35% (Armstrong & Cohen, 1999; Danella & Blattner, 2000; Edlich et al., 2000; Gotuzzo et al., 2000; Levine, Dosik, Joseph, Felton, Bertoni, Cervantes, et al., 1999). Seroprevalence in women is higher than in men after 20–30 years of age. In most of Europe and the United States the incidence is low, about 0.05% overall, although higher levels have been reported in Italy and in persons from endemic population groups who settled in other countries. Higher seroprevalence is also found in injecting drug users and within affected families (Armstrong & Cohen, 1999; Edlich et al., 2000). HTLV-I is transmitted through sexual contact, parenterally through blood and blood products including contaminated needles, and vertically from mother to child transplacentally and through breast milk. The transplacental route is considered rare (Edlich et al., 2000;

Gotuzzo et al., 2000; Siegel, Gartenhaus, & Kuzel, 2001). Detection in blood is by enzyme-linked immunosorbent assay (ELISA) for screening with positive detection followed by Western blot for confirmation (Gotuzzo et al., 2000). Nucleic acid detection using polymerase chain reaction (PCR) is also used and antigen capture assays are being developed (Danella & Blattner, 2000). HTLV-I is also diagnosed through detecting the proviral DNA in tumor cells by using PCR techniques (Armstrong & Cohen, 1999).

ATL was first described in Japan in 1977, and the etiologic connection to HTLV-I was made in 1982. ATL may account for about 50% of all adult lymphoid malignancies, but only less than 5% of HTLV-I carriers develop ATL, and the precise steps leading to cancer development are not known (Tsukasaki, Koeffler, & Tomonaga, 2000). Polymorphisms in the tumor necrosis factor and other genetic factors appear to be involved in susceptibility to ATL development (Tsukasaki, Miller, Kubota, Takeuchi, Fujimoto, Ikeda, et al., 2001). There are four clinical subtypes: acute ATL, chronic ATL, smoldering ATL, and the lymphoma (lymphomatous) type ATL. Acute ATL is seen in 50%–60% of patients. Onset is usually in adults approximately 50 years of age. Clinical features include leukemia, lymphadenopathy, hepatosplenomegaly, and skin and bone lesions. Flower-like lymphocytes may be observed (Centers for Disease Control and Prevention, 1993; Mandell et al., 2000). Hypercalcemia is very frequent in acute ATL causing other pathology and may be the first indication of ATL. ATL is rapidly progressive and a 6-month survival is typical. Treatment approaches using antiretroviral agents have indicated some remissions (Danella & Blattner, 2000; Edlich et al., 2000). For a review see Siegel et al. (2001).

HAM/TSP is a chronic neurodegenerative disease with symmetrical spastic paresis. It is sometimes initially confused with multiple sclerosis. Symptoms include difficulty walking, pain, stiffness, lower back pain, numbness of legs, paresthesias, and impotence. Bladder and bowel dysfunction including urinary retention and incontinence may occur. About one-third have upper limb weakness (Danella & Blattner, 2000; Edlich et al., 2000). Symptoms can begin with a stiff gait only. HAM/TSP can be rapidly progressive in older people or in those who receive HTLV-I contaminated blood but is more typically progressive over a period of about 10 years. Treatment generally consists of supportive therapy, corticosteroids, and antiretroviral agents (Danella & Blattner, 2000; Edlich et al., 2000). Full diagnostic guidelines are given by the World Health Organization (1989).

In an effort to prevent transmission through blood transfusion, screening of blood donors for HTLV-I began in 1988 in the United States and is in place in some other countries such as Japan. Counseling regarding risk and ways to prevent transmission (such as use of latex condoms for sexual relationships, not sharing needles, and avoiding the breastfeeding of infants in developed countries) should be provided to those found to harbor HTLV-I (Centers for Disease Control and Prevention, 1993). Health care workers are at risk through parenteral exposure to infected blood. That risk is estimated to be equal to or lower than that of acquiring HIV (Edlich et al., 2000).

Helicobacter pylori

H. pylori is causally associated with primary peptic ulcer disease both gastric and duodenal, gastric adenocarcinoma, and mucosa-associated lymphoid tissue (MALT) gastric lymphoma as well as gastritis and, in some cases, recurrent abdominal pain of childhood (Leontiadis, Sharma, & Howden, 1999; Vemura, Okamoto, Yamamoto, Matsumura, Yamaguchi, Yamakido, et al., 2001). Each year in the United States, about 7 million people are affected by *H. pylori*-related diseases (Christensen, 1999). Learning the nature of these associations changed therapy for these disorders, allowing cures through the use of antimicrobial agents. Because of its association with gastric cancer, *H. pylori* has been called a class I carcinogen by the World Health Organization (IARC Working Group on the Evaluation of Carcinogenic Risks to Humans, 1994).

It was not until 1982 that this organism was isolated (Marshall, 1983). It was originally named as a member of the *Campylobacter* genus, and was given its present name in 1989. *Helicobacter pylori* is a gram-negative rod shaped, urease producing, microaerophilic bacterium that has multiple unipolar flagella and is thus motile (Fix & Morris, 2000). It is usually spiral shaped but may assume a coccoid form under stress and in this form is difficult to culture. It can remain viable and be cultured from water after 10 days and can live in the coccoid form more than a year. Its urease enzyme allows it to create a favorable microenvironment in the gastric epithelium where it causes gastric inflammation (Parsonnet, 1998).

H. pylori is said to be one of the most common infections worldwide (Fix & Morris, 2000). The organism may have a coexistence with humans that spans over 100,000 years, and was possibly acquired from sheep via milk (Christensen, 1999). In developing areas, infection occurs early in childhood, while in developed areas infection occurs later. Initial infection may be associated with a self-limited illness of nausea, vomiting, abdominal pain, and diarrhea or be asymptomatic (Fix & Morris, 2000). The prevalence of infection with *H. pylori* in the developing world is close to 90% while in developed countries it is about 47%–60% by the seventh decade of life (Fallone, 1999). There is an inverse relationship with socioeconomic status across populations (Fix & Morris, 2000). In the EUROGAST study of 3,000 subjects in 13 countries, the prevalence of *H. pylori* infection for lowest, middle, and higher socioeconomic groups were respectively 85%, 52%, and 11% (EUROGAST Study Group, 1993). Clustering of infection has been noted, for instance among submarine crews, within families, and in institutions (Fix & Morris, 2000). Some of the aggregation of gastric cancer in families may be due to familial clustering of *H. pylori* infection (Brenner, Bode, & Boeing, 2000). Poor sanitation, overcrowded conditions, and contaminated water facilitate infection. Other factors may contribute to *H. pylori* infection that are specific to the host (such as genetic factors, immune status, and sociocultural factors), and the organism (such as strain of organism, virulence factors, degree of infectivity) (Gold & Marty, 1997).

There is uncertainty about how *H. pylori* is transmitted (Parsonnet, Shmuely, & Haggerty, 1999). In humans it is present in vomitus and in stools. Gastroenteritis facilitates exposure to stool and vomitus, perhaps even by aerosolized material that may aid in transmission, especially in countries where such illness is common (Parsonnet et al., 1999). The mode of transmission is believed to be person to person by the fecal-oral, gastrointestinal-oral (documented spread iatrogenically by endoscopy), and possibly by the oral-oral route. The evidence for the latter is inferred by the findings of the organism in dental plaque and saliva; however, there is little concordance between spouses, and patients are not usually reinfected by their spouse. Environmental sources such as water or water-contaminated food may act as vehicles (Parsonnet, 1998; Parsonnet et al., 1999). Other *Helicobacter* species are known and may cause disease in the immunocompromised (Solnick & Schauer, 2001). Humans are the only known reservoir for *H. pylori*, but other species of *Helicobacter* are found in animals (Fallone, 1999), and *H. fennelliae* and *H. cinaedi* reside in the lower gastrointestinal tract causing diarrhea in immunocompromised persons (Gold &

Marty, 1997). *H. pylori* may be acquired by laboratory cats, leading to speculation (but not evidence) that domestic animals could transmit the organisms to humans (Parsonnet, 1998; Parsonnet et al., 1999). In Pennsylvania, one study found that drinking water from wells and other sources containing *H. pylori* was associated with a risk of developing peptic ulcers ("*Helicobacter pylori*, ulcers and drinking water—USA," 1999).

The method of detection and diagnosis depends on the level of specificity necessary. Techniques can be invasive (usually endoscopic) or noninvasive. Invasive techniques depend on histological findings, culture of the organism and/or the rapid urease test for diagnosis. Non-invasive techniques include the carbon-labeled urea breath test based on the characteristic of *H. pylori* to be urease producing, and serologic testing via ELISA (Fix & Morris, 2000; Smith & Parsonnet, 1998).

Not all who are colonized with *H. pylori* develop chronic infection and disease. More than 95% of duodenal and 70%–90% of gastric ulcers are associated with *H. pylori*, and 11%–22% of those infected will develop peptic ulcer disease within 10 years (Unge, 1998). Many factors potentially interact to determine who will remain asymptomatic and who will develop complications such as peptic ulcer and gastric malignancy (Day & Sherman, 1999).

H. pylori has also been associated in the literature with nongastrointestinal chronic conditions such as bronchiectasis, sudden infant death syndrome, coronary artery disease, and chronic urticaria (Mawhorter & Lauer, 2001; Wustlich, Brehler, Luger, Pohle, Domschke, & Foerster, 1999). The evidence for these associations has been carefully reviewed, and has not been found to be convincing when subjected to appropriate controls and evaluated for design flaws. Leontiadis, Sharma, and Howden (1999) establish nine criteria by which to judge such studies: "Is the evidence from true experiments in humans? Is the association strong? Is the association consistent from study to study? Is the temporal relationship correct? Is there a dose-response relationship? Does the association make epidemiological sense? Does the association make biological sense? Is the association specific? Is the association analogous to a previously proven causal association?" (p. 926).

In adults, eradication treatment for peptic ulcers is recommended. Typically this includes a proton pump inhibitor such as omeproazole or lansoprazole plus clarithromycin and amoxicillin or metronidazole twice a day for 7–14 days or a prepackaged triple therapeutic agent (Prevpac, consisting of lansoprazole, amoxicillin, and clarithromycin). Other regimens may be used subsequently for those in whom treatment fails (Graham, Rakel, Fendrick, Go, Marshall, Peura, et al., 1999; Hunt, Fallone, Thomson, & Canadian *Helicobacter* Study Group, 1999). Using ranitidine bismuth citrate, amoxicillin, clarithromycin, and metronidazole twice daily for 5 days is also said to result in high efficacy and higher adherence because of the shorter length of therapy (Gisbert, Marcos, Gisbert, & Pajares, 2001). Eradication of *H. pylori* in MALT lymphomas causes regression in about 60% of patients (Unge, 1998). Regression of a gastric T-cell lymphoma by eradicating *H. pylori* has also been described (Bariol, Field, Vickers, & Ward, 2001). Whether or not to eradicate *H. pylori* in cases of dysphagia or in those who are asymptomatically affected is still the subject of controversy and some have found no benefit in doing so (Talley, Vakil, Ballard, & Fennerty, 1999). Improved living conditions will reduce the prevalence of *H. pylori* worldwide; however, societal changes such as increased day care could alter this (Blaser, 1999). Already there has been a decrease of infection in the United States along with a decreased frequency of peptic ulcer disease and gastric cancer (Christensen, 1999). Oral vaccine development shows promise and, if successful, will provide prevention at the population level (Fix & Morris, 2000).

Human Herpesvirus Type 8 (HHV-8)

Experience with Kaposi's sarcoma (KS) in the context of the HIV epidemic had led to the suspicion that an infectious agent was responsible for the disease because of epidemiological observations about the spread and transmission. KS is considered an endothelial cell tumor that occurs in four epidemiological groups: 1) classical KS, which occurs in older men of Mediterranean and Eastern European Jewish origin and has an indolent course; 2) endemic KS, which occurs in equatorial Africa across age groups but mainly in children and adults under 40 years of age and which can be aggressive; 3) iatrogenic KS, which is seen in immunosuppressed non-AIDS patients, mainly those who are organ transplant recipients; and 4) HIV/AIDS-associated KS. In all age and epidemiological groupings, men are preferentially affected (Ensoli, Sgadari, Barillari, Sirianni, Sturzl, & Monini, 2001; Lashley, 2000).

HHV-8 is also known as Kaposi's sarcoma-associated herpesvirus (KSHV), and was discovered in material from a Kaposi's sarcoma (KS) lesion in a patient with AIDS in 1994 (Chang, Cesarman, Pessin, Lee, Culpepper, Knowles, et al., 1994). It was quickly linked to a causal relationship with KS, however many researchers believe that HHV-8 is necessary but not sufficient to cause KS (Iscovich, Boffetta, Franceschi, Azizi, & Sarid, 2000; Jaffe & Pellett, 1999). Since that time it has also been linked to primary effusion lymphoma (formerly called body cavity-based lymphoma) which is a non-Hodgkin lymphoma, and some cases of multicentric Castleman's disease, which is a hyperplastic B-cell lymphoproliferative disorder (Olsen & Moore, 2000). Association with multiple myeloma has been postulated but not confirmed (Berenson & Vescio, 1999).

HHV-8 is one of eight herpesviruses known to infect humans. One other, HHV-4 or Epstein-Barr virus, has also been closely linked to malignancy development. HHV-8 is classified in the herpesvirus family in the Gammaherpesviridae subfamily as a rhadinovirus (Armstrong & Cohen, 1999). There are several variants or types (Schulz, 1999; Schulz & Moore, 1999). Transmission occurs horizontally by nonsexual transmission among children and there have been a few cases of parenteral transmission from transplantation and transfusion described as well as vertical transmission from mother to child (Schulz, 1999). Sexual transmission has also been described, particularly in men who have sex with men, and HHV-8 has been found in saliva and in seminal fluid (Schulz, 2000). Orogenital transmission has been described (Dukers et al., 2000). There are still some unknowns regarding transmission, and the reason(s) for the preponderance of KS in males.

KS lesions may appear on the skin as reddish, purple, or brown patches; plaques or nodules and are often multiple. When associated with HIV infection they may affect the oral cavity, lymphatics, gastrointestinal tract, lung, liver, adrenal glands, and the heart, and may be disseminated. Complications can arise because of the size of the tumor. In the classical form, the disease is only slowly progressive and is usually confined to the legs. Treatment may be with radiation or chemotherapy and newer approaches such as anti-angiogenesis compounds are underway (Mitsuyasu, 2000). HIV/AIDS-associated KS was first reported in 1981 in the U.S. as a forecaster of the HIV epidemic, and in recent years has been declining in frequency for unknown reasons (Lashley, 2000). Some believe that the decline is due to decreased viral loads due to protease inhibitor therapy. Information about HHV-8 in Castleman's disease and in primary effusion lymphomas is sparse because of the relative rarity of these conditions. In regard to multiple myeloma, HHV-8 has been found in most of these patients and it has been postulated that pathology might occur by inducing changes in the bone marrow, although criteria for causality have not been met (Berenson & Vescio, 1999). HIV may be involved in the pathogenesis in patients with AIDS (Mitsuyasu, 2000).

HHV-8 is considered causally associated with KS, with the rarer multicentric Castleman's disease and primary effusion lymphoma, and is specific to this subset of lymphomas (Cesarman & Knowles, 1999). However, the mechanism by which causation occurs has not yet been elucidated, nor is whether or not other conditions or cofactors are necessary for malignancy development in addition to HHV-8. Other unknowns exist such as the reason for the preferential infection of males and the decline seen in the U.S. among HIV-infected males in recent years. Antiretroviral therapy, especially HAART, has elicited positive treatment responses.

Chlamydia pneumoniae

Known cardiovascular risk factors such as smoking do not fully explain noted geographical and temporal variations in coronary heart disease. Thus, microbial agents have been suspected of playing a role in etiology and attention has focused on cytomegalovirus, *Helicobacter pylori*, and *Chlamydia pneumoniae* (Mawhorter & Lauer, 2001; Muhlestein, 2000; Ngeh & Gupta, 2001; Ridker et al., 2001). The most attention has centered upon *Chlamydia pneumoniae*, which has been suspected of playing a causative role in the development of atherosclerosis and coronary heart disease, both major causes of morbidity and mortality. The basis for this suspicion has been the recovery of the organism in atherosclerotic plaques, and the long held idea that an infectious agent might trigger the inflammation that occurs during the development of atherosclerosis (Ridker, Kundsin, Stampfer, Poulin, & Hennekens, 1999).

C. pneumoniae is a unique bacterium because it is an obligate intracellular organism that is more characteristic of a virus. It was previously called *Bedsonia* or *Miyagawanella* (Schacter & Alexander, 1998). *Chlamydia* are unable to synthesize adenosine triphosphate and so they have been called energy parasites (Mabey, 2000). The organism is hard to culture, making detection difficult. It has a unique reproductive cycle and contains an elementary body that is the infectious component (Wong, Gallagher, & Ward, 1999). The genus *Chlamydia* is currently known to contain three species that cause disease in humans, one of which, *C. trachomatis*, is responsible for the eye disease trachoma. In fact, it was during a trachoma study in Taiwan in 1965 that *C. pneumoniae* was first found, and it was not until 1983 that its occurrence in a college student with pharyngitis led to the recognition of its major causative niche (Grayston, Kuo, Wang, & Altman, 1986; Mabey, 2000). *C. pneumoniae* is a common cause of bronchitis, pharyngitis, sinusitis, and community-acquired pneumonia. The majority of the population is exposed to the organism early in life with a peak from 5–15 years of age, and infection is often subclinical and unrecognized (Mabey, 2000). Transmission is person to person via respiratory secretions.

Ways that infection might contribute to the development of atherosclerosis include damage to endothelial cells by the microbe or its endotoxins or immune complexes; possible binding of endotoxin to lipoproteins, causing disturbances including alterations of cholesterol metabolism, activation of macrophages leading to cytokine production, upregulation of the major histocompatibility complex, increased synthesis of acute phase proteins such as fibrinogen, enhanced activity of procoagulant mediators leading to a hypercoaguable state, and heat shock protein expression (Gupta & Camm, 1999).

Evidence for the involvement of *C. pneumoniae* in atherosclerosis includes seroepidemiologic studies finding elevated antibodies and immune complexes containing *C. pneumoniae* antigen in patients with acute myocardial infarctions and coronary heart disease, after controlling for confounding factors (Saikku, Leinonen, Mattila, Ekman, Nieminen, Makela, et al., 1988), the presence of *C. pneumoniae* in atherosclerotic plaques observed through electron microscopy studies, immunocytochemical staining, and PCR testing; and in situ hybridization studies. It has been observed that the organism can infect and replicate within macrophages, smooth muscle and endothelial cells, and can be transported to coronary arteries from the respiratory tract. Furthermore, animal model experiments have shown that rabbits infected with *C. pneumoniae* who develop pneumonia can develop atherosclerotic lesions. Other evidence comes from the response to antibiotics (Gupta, 1999; Muhlestein, 2000). The organism is present in many atherosclerotic lesions in viable form and in early lesions associated with pathological changes (Shor & Phillips, 1999). Experimental studies using antibiotics to treat or prevent CHD have been conducted but most have not been prospective and have used a small sample size. In the ROXIS pilot study using roxithromycin in patients with non-Q-wave myocardial infarctions and angina, results appear promising (Gurfinkel, Bozovich, Beck, Testa, Livellara, & Mautner, 1999). Large-scale prospective randomized studies in various populations are needed. The WIZARD study examines outcomes in coronary patients who have an antibiotic added to their regimen (Gurfinkel & Bozovich, 1999). Overall, seroepidemiologic studies demonstrated that having *C. pneumoniae* antibodies conferred a twofold risk for heart disease (Shor & Phillips, 1999); however, negative reports also are found in the literature (Caligiuri, Rottenberg, Nicoletti, Wigzell, & Hansson, 2001; Hoffmeister, Rothenbacher, Wanner, Bode, Persson, Brenner, et al., 2000). *C. pneumoniae* has also been linked to Alzheimer disease, asthma, multiple sclerosis, sarcoidosis, abdominal aortic aneurysm, and reactive arthritis, but no strong causal evidence has yet been presented (Allegra & Blasi, 1999; Blanchard, Armenian, Peeling, Friesen, Shen, & Brunham, 2000; Centers for Disease Control and Prevention, 1999; Stratton, Mitchell, & Sriram, 2000). At this time, it can be said that there is a strong association between *C. pneumoniae* and atherosclerosis but that all criteria for causality have not been completely fulfilled (Shor & Phillips, 1999). If *C. pneumoniae* causes, substantially contributes to, or exacerbates CHD it opens new avenues for both prevention and treatment in at least some cases.

SUMMARY

Links between chronic diseases and microbial agents have been clearly established in a few instances. Many of these agents are newly emergent, having been recognized in the past 30 years. Further work is needed to more clearly delineate other causative relationships. Such work holds promise for new approaches to prevention and treatment.

REFERENCES

Allegra, L., & Blasi, F. (Eds.). (1999). Chlamydia pneumoniae. *The lung and the heart.* Milano: Springer.

Armstrong, D., & Cohen, J. (Eds.). (1999). *Infectious diseases*. London: Mosby.
Bariol, C., Field, A., Vickers, C. R., & Ward, R. (2001). Regression of gastric T cell lymphoma with eradication of *Helicobacter pylori*. *Gut, 48*, 269–271.
Berenson, J. R., & Vescio, R. A. (1999). HHV-8 is present in multiple myeloma patients. *Blood, 93*, 3157–3159.
Blanchard, J. F., Armenian, H. K., Peeling, R., Friesen, P. P., Shen, C., & Brunham, R. C. (2000). The relationship between *Chlamydia pneumoniae* infection and abdominal aortic aneurysm: Case-control study. *Clinical Infectious Diseases, 30*, 946–947.
Blaser, M. J. (1999). Where does *Helicobacter pylori* come from and why is it going away? *Journal of the American Medical Association, 282*, 2260–2262.
Brenner, H., Bode, G., & Boeing, H. (2000). *Helicobacter pylori* infection among offspring of patients with stomach cancer. *Gastroenterology, 118*, 222–224.
Brown, K. E. (2000). Haematological consequences of parvovirus B19 infection. *Baillière's Clinical Haematology, 13*, 245–259.
Caligiuri, G., Rottenberg, M., Nicoletti, A., Wigzell, H., & Hansson, G. K. (2001). *Chlamydia pneumoniae* infection does not induce or modify atherosclerosis in mice. *Circulation, 103*, 2834–2838.
Campadelli-Fiume, G., Mirandola, P., & Menotti, L. (1999). Human herpesvirus 6: An emerging pathogen. *Emerging Infectious Diseases, 5*, 353–356.
Centers for Disease Control and Prevention. (1993). Recommendations for counseling persons infected with human T-lymphotrophic virus, types I and II. *Morbidity and Mortality Weekly Report, 42*(No. RR-9), 1–13.
Centers for Disease Control and Prevention. (1999, January). *Chlamydia pneumoniae—technical information* [On-line]. Available: http://www.cdc.gov/ncidod/dbmd/diseaseinfo/ and select *Chlamydia pneumoniae*.
Cesarman, E., & Knowles, D. M. (1999). The role of Kaposi's sarcoma-associated herpesvirus (KSHV/HHV-8) in lymphoproliferative diseases. *Seminars in Cancer Biology, 9*, 165–174.
Chang, Y., Cesarman, E., Pessin, M. S., Lee, F., Culpepper, J., Knowles, D., et al. (1994). Identification of herpesvirus-like DNA sequences in AIDS-associated Kaposi's sarcoma. *Science, 266*, 1865–1869.
Christensen, D. (1999). Is your stomach bugging you? *Science News, 156*, 234–235.
Connor, B. A., Johnson, E. J., & Soave, R. (2001). Reiter syndrome following protracted symptoms of *Cyclospora* infection. *Emerging Infectious Diseases, 7*, 453–454.
Danella, R. D., & Blattner, W. A. (2000). Human T-lymphotropic virus type I/II infection. In G. T. Strickland (Ed.), *Hunter's tropical medicine and emerging infectious diseases* (8th ed., pp. 192–196). Philadelphia: WB Saunders Co.
Day, A. S., & Sherman, P. M. (1999). Understanding disease outcome following acquisition of *Helicobacter pylori* infection during childhood. *Canadian Journal of Gastroenterology, 13*, 229–234.
Del Mistro, A., & Chieco Bianchi, L. (2001). HPV-related neoplasias in HIV-infected individuals. *European Journal of Cancer, 37*, 1227–1235.
Dukers, N. H., Renwick, N., Prins, M., Geskus, R. B., Schulz, T. F., Weverling, G. J., et al. (2000). Risk factors for human herpesvirus 8 seropositivity and

seroconversion in a cohort of homosexual men. *American Journal of Epidemiology, 151*, 213–224.
Edlich, R. F., Arnette, J. A., & Williams, F. M. (2000). Global epidemic of human T-cell lymphotropic virus type-I (HTLV-I). *Journal of Emergency Medicine, 18*, 109–119.
Enbom, M. (2001). Human herpesvirus 6 in the pathogenesis of multiple sclerosis. *Acta Pathologica, Microbiologica et Immunologica Scandinavica, 109*, 409–411.
EUROGAST Study Group. (1993). Epidemiology of, and risk factors for, *Helicobacter pylori* infection among 3194 asymptomatic subjects in 17 populations. *Gut, 34*, 1672–1676.
Fallone, C. A. (1999). Determinants of ethnic or geographical differences in infectivity and transmissibility of *Helicobacter pylori*. *Canadian Journal of Gastroenterology, 13*, 251–255.
Fix, A. D., & Morris, J. G., Jr. (2000). *Helicobacter pylori* infections. In G. T. Strickland (Ed.), *Hunter's tropical medicine and emerging infectious diseases* (8th ed., pp. 345–348). Philadelphia: WB Saunders.
Fredricks, D. N., & Relman, D. A. (1998). Infectious agents and the etiology of chronic idiopathic diseases. *Current Clinical Topics in Infectious Diseases, 18*, 180–200.
Gallo, R. C., & Thomson, M. M. (1996). Introduction. In P. Höllsberg & D. A. Hafler (Eds.), *Human T-cell lymphotropic virus type I* (pp. 1–10). New York: John Wiley.
Gisbert, J. P., Marcos, S., Gisbert, J. L., & Pajares, J. M. High efficacy of ranitidine bismuth citrate, amoxicillin, clarithromycin and metronidazole twice daily for only five days. *Helicobacter, 6*(2), 81–83.
Gold, B. D., & Marty, A. (1997). *Helicobacter pylori*. In C. R. Horsbaugh, Jr., & A. M. Nelson (Eds.), *Pathology of emerging infections* (pp. 225–241). Washington, DC: American Society for Microbiology.
Gotuzzo, E., Arango, C., deQueiroz-Campos, A., & Istúriz, R. (2000). HTLV-1 in Latin America. *Infectious Disease Clinics of North America, 14*, 211–240.
Graham, D. Y., Rakel, R. E., Fendrick, A. M., Go, M. E., Marshall, B. J., Peura, D. A., et al. (1999). Practical advice on eradicating *Helicobacter pylori* infection. *Postgraduate Medicine, 105*, 137–148.
Grayston, J. T., Kuo, C. C., Wang, S. P., & Altman, J. (1986). A new *Chlamydia psittaci* strian, TWAR, isolated in acute respiratory tract infections. *New England Journal of Medicine, 315*, 161–168.
Guerrant, R. L., Walker, D. H., & Weller, P. F. (Eds.). (1999). *Tropical infectious diseases*. Philadelphia: Churchill Livingstone.
Gupta, S. (1999). Chronic infection in the aetiology of atherosclerosis—focus on *Chlamydia pneumoniae*. *Atherosclerosis, 143*, 1–6.
Gupta, S., & Camm, A. J. (1999). Chronic infection, *Chlamydia*, and heart disease. *Developments in Cardiovascular Medicine, 218*, 1–127.
Gurfinkel, E. P., & Bozovich, G. (1999). Emerging role of antibiotics in atherosclerosis. *American Heart Journal, 138*, S537–S538.
Gurfinkel, E. P., Bozovich, G., Beck, E., Testa, E., Livellara, B., & Mautner, B. (1999). Treatment with the antibiotic roxithromycin in patients with acute non-

Q-wave coronary syndromes: The final report of the ROXIS study. *European Heart Journal, 20,* 121–127.

Helicobacter pylori, ulcers and drinking water—USA. (1999). *ProMED Digest, 99*(133), unpaginated.

Heyll, A., Meckenstock, G., Aul, C., Sohngen, D., Borchard, F., Hadding, U., et al. (1994). Possible transmission of sarcoidosis via allogeneic bone marrow transplantation. *Bone Marrow Transplant, 4,* 161–164.

Hoffmeister, A., Rothenbacher, D., Wanner, P., Bode, G., Persson, K., Brenner, H., et al. (2000). Seropositivity to chlamydial lipopolysaccharide and *Chlamydia pneumoniae,* systemic inflammation and stable coronary artery disease: Negative results of a case-control study. *Journal of the American College of Cardiology, 35,* 112–118.

Hunt, R. H., Fallone, C. A., Thomson, A. B. R., & Canadian *Helicobacter* Study Group. (1999). Canadian *Helicobacter pylori* Consensus Conference update: Infections in adults. *Canadian Journal of Gastroenterology, 13,* 213–217.

IARC Working Group on the Evaluation of Carcinogenic Risks to Humans. (1994). *Schistosomes, liver flukes and* Helicobacter pylori*: Views and expert opinions of an IARC Working Group on the Evaluation of Carcinogenic Risks in Humans,* Monograph 61. Lyon, France: International Agency for Research on Cancer.

Iscovich, J., Boffetta, P., Francheschi, S., Azizi, E., & Sarid, R. (2000). Classic Kaposi sarcoma: Epidemiology and risk factors. *Cancer, 88,* 500–517.

Jaffe, H. W., & Pellett, P. E. (1999). Human herpesvirus 8 and Kaposi's sarcoma—some answers, more questions. *New England Journal of Medicine, 340,* 1912–1913.

Karlsson, H., Bachmann, S., Schröder, J., McArthur, J., Torrey, E. F., & Yolken, R. H. (2001). Retroviral RNA identified in the cerebrospinal fluids and brains of individuals with schizophrenia. *Proceedings of the National Academy of Sciences of the United States of America, 98,* 4634–4639.

Kuper, H., Adami, H.-O., & Trichopoulos, D. (2000). Infections as a major preventable cause of human cancer. *Journal of Internal Medicine, 248,* 171–183.

Lashley, F. R. (2000). The clinical spectrum of HIV infection and its treatment. In J. D. Durham & F. R. Lashley (Eds.), *The person with HIV/AIDS: Nursing perspectives* (3rd ed., pp. 167–270). New York: Springer Publishing Co.

Lauer, G. M., & Walker, B. D. (2001). Hepatitis C virus infection. *New England Journal of Medicine, 345,* 41–52.

Leontiadis, G. I., Sharma, V. K., & Howden, C. W. (1999). Non-gastrointestinal tract associations of *Helicobacter pylori* infection. *Archives of Internal Medicine, 159,* 925–940.

Levine, P. H., Dosik, H., Joseph, E. M., Felton, S., Bertoni, M. A., Cervantes, J., et al. (1999). A study of adult T-cell leukemia/lymphoma incidence in central Brooklyn. *International Journal of Cancer, 80,* 662–666.

Mabey, D. C. W. (2000). Chlamydial infections. In G. T. Strickland (Ed.), *Hunter's tropical medicine and emerging infectious diseases* (8th ed., pp. 349–351). Philadelphia: WB Saunders.

Maiwald, M., & Relman, D. A. (2001). Whipple's disease and *Tropheryma whippelii*: Secrets slowly revealed. *Clinical Infectious Diseases, 32,* 457–463.

Mandell, G. L., Bennett, J. E., & Dolin, R. (Eds.). (2000). *Mandell, Douglas, and Bennett's principles and practice of infectious diseases* (pp. 1862–1873). Philadelphia: Churchill Livingstone.

Manns, A., Hisada, M., & La Grenade, L. (1999). Human T-Lymphotropic virus type I infection. *Lancet, 353*, 1951–1958.

Marshall, B. J. (1983). Unidentified curved bacilli on gastric epithelium in active chronic gastritis. *Lancet, 1*, 1273–1275.

Mawhorter, S. D., & Lauer, M. A. (2001). Is atherosclerosis an infectious disease? *Cleveland Clinic Journal of Medicine, 68*, 449–458.

Mitsuyasu, R. (2000). Update on the pathogenesis and treatment of Kaposi sarcoma. *Current Opinion in Oncology, 12*, 174–180.

Muhlestein, J. B. (2000). Chronic infection and coronary artery disease. *Medical Clinics of North America, 84*, 123–145.

Nachamkin, I., & Blaser, M. J. (2000). *Campylobacter* (2nd ed.). Washington, DC: American Society for Microbiology.

Newman, L. S., Rose, C. S., & Maier, L. A. (1997). Sarcoidosis. *New England Journal of Medicine, 336*, 1224–1234.

Ngeh, J., & Gupta, S. (2001). Inflammation, infection and antimicrobial therapy in coronary disease—where do we currently stand? *Fundamentals of Clinical Pharmacology, 15*(2), 85–93.

Olsen, S. J., & Moore, P. S. (2000). Herpesvirus infections. In G. T. Strickland (Ed.), *Hunter's tropical medicine and emerging infectious diseases* (8th ed., pp. 196–199). Philadelphia: WB Saunders.

Pagano, J. S. (1999). Epstein-Barr virus: The first human tumour virus and its role in cancer. *Proceedings of the Association of American Physicians, 111*, 573–580.

Parkin, D. M., & Ziegler, J. L. (2000). Malignant diseases. In G. T. Strickland (Ed.), *Hunter's tropical medicine and emerging infectious diseases* (8th ed., pp. 94–107). Philadelphia: WB Saunders Co.

Parsonnet, J. (1998). *Helicobacter pylori. Infectious Disease Clinics of North America, 12*, 185–197.

Parsonnet, J., Shmuely, H., & Haggerty, T. (1999). Fecal and oral shedding of *Helicobacter pylori* from healthy infected adults. *Journal of the American Medical Association, 282*, 2240–2245.

Poiesz, B. J., Ruscetti, F. W., Gazdar, A. F., Bunn, P. A., Minna, J. D., & Gallo, R. C. (1980). Detection and isolation of type C retrovirus particles from fresh and cultured lymphocytes of a patient with cutaneous T-cell lymphoma. *Proceedings of the National Academy of Sciences of the United States of America, 77*, 7415–7419.

Ridker, P. M., Danesh, J., Youngman, L., Collins, R., Stampfer, M. J., Peto, R., et al. (2001). A prospective study of *Helicobacter pylori* seropositivity and the risk for future myocardial infarction among socioeconomically similar U.S. men. *Annals of Internal Medicine, 135*, 184–188.

Ridker, P. M., Kundsin, R. B., Stampfer, M. J., Poulin, S., & Hennekens, C. H. (1999). Prospective study of *Chlamydia pneumoniae*, Ig G seropositivity and risks of future myocardial infarction. *Circulation, 99*, 1161–1164.

Saikku, P., Leinonen, M., Mattila, K., Ekman, M. R., Nieminen, M. S., Makela, P. H., et al. (1988). Serological evidence of an association of a novel *Chlamydia*, TWAR, with chronic coronary heart disease and acute myocardial infarction. *Lancet, 2*(8618), 983–986.

Schacter, J., & Alexander, E. R. (1998). Chlamydial infections. In A. S. Evans & P. S. Brachman (Eds.), *Bacterial infections of humans* (3rd ed., pp. 197–222). New York: PlenumMedical Book Co.

Schafer, D. F., & Sorrell, M. F. (1999). Hepatocellular carcinoma. *Lancet, 353*, 1253–1257.

Schulz, T. F. (1999). Epidemiology of Kaposi's sarcoma-associated herpesvirus/ human herpesvirus 8. *Advances in Cancer Research, 76*, 121–160.

Schulz, T. F. (2000). KSVH (HHV8) infection. *Journal of Infection, 41*, 125–129.

Schulz, T. F., & Moore, P. S. (1999). Kaposi's sarcoma-associated herpesvirus: A new human tumor virus, but how? *Trends in Microbiology, 7*, 196–200.

Siegel, R., Gartenhaus, R., & Kuzel, T. (2001). HTLV-I associated leukemia/ lymphoma: Epidemiology, biology and treatment. *Cancer Treatment and Research, 104*, 75–88.

Shor, A., & Phillips, J. I. (1999). *Chlamydia pneumoniae* and atherosclerosis. *Journal of the American Medical Association, 282*, 2071–2073.

Smith, K. L., & Parsonnet, J. (1998). *Helicobacter pylori*. In A. S. Evans & P. S. Brachman (Eds.), *Bacterial infections of humans* (3rd ed., pp. 337–353). New York: Plenum Medical Book Co.

Solnick, J. V., & Schauer, D. B. (2001). Emergence of diverse *Helicobacter* species in the pathogenesis of gastric and enterohepatic diseases. *Clinical Microbiology Reviews, 14*, 59–97.

Stratton, C. W., Mitchell, W. M., & Sriram, S. (2000). Does *Chlamydia pneumoniae* play a role in the pathogenesis of multiple sclerosis? (Editorial). *Journal of Medical Microbiology, 49*(1), 1–3.

Strickland, G. T. (Ed.). (2000). *Hunter's tropical medicine and emerging infectious diseases* (8th ed.). Philadelphia: WB Saunders.

Talley, N. J., Vakil, N., Ballard, E. D. III, & Fennerty, M. B. (1999). Absence of benefit of eradicating *Helicobacter pylori* in patients with nonulcer dyspepsia. *New England Journal of Medicine, 341*, 1106–1111.

Tomsone, V., Logina, I., Millers, A., Chapenko, S., Kozireva, S., & Murovska, M. (2001). Association of human herpesvirus 6 and human herpesvirus 7 with demyelinating diseases of the nervous system. *Journal of Neurovirology, 7*, 564–569.

Tsukahara, M., Tsuneoka, H., Tateishi, H., Fujita, K., & Uchida, M. (2001). *Bartonella* infection associated with systemic juvenile rheumatoid arthritis. *Clinical Infectious Diseases, 32*, E22–E23.

Tsukasaki, K., Koeffler, P., & Tomonaga, M. (2000). Human T-lymphotropic virus type I infection.*Baillière's Clinical Haematology, 13*, 231–243.

Tsukasaki, K., Miller, C. W., Kubota, T., Takeuchi, S., Fujimoto, T., Ikeda, S., et al. (2001). Tumor necrosis factor α polymorphism associated with increased susceptibility to development of adult T-cell leukemia/lymphoma in human T-lymphotropic virus type I carriers. *Cancer Research, 61*, 3770–3774.

Uemura, N., Okamoto, S., Yamamoto, S., Matsumura, N., Yamaguchi, S., Yamakido, M., et al. (2001). *Helicobacter pylori* infection and the development of gastric cancer. *New England Journal of Medicine, 345*, 784–789.

Unge, P. (1998). Are there more clinically important complications of *Helicobacter pylori* infection than peptic ulcer disease? A review of current literature. *Journal of Gastroenterology, 33*(Suppl. 10), 48–52.

Wong, Y-K, Gallagher, P. J., & Ward, M. E. (1999). *Chlamydia pneumoniae* and atherosclerosis. *Heart, 81*, 232–238.

World Health Organization. (1989). Virus diseases: Human T-lymphotropic virus type I, HTLV-I. *Weekly Epidemiological Record, 64*, 382–383.

Wustlich, S., Brehler, R., Luger, T. A., Pohle, T., Domschke, W., & Foerster, E. C. (1999). *Helicobacter pylori* as a possible bacterial focus of chronic urticaria. *Dermatology, 198*, 130–132.

Yuki, N. (2001). Infectious origins of, and molecular mimicry in, Guillain-Barré and Fisher syndromes. *Lancet Infectious Diseases, 1*, 29–37.

22

Travel, Recreation, and Emerging Infectious Diseases

Felissa R. Lashley

Both travel and the seeking of recreational pursuits have increasingly resulted in exposure of persons to emerging infectious diseases they might not otherwise encounter. To some extent, travel and recreation overlap because many engage in recreational activities as part of their travel, and many travel for the specific purpose of recreational pursuits. In regard to travel, tourists increasingly seek more exotic destinations such as tropical rainforests, and business travelers may travel to more remote areas for their activities, which can include private business initiatives, religious or missionary activities, or work on behalf of the government, including the armed services. Virtually any destination can be reached in 36 hours of travel, and many in far less time. This time frame allows for the unrecognized global spread of microbes from one place to another. Ostroff and Kozarsky (1998) state that the "global village of the late 20th century provides global opportunities for disease emergence and transmission" (p. 231). Travel may be daily as in commuting, periodic or seasonal for leisure, tourism or recreation, or long-term for colonization or migration (Martens & Hall, 2000). Increasingly, travel is between developed and developing countries, and vice-versa. It is estimated that among short-term travelers to tropical or subtropical destinations, 50%–75% report some health impairment as a consequence, often due to an infectious agent (Guerrant, Walker, & Weller, 1999). Diarrhea, ranging from self-limited to life-threatening affects 20%–70% of travelers to tropical and subtropical countries. The organisms involved vary and may be bacterial, such as *E. coli*, or parasitic such as microsporidia (see chapter 3) (Müller, Bialek, Kämper, Fatkenheuer, Salzberger, & Franzen, 2001).

TRAVEL

The risk for travel-associated emerging or reemerging infectious diseases is due to several factors:

- New emerging diseases may appear in areas frequented by travelers providing the first information about a new agent outside that region.
- Travelers may encounter infections endemic where they are visiting that are non-endemic for their country of origin, that they then transport back.
- Travelers may seek adventure such as engaging in strenuous or unusual outdoor activities such as cave exploration, eat unusual or local foods sometimes from street vendors, use recreational drugs, come into close contact with animals even in relatively protected environments such as aquariums, or more exposed ones such as when on a safari, or engage in sexual adventures, thus increasing the opportunity to encounter emerging infectious diseases; and
- They may decide to adapt local customs such as walking barefoot and acquiring cutaneous larva migrans, sleeping in exposed areas without mosquito nets and being exposed to mosquitos carrying malaria or dengue, or sleep in accommodations allowing exposure to rodents carrying the agents of hemorrhagic fevers or plague.

People from Asia making the religious pilgrimage to Mecca in 1987 brought an epidemic strain of group A *Neisseria meningitidis* that was transmitted to other pilgrims, who brought it back to sub-Saharan Africa where it caused epidemics (Moore, Reeves, Schwartz, Gellin, & Broome, 1989).

Migrants and immigrants also represent a type of traveller, and at times of turmoil or disaster, large numbers of migrants may be suddenly admitted from developing to developed countries, possibly bringing with them endemic infectious diseases from their countries that are not endemic to their new locale (Gushulak & MacPherson, 2000; Miller, Boyd, Ostrowski, Cooksey, Parise, Gonzaga, et al., 2000). In one report, a woman in Georgia with no risk factors or relevant travel history acquired malaria. It was postulated that resident *Anopheles quadrimaculatus* mosquitoes acted as vectors, and that transmission was related to the woman's housing proximity to that of the housing of seasonal migrant workers who were natives of malaria-endemic countries and who were potentially gametocytemic (MacArthur, Holtz, Jenkins, Newell, Koehler, Parise, et al., 2001). Some of these diseases may be acquired en route, for example if they must traverse or ingest contaminated water to reach their destinations. Frequently, they will then seek unskilled work in restaurants in the developed nation, where the infectious agent they have acquired or harbor is transmitted to residents via a foodborne route (Niler, 2000). Migrants or immigrants may be reexposed to endemic diseases not only when they return to visit in their native country but also when they associate with newly arrived persons from their country or ethnic group (Cookson, Carballo, Nolan, Keystone, & Jong, 2001).

Those migrating or immigrating because of civil unrest or adverse environmental conditions are at high risk for the emergence of disease, because they may be malnourished, stressed, exposed to crowded and unsanitary living conditions where clean water and food may not be available, or vulnerable to sexual predators leading to the acquisition of sexually transmitted diseases. They may not be sheltered from exposure to vectors and animals. An example was the movement of Rwandan refugees into Zaire in 1994 where outbreaks such as cholera swept through refugee camps (Wilson, 1995).

Travelers are both potential victims of an emerging infectious disease and vehicles for further spread, particularly when they return home. When people travel they bring with them pathogens that are in or on their bodies (these can be in an incubation period, latent or chronic); their normal microbiological flora, that may or may not be similar to the new locale; their own vulnerability to infection; their cultural preferences, customs, and behavior that may make them vulnerable to disease; and their baggage, that may also transport organisms, vectors, or contaminated foods (Cookson et al., 2001; Wilson, 1995). Some pathogens can only be transmitted under certain circumstances. For example, if a person infected with schistosomiasis contaminates water in a new region, it still requires a certain kind of snail to establish a disease cycle. Changing weather and climactic conditions are increasing the geographic range of some disease vectors allowing emergence in new areas. Some infectious diseases linked to travel are not considered emerging or reemerging in the context of this book and will not be considered here.

The traveler may also be at risk for acquiring infectious disease during transport to or from their destination. Outbreaks of emerging infectious diseases occurring in persons who have traveled together (such as on the same aircraft) are often difficult to detect once the affected persons have scattered to various geographic locales. Examples of these include malaria, tuberculosis (TB), and legionellosis. Exposure of both passengers and flight crews to TB have been described on commercial aircraft. Those at greatest risk were on longer flights and seated in the same section as the source person (Centers for Disease Control and Prevention, 1995; Ormerod, 2000). Malaria may be acquired by travelers who have been in endemic areas for travel as well as by those who become infected during brief stops at airports in endemic malarial areas (sometimes known as "runway malaria") or who are bitten in flight by infected mosquitos (Isaäcson, 1989; Isaäcson & Frean, 2001). The term airport malaria is used to describe malaria that is acquired through the bite of a mosquito that had been imported to a non-endemic malarial country by air. The first described case was in France in the late 1970s. In a review of the comparatively rare airport malarial cases, a number of them occurred in persons associated occupationally with airports such as cargo handlers and customs officers. Other cases occurred, however, in those who lived or visited near an international airport. In one case, the landlord of a public house near Gatwick airport in London developed malaria, and it was thought that an imported infected mosquito was brought into the pub through a vehicle carrying the aircrew there from the airport (Isaäcson, 1989). Live mosquitos were detected in 12 of 67 airplanes that arrived at Gatwick airport in London in one study, and in 27 airplanes arriving at Nairobi airport in 1986, 150 adult mosquitos were detected. A study conducted in 2000 also found mosquitos on flights from Africa (Karch, Dellile, Guillet, & Mouchet, 2001). Not only are mosquitos carried in the passenger or cargo hold, but they are also carried in the wheel bays. Various disinfection is recommended for vector control but this does not eliminate all risk (Isaäcson, 1989; Karch et al., 2001). Travelers often acquire malaria because of inadequate chemoprophylaxis, especially during travel to areas where the malarial parasite is resistant to chloroquine (Centers for Disease Control and Prevention, 2001b). Malaria is considered in detail in chapter 15.

Outbreaks of infectious diseases may also occur on cruise ships. Gastroenteritis from various sources had been reported to occur on cruise ships from both contaminated water and food because sometimes these ships purchase local foodstuffs or water that are contaminated. Before 1996, however, there were no confirmed reports of waterborne outbreaks of *E. coli* on cruise ships. Today, it is called an emerging waterborne pathogen on cruise ships. Outbreaks are believed to occur from water that is taken on in foreign ports. Recommendations have been made to ensure improved handling practices, careful disinfection, and monitoring of water quality to prevent future outbreaks. Ships docking in U.S. ports are also supposed to report the number of passengers or crew members who have visited the ship's physician for diarrhea 24 hours before arrival. This surveillance is under the auspices of the Vessel Sanitation Program of the CDC (Daniels, Neimann, Karpati, Parashar, Greene, Wells, et al., 2000). The semi-closed air systems on cruise ships have also led to outbreaks of influenza, and CDC has recommended that travelers at high risk for complications should consider receiving influenza vaccine before travel with a large tourist group, to the tropics, or in the Southern hemisphere from April through September. They also suggest that crew members have at least an 80% vaccination rate (Centers for Disease Control and Prevention, 2001a).

Travel-related Legionnaires' disease has also been reported. Legionnaires' disease is caused by *Legionella pneumophila*, a bacterium, and first was noticed among those attending an American Legion convention in Philadelphia in July, 1976. Retrospective studies indicated at least two prior outbreaks. Aerosols from the cooling system were identified as the source of the organism in that outbreak (Breiman & Butler, 1998). Recent reports have described outbreaks among cruise ship passengers who used or spent time near a whirlpool spa. These outbreaks often are undetected because travelers disperse after disembarking. In another outbreak, the water supply system was the source of infection (Castellani Pastoris, Lo Monaco, Goldoni, Mentore, Balestra, Ciceroni, et al., 1999). In one instance in 1994, a New Jersey physician notified the health department that three patients with atypical pneumonia all had been passengers on the same cruise ship. This led to an investigation that detected 50 passengers from that ship with Legionnaires' disease. The investigation of this outbreak led to new CDC guidelines for prevention of Legionnaires' disease aboard cruise ships (Jernigan, Hofmann, Cetron, Genese, Nuorti, Fields, et al., 1996). In another travel-related outbreak, a multistate outbreak of Legionnaires' disease occurred among nine members of tour groups staying at lodges in Vermont where they had gone to observe fall foliage. Most of those affected were senior citizens who presumably were more vulnerable because of disease and underlying illnesses (Mamolen, Breiman, Barbaree, Gunn, Stone, Spika, et al., 1993). Legionnaires' disease is considered in detail in chapter 13.

Souvenirs may be an unwitting source of infection. In one particular incidence, a traveler brought home a camel hair saddle from Pakistan. It was given to a 12-year-old girl. Later, she developed a large carbuncle that turned out to be cutaneous anthrax, a rare disease in developed countries but still a problem in countries such as Iran, Turkey, Pakistan, and the Sudan (Smith, 1995). Food- and waterborne illnesses are a very frequent consequence of travel. Travel to developing countries may put the traveler into contact with contaminated food and water, often by the fecal-oral route. Contamination may occur during growing, harvesting, handling, transporting, storing, or preparation of the foods. When abroad, travelers may wish to try local foods and buy from street vendors whose hygienic practices are unknown. Cholera, cryptosporidiosis, and other infectious agents causing diarrhea have been acquired by travelers in this way. Gnathostomosis, caused by a nematode, has been acquired in Acapulco, Mexico, after eating poorly cooked or raw fish, particularly as ceviche, in which fish salad is "cooked" only in lime juice (Rojas-Molina, Pedraza-Sanchez, Torres-Bibiano, Meza-Martinez, & Escobar-Gutierrez, 1999). Both recreational and drinking water may be contaminated in developing countries. Many of those who were participating in the Eco-Challenge in Borneo in the fall of 2000, acquired leptospirosis, developing after their return home. Participants noted that in the course of their participation, they acquired open sores and leech bites that might have contributed to acquiring infection ("Leptospirosis," 2001). Food- and waterborne infections are considered in more detail in chapter 3, and as specific diseases such as cholera, cyclosporiasis, or cryptosporidiosis (see chapters 4, 5, and 6).

Risks from emerging infectious agents may also result from the need for medical treatment in developing countries where equipment, needles, and syringes may not be sterile. There may also be a risk from blood transfusions, especially where endemic transmissible infections are prevalent in the blood donor population (see chapter 3). For example, a case of HIV infection was acquired by a tourist in Africa by a transfusion received after a bus accident (Hill, 1989). Endemic diseases in local areas pose a risk to travelers. In two recent instances, one in a group from Pennsylvania and one from Washington, coccidioidomycosis was acquired while in Mexico presumably from dust exposure (Cairns, Blythe, Kao, Pappagianis, Kaufman, Kobayashi, et al., 2000; Centers for Disease Control and Prevention, 2000a).

RECREATION

Increasingly, recreational activities both close to home and at near and far distances bring people into greater contact with animals and vectors of emerging infectious diseases. These may occur when people pursue hobbies that expose them to zoonoses such as by close contact with wild animals or pets, during cave exploration, hiking in wilderness areas, hunting, camping, and pursuing recreational water activities such as swimming, boating, or whitewater rafting. Even swallowing a small amount of water while engaging in these activities might prove hazardous. Acquisition of infectious diseases through recreational activities involving water and food are discussed also in chapter 3. In one instance, a female veterinary ophthalmologist fell off her raft during a whitewater excursion in a Costa Rican rain forest. She returned home to Utah where 4 days later she developed fever, shaking chills, diaphoresis, headache, and muscle and eye aches, as well as renal and liver involvement. It was determined that she had acquired leptospirosis, considered to be a reemerging disease in the U.S. (Levitt, 2001). Leptospirosis was also responsible for an outbreak involving triathletes who became ill after swimming in a lake in Springfield, Illinois (Centers for Disease Control and Prevention, 1998). Leptospirosis can be acquired closer to home as well. In 1996, three inner-city residents of Baltimore, Maryland who had flulike illnesses were determined to actually have leptospirosis. It was postulated that they contracted leptospirosis by walking barefoot through alleys contaminated by infected animal urine (Ault, 2000). Close contact between animals and people occur during visits to petting zoos and animal farms. Cases of *E. coli* O157:H7, such as have occurred recently in

Pennsylvania and Washington, may result from such contact (Centers for Disease Control and Prevention, 2001d). Many people keep pets including exotic pets such as reptiles including turtles, snakes, lizards, and iguanas. Over 90% of reptiles may carry *Salmonella enterica* which can cause gastrointeritis, that in children may lead to more severe illness such as meningitis (Ward, 2000). It is believed that salmonellosis from pet reptiles is underreported (Warwick, Lambiris, Westwood, & Steedman, 2001). Those who are immunosuppressed need to exert caution with reptilian pets, avoid close contacts with animals, and take other precautions (USPHS/IDSA, 1999, 2001). Expansion of walking in forested areas, and the expansion of housing into areas formerly inhabited only by wildlife, expose persons to closer proximity with the vectors of emerging infectious diseases. The most well-known example is Lyme disease, discussed in detail in chapter 14. Even lying or walking on the beach in a tropical or subtropical country may result in disease. Cutaneous larva migrans is the most frequent skin disease among travelers returning from tropical countries. This hookworm may be shed by dogs or cats who shed the eggs via feces on sandy beaches or soils where the relaxing tourist who goes barefoot on the sand or who lies on it may acquire the disease (Caumes, 2000; Tremblay, MacLean, Gyorkos, & MacPherson, 2000). Closer to home, cryptosporidiosis can be acquired from swimming pools (Centers for Disease Control and Prevention, 2001e; Puech, McAnulty, Lesjak, Shaw, Heron, & Watson, 2001). Home gardening can occasionally be hazardous. *Legionella longbeachae*-associated pneumonia has been traced to contaminated potting soil in California, Oregon, Washington, Japan, and Australia (Centers for Disease Control and Prevention, 2000b). Malaria may also be acquired during recreational pursuits in the U.S., since there have been a number of cases reported from Suffolk County, New York, acquired during hiking and camping (Centers for Disease Control and Prevention, 2000c).

An example of a reemerging disease associated with travel and/or recreational activity is plague. It is increasingly recognized as problematic in the U.S. and is discussed in more depth in the text that follows. Other diseases are listed in Appendices A and B.

Plague

Although plague is an ancient disease, known as the "black death" and responsible for killing millions during past pandemics, its agent is maintained in nature as a zoonotic infection in Asia, Africa, and the Americas. It is considered by some as an emerging or reemerging infectious disease because its geographic boundary contacts with humans have expanded.

Plague results from the gram-negative bacterium *Yersinia pestis*, which is nonmotile, and nonsporulating, and is a member of the *Enterobacteriaceae* family. There are three biotypes—antiqua, mediaevalis, and orientalis (Dennis, 2000). It is a zoonosis. This agent uses fleas as vectors, and over 150 species of fleas are vectors for it. The major hosts are wild and domestic rodents, although over 200 mammal species have been found to be naturally infected with *Yersinia pestis* (Dennis & Meier, 1997). The chief wild rodent hosts in the U.S. are ground squirrels, prairie dogs, wood rats, deer mice, chipmunks, and moles. Ground squirrel fleas are an important vector because they feed on many types of rodents and mammals (including humans) (Dennis, 1999). Rats are the most dangerous animal host for humans and *Rat rattus* is considered most dangerous because of its proximity to humans due to its lifestyle (Greenberg, 1999). A more recently recognized risk is exposure to *Y. pestis*-infected domestic cats. In a study of human plague in 8 western states during the years 1977 through 1998, 7.7% of the 297 cases reported were from infected cats due to bites, scratches, or other contact without flea bites. It is theorized that these types of cases will increase as residential development continues in plague endemic areas (Gage, Dennis, Orloski, Ettestad, Brown, Reynolds, et al., 2000). In South America, pet rodents such as guinea pigs may facilitate human exposure to infected fleas (Ruiz, 2001). Humans may encounter plague-carrying fleas when hiking, hunting, or camping in endemic areas. In the U.S. this includes the western third of the United States (Centers for Disease Control and Prevention, 2000b; Greenberg, 1999). About 80% of all U.S. cases are from New Mexico, Arizona and Colorado with about 10% from California and the rest from other states (Dennis & Gage, 1999). In 2000, six cases of plague were reported in the United States (Centers for Disease Control and Prevention, 2001c). In Rocky Mountain National Park, near Estes Park, Colorado, there are signs warning visitors not to handle the friendly ground squirrels since they may carry plague. Despite the fact that they go on to explain what plague is, many tourists continue to disregard the warnings and feed and handle the ground squirrels. Currently plague is more of a rural or suburban "fringe" illness in the U.S., and the last known urban outbreak was in Los Angeles in 1924–1925 (Dennis, 1999). *Y. pestis*-infected rats have been found in recent decades, however, in cities such as Tacoma, WA; San Francisco; Los Angeles; and Dallas (Dennis, 1999). Transmission is through handling infected animals, as a result of being bitten by infected fleas, or through inhalation of infected respiratory droplets (pneumonic plague) (Dennis & Gage, 1999). Major outbreaks of pneumonic and bubonic plague occurred in India in 1994, and travelers entering the U.S. were observed for symptoms although no plague cases were identified in the U.S. However, many travelers who were ill were not detected at entry points but came to attention after return to their community physician (Centers for Disease Control and Prevention, 1994).

Plague is usually inapparent in its natural reservoir hosts in its enzootic state. This type of transmission is of low risk to humans. However, epizootic plague with rapid spread may occur resulting in widespread die-offs of infected rodents and natural hosts. When this happens, their fleas disperse, and thus this type poses more of a threat to humans. Other mammals can become incidentally infected, and rabbits have occasionally been a source of infection for hunters. Ungulates such as deer, camel, and goats can become infected, and eating undercooked infected goat and camel meat has been documented as a source of plague outbreaks in northern Africa, the Middle East, and central Asia (Christie, Chen, & Elberg, 1980; Dennis, 1999). Weather and climate changes such as increased rainfall as well as deforestation and new agricultural planting can facilitate wild rodent reproduction and contribute to epizootics (Ruiz, 2001). Other recommendations for prevention of infectious diseases including immunization recommendations that are specific to country of travel or special situations may be obtained from organizations such as the following: Centers for Disease Control and Prevention Traveler's Health [online] Available at http://www.cdc.gov/travel; World Health Organization [online] Available at http://www.who.int/ith; and Travel Medicine Program Health Canada [online] Available at http://www.hc-sc.gc.ca/hpblcdc/osh/mp_e.html as well as local and regional traveler's health clinics.

There are three major clinical pictures: bubonic, septicemic, and pneumonic plague (Ruiz, 2001). The bubonic form accounts for about 85%, and while the other two are usually secondary, they can follow direct exposure (Dennis, 1999). In bubonic plague, the incubation period is usually 2–6 days. Symptoms include chills, fever, myalgia, headache, and weakness. Usually within 24 hours, regional lymph nodes become tender and painful nearest to the site of inoculation (bite), and a bubo forms. Without treatment, agitation, delirium, and prostration occur and adult respiratory distress syndrome (ARDS), sepsis, and disseminated intravascular coagulation (DIC) may occur. The fatality rate if untreated is 50%–60% Treatment is with antimicrobials such as streptomycin, gentamycin, tetracycline, or chloramphenicol (Dennis, 1999, 2000). Patients with the septicemic form may present with diarrhea, nausea, vomiting, and abdominal pain, and are often misdiagnosed with renal disease. Petechiae, ecchymoses, bleeding, DIC, ARDS, endotoxemia, and shock may develop. Pnemonic plague is the form that is transmitted via the respiratory tract from person to person, and may be primary or secondary to bubonic or septicemic plague. An outbreak that occurred in Madagascar in 1997 occurred first in a woodcutter, and then infected his native healer, and others who had stayed in the healer's house as well as family members (Ratsitorahina, Chanteau, Rahalison, Ratsifasoamanana, & Boisier, 2000). The incubation period is 1–4 days. Symptoms include chills, fever, headache, weakness, pains, chest discomfort, cough, tachypnea, and dyspnea with increasing respiratory distress and circulatory collapse. Sputum may be bloody. Sudden death is frequent. If untreated, the fatality rate is virtually 100%. The genome sequence of *Y. pestis* has been determined (Parkhill, Wren, Thomson, Titball, Holden, Prentice, et al., 2001). A vaccine is available but is not recommended for casual use. Detailed information about plague can be found in the plague manual from the World Health Organization (2001). Plague has been suggested as a potential agent for bioterrorism (see chapter 24) (Inglesby, Dennis, Henderson, Bartlett, Ascher, Eitzen, et al., 2000).

CONCLUSION

Travel and leisure time and recreational pursuits bring people into greater contact with the agents of emerging infectious diseases, especially if travel is to developing countries or exotic locales. Depending on the mode of spread, there are a variety of preventive measures that can be taken. These are summarized in Appendix C, Tables C.1–C.6.

REFERENCES

Ault, A. (2000, October 10). Deadly infection re-emerges as people get adventurous. *New York Times* [On-line]. Available: http://www.nytimes.com/2000/10/10/science/10WORM.html

Breiman, R. F., & Butler, J. C. (1998). Legionnaires' disease: Clinical epidemiological, and public health perspectives. *Seminars in Respiratory Infection, 13*(2), 84-89.

Cairns, L., Blythe, D., Kao, A., Pappagianis, D., Kaufman, L., Kobayashi, J., et al. (2000). Outbreak of coccidioidomycosis in Washington state residents returning from Mexico. *Clinical Infectious Diseases, 30*, 61-64.

Castellani Pastoris, M., Lo Monaco, R., Goldoni, P., Mentore, B., Balestra, G., Ciceroni, L., et al. (1999). Legionnaires' disease on a cruise ship linked to the water supply system: Clinical and public health implications. *Clinical Infectious Diseases, 28*, 33-38.

Caumes, E. (2000). Treatment of cutaneous larva migrans. *Clinical Infectious Diseases, 30*, 811-814.

Centers for Disease Control and Prevention. (1994). International notes human plague—India, 1994. *Morbidity and Mortality Weekly Report, 43*, 689-691.

Centers for Disease Control and Prevention. (1995). Exposure of passengers and flight crew to *Mycobacterium tuberculosis* on commercial aircraft, 1992-1995. *Morbidity and Mortality Weekly Report, 44*, 137-140.

Centers for Disease Control and Prevention. (1998). Update: Leptospirosis and unexplained acute febrile illness among athletes participating in triathlons—Illinois and Wisconsin, 1998. *Morbidity and Mortality Weekly Report, 47*, 673-676.

Centers for Disease Control and Prevention. (2000a). Coccidioidomycosis in travelers returning from Mexico—Pennsylvania, 2000. *Morbidity and Mortality Weekly Report, 49*, 1004-1006.

Centers for Disease Control and Prevention. (2000b). Legionnaires' disease associated with potting soil—California, Oregon and Washington May-June 2000. *Morbidity and Mortality Weekly Report, 49*, 777-778.

Centers for Disease Control and Prevention. (2000c). Probable locally acquired mosquito-transmitted *Plasmodium vivax* infection—Suffolk county, New York, 1999. *Morbidity and Mortality Weekly Report, 49*, 495-498.

Centers for Disease Control and Prevention. (2001a). Influenza B virus outbreak on a cruise ship—Northern Europe, 2000. *Morbidity and Mortality Weekly Report, 50*, 137-140.

Centers for Disease Control and Prevention. (2001b). Malaria deaths following inappropriate malaria chemoprophylaxis—United States, 2001. *Morbidity and Mortality Weekly Report, 50*, 597-599.

Centers for Disease Control and Prevention. (2001c). Notifiable diseases/deaths in selected cities. *Morbidity and Mortality Weekly Report, 49*, 1167-1174.

Centers for Disease Control and Prevention. (2001d). Outbreaks of *Escherichia coli* O157:H7 infections among children associated with farm visits—Pennsylvania and Washington, 2000. *Morbidity and Mortality Weekly Report, 50*, 293-297.

Centers for Disease Control and Prevention. (2001e). Protracted outbreaks of cryptosporidiosis associated with swimming pool use—Ohio and Nebraska, 2000. *Morbidity and Mortality Weekly Report, 50*, 406-410.

Christie, A. B., Chen, T. H., & Elberg, S. S. (1980). Plague in camels and goats: Their role in human epidemics. *Journal of Infectious Diseases, 141*, 724-726.

Cookson, S. T., Carballo, M., Nolan, C. M., Keystone, J. S., & Jong, E. C. (2001). Migrating populations—A closer view of who, why, and so what. *Emerging Infectious Diseases*, 7(No. 3 suppl), 551.

Daniels, N. A., Neimann, J., Karpati, A., Parashar, U. D., Greene, K. D, Wells, J. G., et al. (2000). Traveler's diarrhea at sea: Three outbreaks of waterborne enterotoxigenic *Escherichia coli* on cruise ships. *Journal of Infectious Diseases, 181*, 1491–1495.

Dennis, D. T. (1999). Plague. In R. L. Guerrant, D. H. Walker, & P. F. Weller (Eds.), *Tropical infectious diseases* (pp. 506–516). Philadelphia: Churchill Livingstone.

Dennis, D. T. (2000). Plague. In G. T. Strickland (Ed.), *Hunter's tropical medicine and emerging infectious diseases* (pp. 402–411). Philadelphia: WB Saunders Co.

Dennis, D. T., & Gage, K. L. (1999). Plague. In D. Armstrong & J. Cohen (Eds.), *Infectious diseases* (pp. 6:34.5–34.10). London: Mosby.

Dennis, D. T., & Meier, F. A. (1997). Plague. In C. R. Horsburgh, Jr. & A. M. Nelson (Eds.), *Pathology of emerging infections* (pp. 21–47). Washington, DC: American Society for Microbiology.

Gage, K. L., Dennis, D. T., Orloski, K. A., Ettestad, P., Brown, T. L., Reynolds, P. J., et al. (2000). Cases of cat-associated human plague in the Western US, 1997–1998. *Clinical Infectious Diseases, 30*, 893–900.

Greenberg, S. B. (1999). Serious waterborne and wilderness infections. *Critical Care Clinics, 15*, 387–414.

Guerrant, R. L., Walker, D. H., & Weller, P. F. (Eds.). (1999). *Tropical infectious diseases.* Philadelphia: Churchill Livingstone.

Gushulak, B. D., & MacPherson, D. W. (2000). Population mobility and infectious diseases. *Clinical Infectious Diseases, 31*, 776–780.

Hill, D. R. (1989). HIV infection following motor vehicle trauma in central Africa. *Journal of the American Medical Association, 261*, 3282–3283.

Inglesby, T. V., Dennis, D. T., Henderson, D. A., Bartlett, J. G., Ascher, M. S., Eitzen, E., et al. (2000). Plague as a biological weapon. *Journal of the American Medical Association, 283*, 2281–2290.

Isaäcson, M. (1989). Airport malaria: A review. *Bulletin of the World Health Organization, 67*, 737–743.

Isaäcson, M., & Frean, J. A. (2001). African malaria vectors in European aircraft. *Lancet, 357*, 235.

Jernigan, D. B., Hofmann, J., Cetron, M. S., Genese, C. A., Nuorti, J. P., Fields, B. S., et al. (1996). Outbreak of Legionnaires' disease among cruise ship passengers exposed to a contaminated whirlpool spa. *Lancet, 347*, 494–499.

Karch, S., Delille, M-F, Guillet, P., & Mouchet, J. (2001). African malaria vectors in European aircraft. *Lancet, 357*, 235.

Levett, P. N. (2001). Leptospirosis. *Clinical Microbiology Reviews, 14*, 296–326.

Leptospirosis, Eco-Challenge race—Borneo: 2000. (2001). *ProMED Digest 2001*(No. 19), unpaginated.

Lyme disease vaccine. (1999). *The Medical Letter On Drugs and Therapeutics, 41*(Issue 1049), 29–30.

MacArthur, J. R., Holtz, T. H., Jenkins, J., Newell, J. P., Koehler, J. E., Parise, M. E., et al. (2001). Probable locally acquired mosquito-transmitted malaria in Georgia, 1999. *Clinical Infectious Diseases, 32,* E124–E128.

Mamolen, M., Breiman, R. F., Barbaree, J. M., Gunn, R. A., Stone, K. M., Spika, J. S., et al. (1993). Use of multiple molecular subtyping techniques to investigate a Legionnaires' disease outbreak due to identical strains at two tourist lodges. *Journal of Clinical Microbiology, 31,* 2584–1401.

Martens, P., & Hall, L. (2000). Malaria on the move: Human population movement and malaria transmission. *Emerging Infectious Diseases, 6,* 103–109.

Miller, J. M., Boyd, H. A., Ostrowski, S. R., Cookson, S. T., Parise, M. E., Gonzaga, P. S., et al. (2000). Malaria, intestinal parasites, and schistosomiasis among Barawan Somali refugees resettling to the United States: A strategy to reduce morbidity and decrease the risk of imported infections. *American Journal of Tropical Medicine and Hygiene, 62,* 115–121.

Moore, P. S., Reeves, M. W., Schwartz, B., Gellin, B. G., & Broome, C. V. (1989). Intercontinental spread of an epidemic group A *Neisseria meningitidis* strain. *Lancet, 2,* 260–263.

Müller, A., Bialek, R., Kämper, A., Fatkenheuer, G., Salzberger, B., & Franzen, C. (2001). Detection of microsporidia in travelers with diarrhea. *Journal of Clinical Microbiology, 39,* 1630–1632.

Niler, E. (2000). Diseased passage. *Scientific American, 383*(1), 23–24.

Ormerod, P. (2000). Tuberculosis and travel. *Hospital Medicine, 61*(3), 171–173.

Ostroff, S. M., & Kozarsky, P. (1998). Emerging infectious diseases and travel medicine. *Infectious Disease Clinics of North America, 12,* 231–241.

Parkhill, J., Wren, B. W., Thomson, N. R., Titball, R. W., Holden, M. T., Prentice, M. B., et al. (2001). Genome sequence of *Yersinia pestis,* the causative agent of plague. *Nature, 413,* 523–527.

Puech, M. C., McAnulty, J. M., Lesjak, M., Shaw, N., Heron, L., & Watson, J. M. (2001). A statewide outbreak of cryptosporidiosis in New South Wales associated with swimming at public pools. *Epidemiology and Infection, 126,* 389–396.

Ratsitorahina, M., Chanteau, S., Rahalison, L., Ratsifasoamanana, L., & Boisier, P. (2000). Epidemiological and diagnostic aspects of the outbreak of pneumonic plague in Madagascar. *Lancet, 355,* 111–113.

Rojas-Molina, N., Pedraza-Sanchez, S., Torres-Bibiano, B., Meza-Martinez, H., & Escobar-Gutierrez, A. (1999). Gnathostomosis, an emerging foodborne zoonotic disease in Acapulco, Mexico. *Emerging Infectious Diseases, 5,* 264–266.

Ruiz, A. (2001). Plague in the Americas. *Emerging Infectious Diseases,* 7(No. 3, suppl.), 539–540.

Smith, L. (1995). The case of the camel hair carbuncle. *Patient Care, 29*(10), 138–139.

Tremblay, A., MacLean, J. D., Gyorkos, T., & MacPherson, D. W. (2000). Outbreak of cutaneous larva migrans in a group of travellers. *Tropical Medicine and International Health, 5,* 330–334.

USPHS/IDSA. (1999). Appendix. Recommendations to help patients avoid exposure to opportunistic pathogens. *Morbidity and Mortality Weekly Report, 48*(RR-10), 61–66.

USPHS/IDSA Prevention of Opportunistic Infections Working Group. (July 2001). Draft. *2001 USPHS/IDSA guidelines for the prevention of opportunistic infections in persons infected with human immunodeficiency virus.* [Online]. Available: http://www.hivatis.org/trtgdlns.html

Ward, L. (2000). *Salmonella* perils of pet reptiles. *Communicable Disease and Public Health,* 3(1), 2–3.

Warwick, C., Lambiris, A. J. L., Westwood, D., & Steedman, C. (2001). Reptile-related salmonellosis. *Journal of the Royal Society of Medicine, 94,* 124–126.

Wilson, M. E. (1995). Travel and the emergence of infectious diseases. *Emerging Infectious Diseases, 1,* 39–46.

World Health Organization. (2001). *Plague manual: Epidemiology, distribution, surveillance and control.* [Online]. Available: http://www.who.int/emc-documents/plague/whocdscsredc992c.htm

23

Immunocompromised Persons and Emerging Infectious Diseases

Victoria Davey

Immunocompromised persons have one or more conditions that lead to defective immune system function. Impaired immune system function can range from temporary and mild immunosuppression to permanent and life-limiting immunodeficiency diseases. In 1992, the Institute of Medicine included immunocompromised persons as a group at risk for emerging infections (Lederberg, Shope, & Oaks, 1992). The Centers for Disease Control and Prevention (CDC) (1998) include persons with host defense defects as a target population for control of emerging infectious organisms. Increasing numbers of people are living with defects in immune system function for several reasons: life-prolonging treatment of inherited or acquired immunodeficiency diseases; improved therapies for malignancies and related diseases resulting in short- or long-term immunosuppression; increased frequency of tissue and organ transplantaion; and, an aging population experiencing immune system decline as a function of accumulated years of life and comorbidities. Emerging and reemerging pathogens will present new risks to this diverse group that will require special vigilance and development of treatment strategies (Osterholm, 2000).

Primary, or inherited immunodeficiency diseases, such as common variable immunodeficiency and severe combined immunodeficiency

(SCID), are rare and have a genetic basis. More than 80 such diseases are known to date (Vihinen, Arredondo-Vega, Casanova, Etzioni, Giliani, Hammarström, et al., 2001). They have become increasingly treatable, with aggressive use of prophylactic antibiotic regimens, treatment of infection, and administration of immunomodulatory agents (Grimbacher, Holland, Gallin, Greenberg, Hill, Malech, et al., 1999; Holland & Gallin, 2000). Bone marrow transplantation has, in some cases, proved curative. It is possible that gene therapy will further increase the cure rate for these rare conditions (Lashley, 1998).

Acquired immunodeficiency may also be called secondary immunodeficiency. The best known infectious type is probably the acquired immunodeficiency syndrome (AIDS), caused by the human immunodeficiency virus (HIV) types 1 and 2. Other reasons for lesser degrees of secondary immunodeficiency are part of day-to-day life, such as trauma (e.g., asplenia), pregnancy, and aging. Still others are caused by an accumulation of host defense defects such as diabetes mellitus and chronic renal failure. Immune system suppression is a well-described side effect of many drugs, such as cancer chemotherapeutic agents and corticosteroids. Deliberate drug-induced immune system suppression is employed as part of a treatment strategy for malignancies and autoimmune diseases and to prevent rejection of transplanted organs.

Human interactions with the environment as seen with global travel, with changes in food and water acquisition and distribution, with new and more aggressive medical therapies, with a longer life span, and with changes in social patterns, such as urbanization, lead to the likelihood that previously undescribed pathogens may cause human disease in the susceptible immunocompromised hosts, as they do in the normal host. Protective measures to decrease risk of food and waterborne infections are found in Appendix C, Tables C.1–C.3.

Organisms infecting persons who are immunosuppressed may be opportunistic or pathogenic in both the immunocompromised and the immunocompetent. Infections seen in those who are immunosuppressed, especially in HIV infection, tend to have certain characteristics including differences in presentation, atypical location, dissemination, more rapid progression, and greater severity, and are more difficult to treat (Lashley, 2000).

All of these reasons—increasing survivability of persons with inherited and acquired defects, treatments that employ immune system manipulation, and changing interactions of the immunocompromised person with the environment—heighten the need for vigilance for emerging pathogens particular to the immunocompromised patient. This chapter will describe various causes of immunocompromise, and delineate known or potential emerging infectious diseases that may pose a threat to this growing population.

THE SUPPRESSED OR DEFICIENT IMMUNE SYSTEM

Even the briefest overview of the immune system illustrates the remarkable orchestration of its molecular, cellular, and chemical components. Primary or secondary immunodeficiency may result from failure of a single component, but it is important to remember that the resultant immune defects are usually multiple. Table 23.1 delineates some of the major human immunodeficiency diseases and immunosuppressive conditions. Of these, the more frequently encountered are in the secondary immune defect category: 1) immune dysfunction resulting from cancer therapies, preparation for bone marrow transplantation, or immunosuppression after organ transplantation; 2) HIV infection; 3) diabetes mellitus; 4) pregnancy; and 5) aging. The immunocompromise resulting from these entities will be discussed in more detail below. Table 23.2 lists reported emerging pathogens in these immunocompromised populations.

Immune Suppression Caused by Cancer and Cancer Therapy

Malignancies can cause immune system dysfunction in the absence of the suppressive effects of medication. In leukemias and lymphomas, the physical replacement of normal bone marrow stem cells with malignant cells causes at least partial dysfunction (De Pauw & Meunier, 2000). Defects in production of antibodies occur with multiple myeloma and with chronic lymphocytic leukemia (Heinzel, 2000). Malignant lymphomas are associated with decreased cellular immunity (De Pauw & Donnelly, 2000). Chemotherapy with cytotoxic drugs can cause neutropenia, and B and T lymphocyte dysfunction (Collin & Ramphal, 1998), although the most frequently encountered deleterious effect of cytotoxic drugs and therapeutic radiation is neutropenia and neutrophil dysfunction. Chemotherapy and radiation decrease phagocytic activity of neutrophils, decrease their ability to move to and

TABLE 23.1 Categories of Immunocompromise and Associated Diseases

Cause of Immunocompromise	Recognized Diseases/ Clinical Entities	Major Susceptibilities and Comments
Barrier or mechanical		
Defects of skin	Major surgery, burns, trauma Dermatologic conditions Decubitus, vascular, or diabetic ulcers IV catheters	Coagulase negative staphylococci; *Staphylococcus aureus*; *Stenotrophomonas maltophilia*; *Pseudomonas aeruginosa*; *Acinetobacter spp*; *Corynebacterium* and *Bacillus* spp; *Candida* spp; Mucormycosis
Defects of mucous membranes	Mucositis induced by radiation or chemotherapy Inhalation injuries Endotracheal intubation	Viridans streptococci; *Enterococcus* spp; *Capnocytophaga* spp; *Stomatococcus mucilaginosus*; *Candida* spp; Herpes simplex virus
Obstruction of body passages	Tumor Cystic fibrosis	Gram-negative and anaerobic bacteria; fungi including *Aspergillus* and *Candida*
Primary		
Primary B cell immunodeficiency diseases	X-linked agammaglobulinemia IgA deficiency IgG subclass deficiency X-linked hyperIgM syndrome Common variable immunodeficiency	Chronic sinopulmonary infections, meningitis, or bacteremia with encapsulated bacteria; *Streptococcus pneumoniae* or *Hemophilus influenzae*; enterovirus infections
Primary T cell immunodeficiency diseases	Severe combined immunodeficiency (SCID) Adenosine deaminase deficiency (ADA deficiency) Purine nucleoside phosphorylase deficiency MCH Class II deficiency DiGeorge Anomaly Hereditary ataxia telangiectasia Wiskott-Aldrich syndrome	Bacteria: *Mycobacteria* Fungi: *Aspergillus*, *Cryptococcus*, *Histoplasma*, *Coccidioides*, *Pneumocystis carinii* Protozoa: *Toxoplasma* Viruses: *Cytomegalovirus*, Herpes simplex virus Helminths: *Strongyloides stercoralis*

TABLE 23.1 *(continued)*

Cause of Immunocompromise	Recognized Diseases/ Clinical Entities	Major Susceptibilities and Comments
Defects in complement proteins	Hereditary angioedema (HAE)	Encapsulated bacteria; especially meningococci
Defects in phagocyte number or function	Chronic granulomatous disease Job's syndrome or Hyper-IgE recurrent infection syndrome (HIERIS)	*Staphylococcus aureus*; coagulase negative staphylococci; Viridans streptococci; *Enterococcus* spp; *Escherichia coli*; *Pseudomonas aeruginosa*; *Klebsiella pneumoniae*; *Enterobacter* and *Citrobacter* spp; *Serratia* spp; *Paecilomyces lilacinus*; *Aspergillus* spp; *Fusarium* spp
Secondary or acquired		
Defects in phagocyte number or function	Cancer chemotherapy or irradiation Acute leukemia	*Staphylococcus aureus*; coagulase negative staphylococci; viridans streptococci; *Enterococcus* spp; *Escherichia coli*; *Pseudomonas aeruginosa*; *Klebsiella pneumoniae*; *Enterobacter* and *Citrobacter* spp; *Aspergillus* spp; *Fusarium* spp
Drug-induced	Corticosteroids Cyclophosphamide Azathioprine Mycophenolate mofetil Methotrexate Cyclosporine	
Environmental or treatment induced	Malnutrition Pregnancy Solid organ transplantation Bone marrow transplantation	Can cause phagocytic, B and T cell defects; *Listeria monocytogenes*

(continued)

TABLE 23.1 *(continued)*

Cause of Immuno-compromise	Recognized Diseases/ Clinical Entities	Major Susceptibilities and Comments
Infectious	HIV-1 Infection	Bacteria: *Mycobacteria, Pneumococcus, Pseudomonas* Fungi: *Aspergillus, Cryptococcus, Histoplasma, Coccidioides, Pneumocystis carinii* Protozoa: *Toxoplasma,* microsporidia, *Cryptosporidium* Viruses: Cytomegalovirus, Herpes simplex virus, JD virus Helminths: *Strongyloides stercoralis*
	Cytomegalovirus (CMV)	*Pneumocystis carinii; Aspergillus fumigatus; Candida* spp
	Human herpesvirus 6 (HHV 6)	May activate Epstein Barr virus (EBV); CMV; HIV

Sources: Collin & Ramphal, 1998; Risi & Tomascak, 1998; Rosen & Seligman, 1993; Waldmann & Nelson, 1995

gather at the site of inflammation (chemotaxis), and decrease intracellular killing (DePauw & Donnelly, 2000). The use of more aggressive cytotoxic chemotherapy protocols in leukemia have led to a higher prevalence of fungal and yeast infections such as non-albicans *Candida, Malassezia furfur, Trichosporon* species, *Blastoschizomyces capitatus, Rhodotorula rubra, Saccharomyces cerevisiae, Clavispora lusitaniae, Cryptococcus laurentii,* and *Hansenula anomala* (Krcmery, Krupova, & Denning, 1999). In patients with hematological malignancies and bone marrow transplant, invasive aspergillosis, most commonly manifesting as pulmonary disease followed by disseminated infection, is of increasing concern (Patterson, Kirkpatrick, While, Hiemenz, Wingard, Dupont, et al., 2000).

In some observational studies, gram-positive organisms have been shown to replace gram-negative organisms as the most common cause of infection in the neutropenic host (Fenelon, 1998). Bacterial infec-

TABLE 23.2 Emerging Pathogens in the Immunocompromised Person

Pathogen	Potential Source	Particular Risk Groups	Clinical Information	Selected References
Fungi				
Fusarium spp	Skin, sinuses, respiratory tract, spider bite	Neutropenia, chemotherapy, BMT	Assess for fungal skin lesions prior to chemotherapy or BMT preparation	Boutati & Anaissie, 1997
Aspergillus spp	Ventilation systems; increased risk near building construction; exposure to broad-spectrum antibiotics, presence of indwelling catheters	Acute leukemia, BMT, HIV infection	Causes invasive pulmonary or other site infections; in HIV infection risk increase with steroid use or concomitant pulmonary infections	Viscoli & Castagnolo, 1999; Nash, et al., 1997
Rhodotorula rubra	IV catheter-associated	Neutropenia, chemotherapy	Cause of sepsis in hospitalized patients	Kiehn et al., 1992
Non-*albicans Candida* spp	Oral flora; skin; IV catheter-associated	Neutropenia, chemotherapy, BMT; past fungal infection prophylaxis	Candidemia, fever, ascites, disseminated disease	Meis et al., 1999; Krcmery, 1996
Coccidioides immitis	Desert soil; increasing incidence w/climatic changes, exposure to dust in endemic areas	Pregnant women; HIV; solid organ transplant recipients	Disseminated disease in immunocompromised	Kirkland & Fierer, 1996

(continued)

TABLE 23.2 *(continued)*

Pathogen	Potential Source	Particular Risk Groups	Clinical Information	Selected References
Gram-positive pathogens				
Streptococcus mitis	Oral flora	Chemo, mucositis	Bacteremia, adult respiratory distress syndrome	Zinner, 1995
Leuconostoc sp	Plants, vegetables, dairy products; IV catheter-associated	Neonates	Bacteremia, meningitis	Moellering, 2000
Corynebacterium jeikeium or "J–K corynebacterium"	Colonize skin, rectum; IV catheter-associated	Neutropenia; skin breakdown, patients with various malignancies, especially in patient who have had 3rd generation cephalosporins	Sepsis	Zinner, 1995; Wang, Mattson, & Wald, 2001
Rhodococcus equi	Soil organism; pathogen in animals	HIV, others with impaired T cell immunity	Pneumonitis, abscess, empyema	Prescott, 1991
Stomatococcus mucilaginosus	IV catheter-associated	Chemo, mucositis	Formerly thought to be nonpathogenic	Zinner, 1995
Bacillus cereus	Found in skin vesicles or pustules on a limb or digit	Malignancy, neutropenia, HIV, corticosteroids	Necrotizing fasciitis, meningitis	Zinner, 1995

TABLE 23.2 ***(continued)***

Pathogen	Potential Source	Particular Risk Groups	Clinical Information	Selected References
Gram-negative pathogens				
Stenotrophomonas maltophilia and *Pseudomonas cepacia*	Soil, water, plants, decaying organic material, tap water, nebulizers, water baths, dialyzers; central venous catheters	Chronic granulomatous disease, malignancies	Pneumonia, septic shock, Resistant to imipenem, beta-lactams, aminoglycosides	Zinner, 1995
Capnocytophaga spp	Oral flora of dogs; normal flora of human mouth, vagina, GI tract	Mucositis, acute leukemia, BMT	Bacteremia	Gill, 2000
Achromobacter xylosoxidans	IV catheter associated	Mucositis	Bacteremia	Zinner, 2000
Agrobacterium radiobacter	Plant pathogen; IV-catheter associated	Advanced HIV infection; malignancies	Sepsis and pneumonia	Manfredi et al., 1999
Bartonella spp	May be animal-associated; especially cats	HIV, Neutropenia	Cause of bacillary angiomatosis; cat scratch disease; fever, bacteremia, endocarditis	Anderson & Neuman, 1997; Grant & Olsen, 1999; Zinner, 1995

(continued)

TABLE 23.2 ***(continued)***

Pathogen	Potential Source	Particular Risk Groups	Clinical Information	Selected References
Anaerobic organisms				
Fusobacterium nucleatum	Normal oral flora	Leukemia	Ulcerative pharyngitis	Zinner, 1995
Parasites				
Isospora belli	Oocyst contaminated food or water; possibly sexually transmitted	HIV infection	Diarrheal disease	Curry & Smith, 1998
Cyclospora cayetanensis	Oocyst contaminated food (raspberries, basil) or water	HIV infection	Diarrheal disease	Collins & Wright, 1997; Curry & Smith, 1998
Microsporidia	Largely unknown—likely waterborne; possibly food (poorly cooked fish or crustaceans); possibly animals, arthropods	HIV infection	Diarrheal disease; ocular infection; urethritis	Collins & Wright, 1997; Curry & Smith, 1998; Franzen & Müller, 1999

TABLE 23.2 *(continued)*

Pathogen	Potential Source	Particular Risk Groups	Clinical Information	Selected References
Cryptosporidium parvum	Food and water contaminated with animal feces	HIV infection	Diarrheal disease; some extraintestinal disease	Collins & Wright, 1997; Franzen & Müller, 1999; Guerrant, 1997
Other "new" pathogens				
Prototheca spp	An algae; previously not thought to be pathogenic	Hodgkin's lymphoma, IV catheter-associated	Bacteremia and peritonitis	Zinner, 1995
Viruses				
Parvovirus B19	Ubiquitous; cause of fifth disease of childhood	Various malignancies, HIV	Bone marrow suppression in leukemics, neonates; pure red cell aplasia in HIV	Naides, 1998
Human herpesvirus 6	Ubiquitous; cause of sixth disease of childhood (roseola exanthem)	BMT; kidney, liver transplant recipients	Bone marrow suppression, pneumonitis; encephalitis	Campadelli-Fiume et al., 1999; Rodrigues et al., 1999

Abbreviations: Chemo = patients on chemotherapy; BMT = bone marrow transplantation; HIV = human immunodeficiency virus type I tions predominate in the first days post-chemotherapy or radiation, but with persistent neutropenia, invasive and cutaneous infections with fungi can also occur (Collin & Ramphal, 1998; Walsh, 1998). Table 23.2 describes some of the emerging pathogens associated with malignancies and their treatment effects.

Immune Suppression After Bone Marrow Transplantation

Bone marrow transplantation (BMT) has been employed as a definitive treatment for leukemias, malignant lymphomas, aplastic anemia, congenital immunodeficiency diseases, and inborn errors of metabolism (Storb & Thomas, 1995). Preparative or conditioning regimens ablate or partially ablate the recipient's marrow with radiation or a variety of cytotoxic and immunomodulatory agents, the choice of which is influenced by the underlying disease. In the immediate post-transplant period, there is generally severe pancytopenia lasting 2 to 4 weeks that may require aggressive supportive care, including red cell transfusion, colony stimulating factor administration, antibiotics, hyperalimentation, and possibly, a protective environment (Storb & Thomas, 1995). As they do in neutropenia, gram-positive and gram-negative bacteremias and sepsis can occur, particularly when the neutrophil count falls below 500/mm^3. Among gram-positive organisms, coagulase-negative staphylococci and viridans streptococci often predominate, and among gram-negative organisms, *Escherichia coli*, *Klebsiella*, *Enterobacter*, and *Pseudomonas* species are seen most commonly (Van Burik & Weisdorf, 2000). As the neutropenia reverses with donor marrow engraftment, infections with certain viruses, such as respiratory syncytial virus (RSV), become more prevalent as humoral, cellular, and pulmonary alveolar macrophage function may be impaired for up to a year or more (Collin & Ramphal, 1998). Invasive fungal infections, such as aspergillosis and pseudomembranous asperigillosis, may be seen (Nichod, Pache, & Howarth, 2001; Patterson et al., 2000). Graft versus host disease (GVHD) occurs frequently in patients who have undergone allogeneic transplants. This condition—in which donor T lymphocytes recognize the recipient's cells as foreign and mount an immune response directed against them—is treated with immunosuppressive drugs, such cyclosporine and corticosteroids, that further increase risks for infectious complications (Storb & Thomas, 1995; Van Burik & Weisdorf, 2000). Finally, even after transplant recovery, there may be ongoing immunosuppression from such factors as poor granulocyte chemotaxis and reduced immune system precursor cells in bone marrow (Storb & Thomas, 1995).

Immune Suppression After Solid Organ Transplantation

There are approximately 16,000 organ transplantation operations performed in the U.S. annually. Included in this figure are kidney, kidney-pancreas, heart, heart-lung, and liver transplants. Infection after transplantation is a major problem, ranking third in incidence after surgical events and graft rejection (Dumler & Ho, 2000). Factors important in the development of infection and the types of infection are 1) the patients' underlying illness(es)—for example, diabetes mellitus or hepatitis C (see chapter 11)—confer their own infection risks; 2) surgical—for example, the type of anastomoses required, amount of time spent in the operating room, and/or development of lymphoceles from inadequate lymphatics drainage; 3) susceptibility of the grafted organ to cytomegalovirus, a greater risk in lung transplants than others; and 4) the type and duration of immunosuppression required (Dumler & Ho, 2000). In the early post-transplant period (days to weeks) the patient is at most risk from bacterial infection (most commonly gram-negative bacteria), reflecting the general postoperative state. From the second to sixth months, opportunistic infections (e.g., *Pneumocystis carinii* and *Nocardia*) predominate. After 6 months, community-acquired infections and latent viral infections most commonly occur. Prophylactic regimens can anticipate and prevent many of these infections (Dumler & Ho, 2000; Kahan & Clark, 1995).

Post-transplant immunosuppression required for graft retention is accomplished by a variety of drugs. Most of these blunt cell-mediated immunity, but can also cause decreased antibody production and neutropenia. The goal of transplanted graft maintenance is immunologic tolerance—allowing the recipient to retain the functioning organ, without incurring too high a risk of infection from immunosuppression (Sia & Patel, 2000).

Immunocompromise in HIV/AIDS

The HIV/AIDS epidemic was recognized in 1981 when unusual cases of *Pneumocystis carinii* pneumonia and Kaposi's sarcoma were seen in homosexual men from New York and California (Centers for Disease Control, 1981). Because of the average 10-year period between infection and development of AIDS, the epidemic's beginnings had most likely occurred many years earlier. The global spread of HIV has been assisted by a profusion of human and environmental factors. They include ecologic changes that brought humans and animals into closer contact; social patterns and behavior changes like urban migration, sexual practices, drug use, and transfusion of blood products; the ease of international travel; and viral factors, including the long period of asymptomatic illness that allows HIV to be transmitted before the host is debilitated by AIDS (Quinn & Fauci, 1998). The cumulative number of persons, adults and children, living with AIDS is estimated by the World Health Organization as 36.1 million. An additional 21.8 million have died from the disease (World Health Organization, 2000). At the end of December 2000, there were 774,467 cumulative reported cases of AIDS in the U.S. (Centers for Disease Control and Prevention, 2000). HIV/AIDS provides a model of the potential devastation of an emerging infectious disease, but with its huge number of victims it is also responsible for the large population of immunocompromised people at risk for other emerging infections. In fact, many infections that now fit the definition of "emerging" have been identified in people with HIV/AIDS.

HIV causes dysfunction of nearly all components of the immune system. After infection with HIV, the immune system mounts a vigorous response, as it would to any invading microorganism, but untreated HIV eventually overcomes the normal host's defenses, ultimately leading to death, usually from opportunistic infections and cancers (Cohen, Cicala, Vaccarezza, & Fauci, 2000). HIV preferentially infects CD4+ lymphocytes, as well as monocytes and macrophages. The progressive decline in numbers and the dysfunction of the CD4+ lymphocyte that accompanies infection constitute the cornerstones of the immune system dysfunction caused by HIV. HIV causes death or dysfunction of the CD4+ lymphocytes through a variety of mechanisms: direct infection (use of the CD4+ lymphocyte to produce new viral particles); clumping of infected and uninfected CD4+ lymphocytes (syncytia formation); changing the normal "programmed" cell life cycle (apoptosis); and possibly causing an autoimmune phenomenon where the activated immune system kills uninfected CD4+ lymphocytes as well as those infected with HIV. HIV is not as lethal to macrophages—they remain a chronically-infected reservoir of HIV that is less susceptible to any of the currently available antiviral medications (Cohen et al., 2000). Other effects of HIV on immune system elements lead to broad dysfunction: B lymphocytes have decreased ability to respond to antigen, neutrophils experience dysregulation, and cytokine/lymphokine production and activity are disrupted. There is a progressive loss of ability to produce IL-2 and IL-12, which stimulate proliferation and lytic activity of cytotoxic T lymphocytes and natural killer cells (Cohen et al., 2000).

HIV-infected persons with advanced disease are susceptible to a variety of bacterial, viral, fungal, and parasitic infections as a consequence of their broad immune system defects. Without treatment with highly active antiretroviral therapy (HAART) that protects against HIV/AIDS-associated infections by preserving or returning a degree of immune system function, there are characteristic infections associated with specific levels of immune system decline in HIV infection. These include *Pneumocystis carinii* pneumonia, recurrent oral candidiasis, perirectal herpes simplex, and *Mycobacterium avium* complex bacteremia. Others occurring in high frequency are tuberculosis, cerebral toxoplasmosis, *Cryptococcus neoformans*, persistent cryptosporidiosis, and microsporidiosis. Many were formerly rare disorders in humans, having mostly been zoonotic or of limited prevalence. These uncommon infections include isosporiasis, JC virus, *Rhodococcus equi*, *Bartonella*, non-albicans *Candida*, *Penicillium marneffei*, and *Sporothrix schenckii* (Lashley, 2000; Masur, 2000). Table 23.2 lists some of the emerging pathogens of particular concern in HIV-infected patients. Also see Appendix A and chapter 12.

Immunosuppression in Diabetes Mellitus

According to the CDC (2001), diabetes in the U.S. increased by about 6% in 1999, leading government researchers to call diabetes mellitus an unfolding epidemic. This increase has been attributed primarily to obesity, which has increased 57% among Americans from 1991. Approximately 800,000 new cases of diabetes mellitus are diagnosed each year. It is the seventh leading cause of death in this country and a major contributor to serious health problems. The 1999 rise crossed races and age groups but was greatest among people aged 30–39 years. Diabetes mellitus is more prevalent in African Americans, Hispanics, certain Native Americans, and in other ethnic minority groups than in Caucasian Americans.

Diabetes mellitus causes suppression of cell-mediated immunity and phagocyte function as a result of hyperglycemia (Eisenbarth & Castano, 1995). Type 1 diabetics may also have impaired production of IL-2 (Eisenbarth & Castano, 1995). Susceptibility to infection appears to improve with glycemic control (Foster, 2000). Immunosuppression in diabetes mellitus leads to an increase in common infections like urinary tract and wound infections, as well as more serious infections. Rhinocerebral mucormycosis, a devastating fungal infection originating in the nasal mucosa, occurs classically after an episode of diabetic ketoacidosis. Malignant external otitis, often caused by *Pseudomonas aeruginosa*, tends to occur in older diabetics (Eisenbarth & Castano, 1995; Foster, 2000). *Coccidioides immitis*, an emerging human pathogen, is a fungus endemic to desert areas of California, Arizona, New Mexico, and west Texas. In diabetics, it can cause pulmonary infection characterized by multiple thin-walled pulmonary cavities (Kirkland & Fierer, 1996). Diabetics may also be at greater risk for development of disease after exposure to *Mycobacterium tuberculosis* (Washington & Miller, 1998).

Immunosuppression in Pregnancy

Pregnancy results in a mild state of immunosuppression. Hormonal changes brought about by the pregnant uterus, including elevated serum levels of endogenous corticosteroids and progesterone, can lead to poor lymphocyte function. Decreased levels of the immunoglobulin IgG have been described (Claman, 1995), and, in general, pregnancy may produce an immune response directed more towards Th2-like functions (regulation of B cell functions) rather than Th1 activity (regulation of T cell functions) (Kirkland & Fierer, 1996). Infections reported to be worse in the pregnant woman include: hepatitis (see chapter 11), influenza, cholera (see chapter 4), scarlet fever, malaria (see chapter 15), gonorrhea, typhoid, leprosy, and listeriosis (see chapter 3) (Claman, 1995). A recent report describes a case of psittacosis in a pregnant woman after contact with blood and membranes of parturient sheep. The normal hosts of *Chlamydia psittaci* are psittacine birds that may shed bacteria even when they are asymptomatic. *C. psittaci* is also a known infectious cause of abortion in sheep and goats. One author recommends pregnant women avoid contact with parturient sheep or goats and psittacine birds to prevent a serious febrile illness associated with pregnancy loss (Jorgensen, 1997). *Coccidioides immitis* infection in pregnancy may be associated with rapid growth of the organism, a process thought to be influenced by hormonal change (Kirkland & Fierer, 1996).

Immune System Decline in Aging

Cellular and humoral immunity decline with age. This fact, combined with impairment of certain physical aspects of host defense (e.g., normal blood circulation, a vigorous cough reflex, and normal wound healing), leaves the elderly susceptible to a variety of infections. For example, bacteriuria and urinary tract infections are seen with high frequency in men with obstructed urine flow as a consequence of prostatic hypertrophy. Pneumonias from all causes are 50 times more common in persons over 75 years old than in teenagers. Institutionalized elderly persons are at greater risk for person-to-person transmitted nosocomial infections, such as tuberculosis and diarrheal disease from enteric pathogens, many of which may be resistant strains. The physiologic response to infection can also be diminished, with less fever, less leukocytosis, and blunted clinical signs and symptoms. Because of this, elderly persons with pneumonia or sepsis may present with only confusion as their major clinical manifestation of infection (Crossley & Peterson, 2000; Tramont & Hoover, 2000).

CONCLUSIONS

The immunocompromised state includes a wide range of inherited and acquired immune system defects. There is a growing body of knowledge concerning susceptibility to infection in this diverse group, but there is also increasing recognition that the person with a defective or suppressed immune system may be at risk for infections from an untold number of unrecognized organisms. These include animal and plant pathogens, organisms thought to be nonpathogenic, and recurrence of latent infections. Study of the types of infections that occur in the immunocompromised person have certainly led to a greater understanding of the workings of the human immune system. Such study may also serve to enhance our ability to protect the population with normal immune systems. A good example is the emergence of

Cryptosporidium parvum. C. parvum was first recognized as an uncommon pathogen in immunosuppressed persons, but then was noted to be a frequent cause of diarrhea in HIV/AIDS patients. Soon after the AIDS epidemic began, it was identified as causing disease in normal hosts, as well as emerging in the Milwaukee outbreak in 1993 (see chapter 5). Understanding of cryptosporidial disease in immunocompromised patients led to its early detection in widespread outbreaks, and an enhanced ability to prevent future outbreaks through public education, water purification, and food handling techniques (Guerrant, 1997). Further, it is important to have good environmental surveillance for contamination with preventive measures in place (Alberti et al., 2001).

REFERENCES

Alberti, C., Bouakline, A., Ribaud, P., Lacroix, C., Rousselot, P., Leblanc, T., et al. (2001). Relationship between environmental fungal contamination and the incidence of invasive aspergillosis in haematology patients. *Journal of Hospital Infection, 48*, 198–206.

Anderson, B. E., & Neuman, M. A. (1997). *Bartonella* spp. as emerging human pathogens. *Clinical Microbiology Reviews, 10*, 203–219.

Boutati, E. I., & Anaissie, E. J. (1997). *Fusarium*, a significant emerging pathogen in patients with hematologic malignancy: Ten years' experience at a cancer center and implications for management. *Blood, 90*, 999–1008.

Campadelli-Fiume, G., Mirandola, P., & Menotti, L. (1999). Human herpesvirus 6: An emerging pathogen. *Emerging Infectious Diseases, 5*, 243–245.

Centers for Disease Control. (1981). Kaposi's sarcoma and pneumocystis pneumonia among homosexual men—New York and California. *Morbidity and Mortality Weekly Report, 31*, 507–515.

Centers for Disease Control and Prevention. (1998). *Preventing emerging infectious diseases: A strategy for the 21st century.* Atlanta: Department of Health and Human Services.

Centers for Disease Control and Prevention. (2000). *HIV/AIDS surveillance report. Year-end edition, 12*(2), 1–43.

Centers for Disease Control and Prevention. (2001, January 26). *Diabetes rates rise another 6 percent in 1999* [News Release]. Atlanta: Department of Health and Human Services.

Claman, H. N. (1995). Immunology of reproduction and infertility. In M. M. Frank, F. K. Austen, H. N. Claman, & E. R. Unanue (Eds.), *Samter's immunologic diseases* (Vol. II, pp. 999–1007). Boston: Little, Brown.

Cohen, O., Cicala, C., Vaccarezza, M., & Fauci, A. S. (2000). The immunology of human immunodeficiency virus infection. In G. L. Mandell, J. E. Bennett, &

R. E. Dolin (Eds.), *Mandell, Douglas, and Bennett's principles and practice of infectious diseases* (pp. 1374–1398). Philadelphia: Churchill Livingstone.

Collin, B. S., & Ramphal, R. (1998). Pneumonia in the compromised host including cancer patients and transplant patients. *Infectious Disease Clinics of North America, 12*, 781–805.

Collins, P. A., & Wright, M. E. (1997). Emerging intestinal protozoa: A diagnostic dilemma. *Clinical Laboratory Science, 10*, 273–278.

Crossley, K. B., & Peterson, P. K. (2000). Infections in the elderly. In G. L. Mandell, J. E. Bennett, & R. E. Dolin (Eds.), *Mandell, Douglas, and Bennett's principles and practice of infectious diseases* (pp. 3164–3169). Philadelphia: Churchill Livingstone.

Curry, A., & Smith, H. V. (1998). Emerging pathogens: *Isospora, Cyclospora* and Microsporidia. *Parasitology, 117*, S143–S159.

De Pauw, B. E., & Donnelly, J. P. (2000). Infections in the immunocompromised host: General principles. In G. L. Mandell, J. E. Bennett, & R. E. Dolin (Eds.), *Mandell, Douglas, and Bennett's principles and practice of infectious diseases* (pp. 3079–3090). Philadelphia: Churchill Livingstone.

De Pauw, B. E., & Meunier, F. (2000). Infections in patients with leukemia and lymphoma. In G. L. Mandell, J. E. Bennett, & R. E. Dolin (Eds.), *Mandell, Douglas, and Bennett's principles and practice of infectious diseases* (pp. 3090–3102). Philadelphia: Churchill Livingstone.

Dumler, J. S., & Ho, M. (2000). Risk factors and approaches to infections in transplant recipients. In G. L. Mandell, J. E. Bennett, & R. E. Dolin (Eds.), *Mandell, Douglas, and Bennett's principles and practice of infectious diseases* (pp. 3126–3136). Philadelphia: Churchill Livingstone.

Eisenbarth, G. S., & Castano, L. (1995). Diabetes mellitus. In M. M. Frank, F. K. Austen, H. N. Claman, & E. R. Unanue (Eds.), *Samter's immunologic diseases* (Vol. II, pp. 1007–1026). Boston: Little, Brown.

Fenelon, L. (1998). Unusual infections and new diagnostic methods in immunocompromised host. *Current Opinion in Infectious Diseases, 11*, 437–440.

Foster, D. W. (2000). Diabetes mellitus: Late complications of diabetes. In *Harrison's On Line* [On-line]. Available: http://www.harrisonsonline.com/server-java/Arknoid/harrisons/1096-7133 /Ch.../Page9.htm

Franzen, C., & Müller, A. (1999). *Cryptosporidia* and *Microsporidia*—waterborne diseases in the immunocompromised host. *Diagnosis of Microbiologic and Infectious Diseases, 34*, 245–262.

Gill, V. J. (2000). *Capnocytophaga.* In G. L. Mandell, J. E. Bennett, & R. E. Dolin (Eds.), *Mandell, Douglas, and Bennett's principles and practice of infectious diseases* (pp. 2441–2444). Philadelphia: Churchill Livingstone.

Grant, S., & Olsen, C. W. (1999). Preventing zoonotic diseases in immunocompromised persons: The role of physicians and veterinarians. *Emerging Infectious Diseases, 5*, 159–163.

Grimbacher, B., Holland, S. E., Gallin, J. I., Greenberg, F., Hill, S. C., Malech, H. L., Miller, J. A., O'Connell, A. C., & Puck, J. M. (1999). Hyper-IgE syndrome with recurrent infections—an autosomal dominant multisystem disorder. *New England Journal of Medicine, 340*, 692–702.

Guerrant, R. L. (1997). Cryptosporidiosis: An emerging, highly infectious threat. *Emerging Infectious Diseases, 3*, 51–57.

Heinzel, F. P. (2000). Antibodies. In G. L. Mandell, J. E. Bennett, & R. E. Dolin (Eds.), *Mandell, Douglas, and Bennett's principles and practice of infectious diseases* (pp. 45–66). Philadelphia: Churchill Livingstone.

Holland, S. E., & Gallin, J. I. (2000). Evaluation of the patient with suspected immunodeficiency. In G. L. Mandell, J. E. Bennett, & R. E. Dolin (Eds.), *Mandell, Douglas, and Bennett's principles and practice of infectious diseases, and practice of infectious diseases* (pp. 146–155). Philadelphia: Churchill Livingstone.

Jorgensen, D. M. (1997). Gestational psittacosis in a Montana sheep rancher. *Emerging Infectious Diseases, 3*, 191–194.

Kahan, B. D., & Clark, J. H. (1995). Transplantation of solid organs. In M. M. Frank, F. K. Austen, H. N. Claman, & E. R. Unanue (Eds.), *Samter's immunologic diseases* (Vol. II, pp. 1495–1509). Boston: Little, Brown.

Kiehn, T. E., Gorey, E., Brown, A. E., Edwards, F. F., & Armstrong, D. (1992). Sepsis due to *Rhodotorula* related to use of central venous catheters. *Clinical Infectious Diseases, 14*, 841–846.

Kirkland, T. N., & Fierer, J. (1996). Coccidioidomycosis: A reemerging infectious disease. *Emerging Infectious Diseases, 2*, 192–199.

Krcmery, V. (1996). Emerging fungal infections in cancer patients. *Journal of Hospital Infection, 33*, 109–117.

Krcmery, V., Krupova, I., & Denning, D. W. (1999). Invasive yeast infections other than *Candida* spp. in acute leukaemia. *Journal of Hospital Infection, 41*, 181–194.

Lashley, F. R. (1998). *Clinical genetics in nursing practice* (2nd ed.). New York: Springer Publishing.

Lashley, F. R. (2000). The clinical spectrum of HIV infection and its treatment. In J. D. Durham & F. R. Lashley (Eds.), *The person with HIV/AIDS: Nursing perspectives* (3rd ed., pp. 167–269). New York: Springer Publishing Co.

Lederberg, J., Shope, R., & Oaks, S. C. (1992). *Report: Institute of Medicine. Emerging infections: Microbial threats to health in the United States*. Washington, DC: National Academy Press.

Manfredi, R., Nanetti, A., & Ferri, M. (1999). Emerging gram-negative pathogens in the immunocompromised host: *Agrobacterium radiobacter* septicemia during HIV disease. *Microbiologica, 22*, 375–382.

Masur, H. (2000). Management of opportunistic infections associated with human immunodeficiency virus infection. In G. L. Mandell, J. E. Bennett, & R. E. Dolin (Eds.), *Mandell, Douglas, and Bennett's principles and practice of infectious diseases* (pp. 1500–1519). Philadelphia: Churchill Livingstone.

Meis, J. F. G. M., Ruhnke, M., DePauw, B. E., Odds, F. C., Siegert W., & Verweij, P. E. (1999). *Candida dubliniensis* candidemia in patients with chemotherapy induced neutropenia and bone marrow transplantation. *Emerging Infectious Diseases, 5*, 150–153.

Moellering, R. C. (2000). *Enterococcus* species, *Streptococcus* species, and *Leuconostoc* species. In G. L. Mandell, J. E. Bennett, & R. E. Dolin (Eds.), *Mandell, Douglas, and Bennett's principles and practice of infectious diseases* (pp. 2147–2156). Philadelphia: Churchill Livingstone.

Naides, S. J. (1998). Rheumatic manifestations of parvovirus B19 infection. *Rheumatic Disease Clinics of North America, 24,* 375–401.

Nash, G., Irvine, R., Kerschmann, R. L., & Herndier, B. (1997). Pulmonary aspergillosis in acquired immune deficiency syndrome: Autopsy study of an emerging pulmonary complication of human immunodeficiency virus infection. *Human Pathology, 28,* 1268–1275.

Nicod, L. P., Pache, J. C., & Howarth, N. (2001). Fungal infections in transplant recipients. *European Respiratory Journal, 17,* 133–140.

Osterholm, M. T. (2000). Emerging infections—another warning. *New England Journal of Medicine, 342,* 1280–1282.

Patterson, T. F., Kirkpatrick, W. R., White, M., Hiemenz, J. W., Wingard, J. R., Dupont, B., et al. (2000). Invasive aspergillosis. Disease spectrum, treatment practices, and outcomes. *Medicine, 79,* 281–282.

Prescott, J. F. (1991). *Rhodococcus equi*: An animal and human pathogen. *Clinical Microbiological Reviews, 4,* 20–34.

Quinn, T. C., & Fauci, A. S. (1998). The AIDS epidemic: Demographic aspects, population biology, and virus evolution (pp. 327–363). In R. M. Krause (Ed.), *Emerging infections.* New York: Academic Press.

Risi, G. F., & Tomascak, V. (1998). Prevention of infection in the immunocompromised host. *American Journal of Infection Control, 26,* 596–604.

Rodrigues, G. D. A., Nagendra, S., Lee, C-K., & de Magalhaes-Silverman, M. (1999). Human herpes virus 6 fatal encephalitis in a bone marrow recipient. *Scandinavian Journal of Infectious Diseases, 31,* 313–315.

Rosen, F. S., & Seligman, M. (1993). *Immunodeficiencies.* Chur, Switzerland: Harwood.

Sia, I. G., & Patel, R. (2000). New strategies for prevention and therapy of cytomegalovirus infections and disease in solid-organ transplant recipients. *Clinical Microbiology Reviews, 13,* 83–121.

Storb, R., & Thomas, E. D. (1995). Transplantation of bone marrow. In M. M. Frank, F. K. Austen, H. N. Claman, & E. R. Unanue (Eds.), *Samter's immunologic diseases* (Vol. II, pp. 1471–1493). Boston: Little, Brown.

Tramont, E. C., & Hoover, D. L. (2000). Innate (general or nonspecific) host defense mechanisms. In G. L. Mandell, J. E. Bennett, & R. E. Dolin (Eds.), *Mandell, Douglas, and Bennett's principles and practice of infectious diseases* (pp. 31–39). Philadelphia: Churchill Livingstone.

Van Burik, J., & Weisdorf, D. (2000). Infections in recipients of blood and marrow transplantation. In G. L. Mandell, J. E. Bennett, & R. E. Dolin (Eds.), *Mandell, Douglas, and Bennett's principles and practice of infectious diseases* (pp. 3136–3148). Philadelphia: Churchill Livingstone.

Vihinen, M., Arredondo-Vega, F. X., Casanova, J. L., Etzioni, A., Giliani, S., Hammarström, L., et al. (2001). Primary immunodeficiency mutation databases. *Advances in Genetics, 43,* 103–188.

Viscoli, C., & Castagnolo, E. (1999). Emerging fungal pathogens, drug resistance and the role of lipid formulations of amphotericin B in the treatment of fungal infections in cancer patients: A review. *International Journal of Infectious Diseases, 3,* 109–118.

Waldmann, T. A., & Nelson, D. (1995). Inherited immunodeficiencies. In M. M. Frank, F. K. Austen, H. N. Claman, & E. R. Unanue (Eds.), *Samter's immunologic diseases* (Vol. II, pp. 1471–1493). Boston: Little, Brown.

Walsh, T. J. (1998). Primary cutaneous aspergillosis—an emerging infection among immunocompromised patients. *Clinical Infectious Diseases, 27,* 453–457.

Wang, C. C., Mattson, D., & Wald, A. (2001). *Corynebacterium jeikeum* bacteremia in bone marrow transplant patients with Hickman catheters. *Bone Marrow Transplantation, 27,* 445–449.

Washington, L., & Miller, W. T. (1998). Mycobacterial infection in immunocompromised patients. *Journal of Thoracic Imaging, 13,* 271–281.

World Health Organization. (2000). Global AIDS surveillance. Part 1. *Weekly Epidemiological Record, 75*(No. 47), 379–383.

Zinner, S. H. (1995). New and unusual infections in neutropenic patients. *Cancer Treatment and Research, 79,* 173–184.

24

Bioterrorism

Dennis M. Perrotta

A FICTIONAL, BUT PLAUSIBLE SCENARIO

It had been a hard-fought victory. The candidate came from behind to beat the incumbent and now it was time to celebrate and thank thousands of supporters that made his bid for political office a success. Nearly 12,000 thousand campaign workers, supporters, family, and friends were in Memorial Auditorium to witness the beginning of a new political era.

Preparations had been underway for this gala event for weeks and a large number of workers had set the final touches for the stage, the entertainment, the banquet, and the speeches. Unnoticed among the hundreds of busy workers were four individuals who seemed to focus their attention on the air-conditioning system.

As the gala event reached the grand finale, the revelers witnessed hundreds of colorful balloons being released from the auditorium ceiling. What they did not notice was an ultra-fine powder simultaneously released from four parts of the auditorium air-handling system, creating an invisible cloud that enveloped the jubilant crowd. An hour later, the last of the crowd had left, and an hour after that, the four air-conditioning workers were crossing the state line.

Later that week, hospitals throughout the region began to see an alarming influx of patients presenting with malaise, high fever, chills, headache, cough with production of bloody sputum, and toxemia. Radiographic examination revealed patchy or consolidated bronchopneumonia that clinically progressed into dyspnea, stridor, and cyanosis. In the cases that first arrived, death was due to respiratory failure, circulatory collapse, and a bleeding diathesis. This course was seen in nearly every patient presenting in this fashion. They were arriving in ever-increasing numbers now. Make-shift morgues to handle the growing number of dead were established in refrigerated trailers. No one knew what they were dealing with.

Epidemiologists determined that there was one event in common among all the cases, and that was attendance at the political gala. Microbiologists ran their tests three times to make sure of their unprecedented results. Yersinia pestis, *the etiologic agent of plague, was identified by immunofluorescent staining of material from sputum of a dozen of the first patients.*

By the end of the second week, nearly all of the 4,000 persons who did not receive appropriate antibiotic therapy in time had died. A small number of nurses, physicians, and other health care providers exposed in the beginning of the epidemic also died. Many died before the diagnosis of primary pneumonic plague was established. The state police and Federal Bureau of Investigation, in spite of 10 days of intensive investigation, had no leads identifying the perpetrators of this act of biological terrorism.

INTRODUCTION

The bombings of the World Trade Center in New York City and the Alfred P. Murrah Federal Building in Oklahoma City catalyzed an awakening of American society to the reality of terrorism on its own soil. The September 11, 2001 airplane hijackings and subsequent suicide attacks on the World Trade Center and the Pentagon brought home the possibility of terrorism on American soil with tragic punctuation. The 1995 nerve agent attack in the Tokyo subway system by the Aum Shinrikyo, an apocalyptic religious cult, added a new and frightening dimension about terrorism—the use of chemical and biological weapons as agents of mass destruction. In the fall of 2001, the United States experienced its first multistate bioterrorism event with the delivery of anthrax spores in a powdered form through the mail. Franz, Jahrling, Friedlander, McClain, Hoover, Byrne, and colleagues (1997) point out that international changes, including the breakup of the Soviet Union and the perceived dominance of the United States as a conventional military world power, have raised concerns about the use of biological weapons as a new tool of warfare and terrorism against civilians.

A BRIEF HISTORY OF BIOLOGICAL WEAPON USE

The use of pathogenic microorganisms as weapons is not a 20th century phenomenon. For centuries, militaries developed and used crude methods for dispersing these agents as weapons of warfare. The Center for Nonproliferation Studies (1999) has chronicled major uses of these agents in warfare. In 1346–1347, the Mongols reportedly catapulted corpses of plague victims over the walls into Kaffa (now in the Ukraine), forcing the weary Genoans to flee. Christopher, Cieslak, Pavlin, and Eitzen (1999) related that during the French and Indian Wars, Sir Jeffrey Amherst, a British commander in North America, suggested the deliberate use of smallpox against hostile Indian tribes. On June 24, 1763, an officer under Amherst's direction gave blankets and a handkerchief from the smallpox hospital to Indians as "gifts." Smallpox epidemics in the immunologically naïve tribes followed, though other contacts with Europeans may have also served to transmit smallpox to the tribes.

In 1932, the Imperial Japanese Army began systematic development and testing of biological agents at Ping Fan in Manchuria. Harris (1997) thoroughly examined the activities of the infamous Unit 731, responsible for the majority of these activities. During the years up to the end of World War II, the leaders of Unit 731 conducted an extensive array of live human experiments, including exposures to cold and to a long list of highly toxic agents, including *Y. pestis*, *B. anthracis*, *Vibrio cholerae*, and *Neisseria meningitidis*. Over the course of the program, an estimated 3,000 prisoners, mostly Chinese, died in these experiments.

Two more recent incidents illustrate the potential use of biological weapons. In April 1979, within the city of Sverdlovsk (now Yekaterinburg) in Russia's Ural Mountains, a mysterious outbreak of anthrax took the lives of nearly 70 local citizens. Russian officials attributed the outbreak to consumption of tainted meat sold on the black market. U.S. officials thought differently, believing that the epidemic was due to an explosion at the nearby Soviet Institute of Microbiology and Virology, believed to be a military biological weapons plant. In 1992, Boris Yeltsin, then president of Russia, admitted that there had been an accident at the Institute that resulted in the release of spores of weaponized *Bacillus anthracis*. Meselson, Guillemin, Hugh-Jones, Langmuir, Popova, Shelokov, and Yampolskaya (1994), using exquisite epidemiologic reasoning and evidence, convincingly concluded that the escape of an aerosol of anthrax bacilli from the military facility caused the outbreak.

In 1978, Bulgarian Secret Police agents reportedly assassinated Georgi Markov, a Bulgarian in exile in London. As described by Simon (1999), Markov was attacked by an unknown assailant with a weapon disguised as an umbrella. A pellet, no larger than the head of a pin, was discharged into the subcutaneous tissue of his leg while he waited for a bus. He died 3 days later and, upon autopsy, the pellet was found. The pellet was machined to contain a toxin (in this case, ricin) that would be released when body heat melted the coat of wax encasing the toxin. A similar assassination was attempted just weeks later, but fortunately the toxin was not released as planned.

TERRORISM

O'Neill (1995) defines terrorism as "the unlawful use of force against persons or property to intimidate or coerce a government, the civilian population, or any segment thereof, in the furtherance of political or social objectives" (p. 1.20). Extrapolating to chemical or biological terrorism, Perrotta, Rawlings, and Eckman (1998) suggested that the use of harmful chemicals, pathogenic microbes, or plant or microbial toxins as weapons of terrorism should be known as bioterrorism. That the act is executed in the furtherance of political or social objectives serves to differentiate it from criminal assault.

It is important to understand the variety of categories of terrorist groups because such knowledge helps predict the kind and size of weapons such groups are generally likely to use or are capable of using. Generally, terrorist groups are classified as foreign, domestic, or religious. Foreign terrorist groups may be state supported or independent (Fainberg, 1997). It is clear that the government of the former Soviet Union supported an enormous offensive biological weapons program as detailed by Alibek (Alibek & Handelman, 1999) who, before his defection to the United States, was among the top leaders of that program. A variety of pathogens, including *Francisella tularensis* (tularemia), variola virus (smallpox), and *Bacillus anthracis* (anthrax) were "weaponized" and made ready for missiles aimed at American targets. It is unclear if terrorists were provided with biological weapons from the Soviet Union's sizeable arsenal. International intelligence information, as described by Cole (1997), suggests that 17 countries are suspected of having active biological weapons research programs.

There is a plethora of domestic antigovernment, neo-Nazi groups within the U.S. that have already made attempts to acquire biological agents and toxins. Tucker (1999) reported that in 1995 Larry Wayne Harris, a purported laboratory technician from Ohio, ordered three vials of *Yersinia pestis* (plague bacillus) from a Maryland biomedical supply firm. Concerned about his impatience and apparent unfamiliarity with laboratory techniques, the company notified federal authorities.

Upon investigation, authorities found the vials in the glove compartment of his car. He was arrested and was later identified as a member of a white supremacy organization. He pleaded guilty to federal charges of mail fraud. Tucker (1999) further describes that later, in 1998, Mr. Harris was again arrested in possession of what he described as "enough military-grade anthrax to wipe out Las Vegas" (p. 284). The vials were later determined to contain harmless veterinary vaccine against anthrax.

O'Neill (1995) reported that the quasi-militia, antitax group, the Patriots Council, headquartered in Minneapolis, was planning to assassinate a deputy U.S. marshal and a local sheriff using ricin, a protein toxin derived from the castor plant, *Ricinus communis*. Plans were progressing until four individuals were caught and convicted of acts against the Biological Weapons Anti-Terrorism Act of 1989. So far, no domestic group has carried out a successful first biological terrorism attack on civilian American populations.

Religious cults vary in sophistication and resources, but at least one group, the Rajneesh, successfully carried out what most consider the first biological terrorism attack on American soil. Török, Tauxe, Wise, Livengood, Sokolow, Mauvais, and associates (1997) investigated a large community-wide outbreak of salmonellosis in Dalles, Oregon in 1984. More than 750 individuals became ill after eating from salad bars in 10 area restaurants. This exhaustive epidemiologic examination initially failed to identify any plausible, naturally occurring source for the contamination. It wasn't until 1 year later that a law enforcement and public health investigation identified the source as a clinical laboratory operated by the Rajneesh. The cult had intentionally seeded area salad bars to influence voter turnout in an upcoming election.

The March 1995 release of the organophosphate nerve agent sarin in the Tokyo subway system is generally regarded as the "wake-up call" regarding the use of chemical or biological agents against civilian populations. Olsen (1995) investigated the incident perpetrated by members of the Aum Shinrikyo and noted that the cult had previously tested a variety of biological agents such as *B. anthracis* and the toxin that causes botulism on unsuspected civilian populations in Japan. In the sarin release, 12 persons died and nearly 5,500 injuries were reported. While most intelligence sources indicate that only foreign state-supported groups would have the resources to execute a credible bioterrorism event, the Rajneesh and Aum Shinrikyo appear to serve as exceptions to that belief.

To date, no comprehensive assessment of the threat and risks of bioterrorism has been conducted for the United States (United States

General Accounting Office, 1999). Osterholm (1999) suggests that, "It is not a matter of if a bioterrorism event will occur in the United States, but rather when, where, and how large" (p. 462). Hughes (1999) considers bioterrorism an emerging infectious disease threat since an attack will manifest as a sizeable epidemic, and the resources necessary to mount an effective response will include the same disease surveillance, epidemiology, and laboratory components as a naturally-occurring outbreak does. McDade and Franz (1998) note that partnerships among health care providers, state and local health agencies, and the Centers for Disease Control and Prevention (CDC) are essential for preparedness. This chapter focuses on the use of pathogenic microbes and their toxins as weapons of terrorism. Readers interested in the use of toxic chemicals are referred to Sidell, Takafuji, and Franz (1997).

REQUIREMENTS FOR AN IDEAL BIOLOGICAL AGENT

Nearly any pathogenic microorganism could be used to cause disease in humans on a limited or small scale. Fortunately, relatively few would be effective if employed as a weapon of terrorism against a large population. Sidell, Takafuji, and Franz (1997) outlined six key factors that make a pathogen or toxin suitable for large-scale biological warfare attack:

- readily available or easy to produce in large quantities;
- highly virulent for lethal or incapacitating effects in humans;
- appropriate particle size in aerosol;
- easy to disseminate with proper technology;
- stable; able to withstand harsh environmental conditions; and
- likely to affect only the target population, not the terrorists.

These characteristics also make them attractive to terrorists.

While the cultivation and growth of pathogenic microbes for these purposes is a relatively simple operation, there remain significant barriers to implementing a biologic weapon of mass destruction. Hinton (1999), in his testimony before the United States Senate, observed that a terrorist group would need "a relatively high degree of sophistication to successfully and effectively process, improvise a weapon, and disseminate biological agents to cause mass casualties" (p. 3). One such technological impediment is the fact that the respiratory system is the most likely target of a widespread attack, and particles must be in the range of 1–5 microns in diameter in order to reach the alveolar spaces where damage first occurs. It has been technologically difficult to meet these specifications. Osterholm and Schwartz (2000) relate discussions with an expert on particle technology who believes the technology is readily available.

Potential Biologic Agents

The Centers for Disease Control and Prevention (CDC) (1999) convened a panel of experts to identify biological agents considered to be of greatest potential concern. Applying a variety of criteria, three categories of agents emerged (see Table 24.1).

Category A includes agents that were determined to represent the greatest threat to public health in terms of producing mortality and morbidity and in terms of the need to increase surveillance and to stockpile antidotes, antibiotics, and vaccines. *Category B* agents possess the ability to cause illness, but require fewer public health preparations. *Category C* agents were determined to be possible emerging public health threats. The entire critical agent list is regularly reviewed to allow for new, emerging infectious threats to be added. Agents that may be potential biological weapons may include those plant and animal diseases that also affect socioeconomic stability. For example, foot-and-mouth disease has been considered as a potential biological weapon (Rath & Bürgel, 2001).

SELECTED BIOLOGICAL AGENTS AND THEIR DISEASES

The intent of the terrorist may not be immediately evident, but experience suggests that striking fear, panic, and dread in a society is at the heart of their actions. To that end, the use of agents with high public recognition value might cause the desired social disruption, even if no one becomes ill. The evidence for this lies in the thousands of recently reported biologic agent releases that all were determined to be hoaxes. Because these high profile agents are well-suited for the desires of the terrorist, brief descriptions of three agents and their diseases—smallpox, anthrax, and plague—are presented.

TABLE 24.1 Critical Biological Agent Categories for Public Health Preparedness

Category A agents

Biologic agent	*Disease(s)*
Variola virus	Smallpox
Bacillus anthracis	Anthrax
Yersinia pestis	Plague
Clostridium botulinum toxin	Botulism
Francisella tularensis	Tularaemia
Ebola virus	Ebola hemorrhagic fever;
Marburg virus	Marburg hemorrhagic fever
Lassa virus	Lassa fever;
Junin virus	Argentine hemorrhagic fever
Other arenaviruses	

Category B agents

Biologic agent	*Disease(s)*
Coxiella burnetti	Q fever
Brucella species	Brucellosis
Burkholderia mallei	Glanders
Venezuelan equine encephalitis virus;	Venezuelan encephalomyelitis;
Eastern equine encephalitis virus;	Eastern equine encephalomyelitis;
Western equine encephalitis virus	Western equine encephalomyelitis

Others include:

Ricin toxin from *Ricinus communis*,
Epsilon toxin of *Clostridium perfringens*,
Staphylococcus enterotoxin B,
Salmonella species,
Shigella dysenteriae,
Escherichia coli O157:H7,
Vibrio cholerae, and
Cryptosporidium parvum.

Category C agents

- Nipah virus
- Hantaviruses
- Tickborne hemorrhagic fever viruses
- Tickborne encephalitis viruses
- Yellow fever
- Multidrug-resistant tuberculosis

Source: Centers for Disease Control and Prevention (2000a).

Smallpox

Recognized as a clinical entity since biblical times, smallpox was eradicated from the globe in 1980 as the result of decades of exhaustive planning and fieldwork (Fenner, Henderson, Arita, Jezel, & Ladnyi, 1988). Since that time, stocks of variola virus were consolidated into two World Health Organization (WHO)-approved repositories. Recently, Alibek and Handelman (1999) expressed concern that other clandestine virus stockpiles, as well as expertise and equipment, may have been recruited from the enormous Soviet biological warfare program, which has sharply declined in recent years due to the dissolution of that union and the severe financial environments in the remaining countries. It is this concern that resurrects the specter of the use of variola virus as a biological weapon. Such a release would have dire consequences for the planet, since nearly all immunity against variola infection has waned in the more than 20 years since the last individual was immunized.

Variola is a member of the virus genus *Orthopoxvirus* and is nearly indistinguishable from the other members—monkeypox, vaccinia, and cowpox. This DNA virus infects only humans, although the origins of human disease are unknown. The Institute of Medicine (1999a) observed that from the time smallpox was first described as a human illness until the end of the 19th century, it was considered a uniformly severe disease with case-fatality rates of up to 40% in unvaccinated individuals. Throughout the remaining 80 years of the virus's uncontrolled existence, case-fatality rates were approximately 30%.

Franz and colleagues (1997) outline the pathogenesis of smallpox as beginning with a small aerosol exposure. From the respiratory system, the virus travels to regional lymph nodes where it replicates, produces a viremia, and results in viral multiplication in the spleen, bone marrow, and lymph nodes. By the eighth day after infection, a second viremia occurs, this time followed by fever and toxemia. At the end of a 12–14 day incubation period, an abrupt onset of systemic toxicity with serious malaise, high fever, rigors, vomiting, headache, and backache occurs. A maculopapular rash first appears on the oral and pharyngeal mucosa. The oropharyngeal lesions ulcerate quickly and release large amounts of virus into the saliva, as first described by Sarkar, Mitra, Mukherjee, and De (1973). Respiratory secretions that contain virus from these lesions are the most important source of exposure to contacts. This step occurs during the first week of illness and corresponds with the period during which patients are most contagious.

The rash progresses to the face and forearms, followed by spread to the lower extremities and then centrally to the trunk. Lesions quickly progress from macules to papules and eventually to pustular vesicles. They are more abundant on the extremities and the face, and this centrifugal distribution is an important, although unexplained, clinical feature. During the second week, the pustules form scabs that leave depressed depigmented scars upon healing. Since the virus can be easily recovered from scabs throughout convalescence, patients should be isolated until all scabs separate (Mitra, Sarkar, & Mukherjee, 1974).

Should the victim succumb to the effects of viral infection, death usually occurs during the second week of illness, most likely the result of toxemia associated with circulating immune complexes and soluble variola antigens (Fenner et al., 1988). There have been two irregularly observed variations of smallpox disease, flat-type and hemorrhagic type. Both of these clinical forms were seen in less than 5% of patients, but they were characterized by severe systemic toxicity and high mortality.

While testing of antiviral drugs is an active field of research and development, few, if any, antiviral agents are suitable for use against smallpox (Institute of Medicine, 1999a). Cidofovir, initially developed as a DNA polymerase inhibitor for the treatment of cytomegalovirus retinitis, was found to have inhibitory properties against variola infection in cell culture. Because of potential renal toxicity and low oral bioavailability, however, cidofovir is of limited utility for treating or preventing variola infection in humans. Other strategies are being examined, but they suffer from a lack of a clinically meaningful animal model and from the inaccessibility of virus stocks for testing of drug effectiveness.

The vaccine used in the historic WHO Smallpox Eradication Program did not contain variola virus, as one might expect. The vaccine, prepared on a large scale by inoculating the shaved abdomens of calves, contained vaccinia virus, another member of the *Orthopox* genus that has little pathogenicity for immunocompetent humans (McClain, 1997). This vaccine was administered through a process called scarification that used a bifurcated needle to intradermally inoculate susceptible populations. Vaccination, targeted by intensive, active surveillance, was the linchpin of the smallpox eradication program. After the eradication program was complete, there was no incentive for vaccine manufacturers to continue to formulate smallpox vaccine, so stores of usable vaccine were diminished. In September, 2000, CDC entered into an agreement with OraVax to manufacture smallpox vaccine (LeDuc & Jahrling, 2001).

The WHO had planned to destroy all stocks of variola virus by 1999, but concerns about terrorist organizations possessing the virus for nefarious purposes resulted in the postponement of this action to be reevaluated in 2002 (LeDuc & Jahrling, 2001). The Institute of Medicine (1999a) conducted an assessment for the future scientific needs for live variola virus and concluded that there are legitimate scientific circumstances that support keeping the virus stocks intact. No further action has been taken. The airborne spread, high communicability, nearly complete sensitivity of human populations, and high lethality of this virus make it an excellent candidate for use as a weapon of mass destruction (Henderson, Inglesby, Bartlett, Ascher, Eitzen, Jahrling, et al., 1999). The intentional release of anthrax spores in fall 2001, sharpened fears about smallpox and other potential agents for use in bioterrorist attacks. Because of its potential for use in a bioterrorist attack, an interim smallpox release plan and guidelines and a revision of vaccine recommendations from the Advisory Committee on Immunization practices were issued in November 2001 (on-line at http://www.cdc.gov/nip/smallpox). Other bioterrorism information is available at http://www.bt.cdc.gov.

Anthrax

Described first in biblical times, this zoonotic disease is caused by the gram-positive, spore-forming rod, *Bacillus anthracis*. Anthrax occurs primarily in herbivores, such as goats, sheep, cattle, and horses. Humans are most often infected by contact with infected animals or contaminated animal products (Friedlander & Longfield, 2000). Outbreaks of anthrax during the 16th and 18th centuries occurred with devastating agricultural consequences. Currently, sporadic cases of naturally occurring human cutaneous anthrax are reported in the United States (Centers for Disease Control, 1988). In one case, doing field autopsies of dead sheep, later culture positive for *B. anthracis*, was the suspected exposure (Taylor, Dimmitt, Ezzel, & Whitford, 1993). In the summer of 2000, one such sporadic case of cutaneous anthrax occurred in North Dakota. The 67-year-old infected man had participated in the disposal of cows that had died of anthrax. He became ill four days later, initially noticing a bump on his cheek. He was treated with ciprofloxacin and recovered (Centers for Disease Control and Prevention, 2001). Anthrax is reported in domestic and wild animals in the United States (Centers for Disease Control and Prevention, 2000c). The first use of *B. anthracis* in warfare is suggested by substantial evidence indicating that Germany used this organism, and others, during World War I (Christopher et al., 1999). The Germans reportedly infected Romanian sheep that were being exported to Russia, in an apparent attempt to infect Russian soldiers.

B. anthracis is a relatively large gram-positive bacillus that is nonmotile and forms spores when infected tissues are exposed to ambient air (Dragon & Rennie, 1995). Microscopic examination shows a "jointed bamboo-rod" cellular appearance of the organism when grown on common laboratory media. The virulence of *B. anthracis* is attributed to four known factors: three protein exotoxin components called the protective antigen, lethal factor, and edema factor; and an antiphagocytic capsule (Dixon, Meselson, Guillemin, & Hanna, 1999). The exotoxin components, which are individually without biologic activity, combine in binary form to create two toxins. Edema factor joins with protective antigen to form edema toxin, which is responsible for increased cellular levels of cyclic AMP that lead to the massive edema observed in anthrax-affected tissues and organs. Lethal toxin consists of lethal factor and protective antigen, and is responsible for increasing macrophage release of tumor necrosis factor and interleukin-1, both of which play a role in the sudden death (shock) observed in the systemic phase of inhalational anthrax (Hanna, Acosta, & Collier, 1993). The role of the antiphagocytic capsule as a general virulence factor was described nearly 100 years ago when strains without this capsule were found to be avirulent (Friedlander, 1997).

There are three clinical manifestations of *B. anthracis* in humans: inhalational, gastrointestinal, and cutaneous anthrax (Chin, 2000). Before October 2001, inhalational anthrax was rarely seen, but was known as Woolsorter's Disease because workers in industrial mills were at highest risk of exposure from the hides, wool, and hair of contaminated animals (Brachman, 1980). The last case of inhalational anthrax from this type of exposure occurred in 1978 (Centers for Disease Control and Prevention, 1994a). In late 2001, 11 cases of inhalational anthrax occurred as a result of the intentional distribution of *B. anthracis* spores in letters delivered by the United States Postal Service (Centers for Disease Control and Prevention, 2001b). Cases occurred in media workers, postal workers, a woman who worked in a nonpatient care area of a hospital, and in a 94-year-old woman in rural Connecticut. The exposure source for the latter two are not know. Gastrointestinal anthrax results from ingestion of contaminated meat that has not been sufficiently cooked. This manifestation is not seen in the United States; it was inaccurately reported to be the cause of the 1979 Sverdlovsk outbreak previously described.

The vast majority of reported cases of anthrax have been cutaneous anthrax where pathogenic endospores of *B. anthracis* have been introduced by cut or abrasion (Friedlander & Longfield, 2000). Within 36 hours of development of a painless, pruritic papule, a vesicle forms and undergoes central necrosis. The black eschar is often surrounded by edema and remains painless. Complications are rare; most cases of cutaneous anthrax are self-limiting but dissemination can occur in about 20% of cases, so antibiotic treatment is indicated (Dixon et al., 1999; Friedlander & Longfield, 2000). Eleven cases (seven confirmed and four suspected) of cutaneous anthrax resulting from deliberate distribution of anthrax spores occurred in the U. S. in the fall of 2001 (Centers for Disease Control and Prevention, 2001c).

The intentional airborne spread of anthrax endospores is of greatest public health concern. In this case, spore-bearing particles are deposited in the alveolar spaces where macrophages phagocytize and transport them to regional lymph nodes. Vegetative anthrax bacilli multiply there and are spread by blood and lymph systems throughout the body leading to severe septicemia. Concentrations of exotoxins increase rapidly and result in severe local effects, thoracic hemorrhagic necrotizing lymphadenitis, hemorrhagic necrotizing mediastinitis, and toxemia (Abramova, Grinberg, Yampolskaya, & Walker, 1993). This rapid onset of shock and respiratory distress is followed by death within 36 hours in nearly all untreated victims.

Clinically, patients first present with flu-like symptoms including fever, dyspnea, cough, headache, vomiting, weakness, and chest pain that persist for 2–3 days (Brachman, 1980). In previous reports (Friedlander, 1997), the incubation period for inhalational anthrax was between 1 and 6 days, but the investigation of the Sverdlovsk release by Meselson and colleagues (1994) suggests cases occurred from 2–43 days after exposure. Nearly all of the cases of inhalational anthrax in Sverdlovsk resulted from the initial release of the anthrax bacillus. Neither secondary aerosols nor person-to-person spread of the organism appear to play a role in spread of the disease. These observations about incubation period and the lack of person-to-person spread have important implications for the public health response to an epidemic of inhalational anthrax.

The patient may experience a period of clinical improvement for 1–2 days, but rapidly deteriorates with the sudden onset of respiratory distress, dyspnea, cyanosis, chest pain, and diaphoresis. The radiographic observation of a widened mediastinum is an important clue to making the diagnosis of inhalational anthrax. Without suspicion from public health or law enforcement sources, it is unlikely that such a diagnosis will otherwise be made in emergency rooms, clinics, or physicians' offices. Autopsy results indicating thoracic hemorrhagic necrotizing lymphadenitis, hemorrhagic necrotizing mediastinitis, or hemorrhagic meningitis should raise strong suspicions of anthrax infection (Inglesby et al., 1999) and may provide the first clue to the identity of the epidemic disease.

Treatment of anthrax is complicated by a lack of clinical trials of treatments for inhalational anthrax, contraindications for use of selected antibiotics in subgroups (children, pregnant women), the extended presence of anthrax spores in the lungs, and the logistic issues of treating very large population groups (Inglesby, Henderson, Bartlett, Ascher, Eitzen, Jahrling, et al., 1999). Intravenous administration of penicillin and doxycycline has most often been recommended, although intravenous ciprofloxicin has been recommended by a consensus group (Dixon et al., 1999; Inglesby et al., 1999). This group, recognizing that there is great risk of recurrence in survivors of inhalational anthrax due to the possibility of delayed germination of spores remaining in alveolar spaces, recommends that treatment continue for 60 days, with oral therapy replacing intravenous therapy as soon as the patient's clinical condition improves. Postexposure prophylaxis may include the use of oral doxycycline or ciprofloxicin. Another approach to treatment for anthrax that is in the exploratory stages is the use of an agent to block the action of bacterial virulence factors (Sellman, Mourez, & Collier, 2001). The 22 cases of anthrax occurring in fall 2001 have led to additional information on clinical signs and symptoms, management and progress, as well as dissemination and spread (Jernigan, Stephens, Ashford, Omenaca, Topiel, Galbraith, et al., 2001; Swartrz, 2001).

A vaccine that protects against anthrax is available, but supplies are currently severely limited, due, in part, to the demand for the vaccine by the United States military, which had inoculated all military personnel. Concerns about adverse effects have not been borne out (Centers for Disease Control and Prevention, 2000b). The capacity to make more vaccine is quite modest, and supplies are expected to remain limited for the foreseeable future. If supplies were available, administration of vaccine would require concurrent antibiotic administration to protect individuals exposed to anthrax spores from a bioterrorist attack. Routine vaccination of civilian U.S. populations is not recommended (Centers for Disease Control and Prevention, 2000c).

In the face of hundreds of anthrax hoaxes in the United States and the accompanying variation in decontamination strategies, the CDC released interim guidelines for management of these situations (Centers for Disease Control and Prevention, 1999). Decontamination of individuals is not generally recommended or necessary but if it is undertaken, it requires only showering with copious amounts of water and soap and the routine laundering of clothes. Physical surfaces may be cleaned with a 0.5% hypochlorite solution following a crime scene investigation. Additional recommendations for avoiding exposure and for decontamination may be found in Centers for Disease Control and Prevention (2001c).

Plague

Few human diseases generate as much fear and emotion as plague does and much has been written about its impact on human populations. This zoonotic infection is caused by *Yersinia pestis*, a relatively small gram-negative coccobacillus that does not form spores. This organism has been the cause of three great pandemics in the 6th, 14th, and 20th centuries. The second pandemic, known as the Black Death, took the lives of more than 40 million people from 1346 through the end of the 14th century (McGovern & Friedlander, 1997).

In more modern times, nearly 700 persons with plague, including 56 fatal cases, were reported from India in a 2-month period of 1994 (Centers for Disease Control and Prevention, 1994a, 1994b). In 1997, a plague patient in Madagascar transmitted pneumonic plague to 18 persons, including 8 persons who died (Ratsitorahina, Chanteau, Rahalison, Rastisofasoamanana, & Biosier, 2000). In the U.S., an average of 10–15 human infections are reported yearly from 13 western states, predominantly New Mexico, Arizona, Colorado, and California (Centers for Disease Control and Prevention, 1994a, 1994b).

There are three clinical presentations of plague: bubonic, septicemic, and pneumonic. Naturally occurring plague is most commonly transmitted by the bite of a flea infected with *Y. pestis* and results in bubonic plague. This happens usually when humans encroach on the mostly rural habitat of rats of the genus *Rattus*, where they are likely to come into contact with infected fleas from those rats. Infection causes a severe febrile illness that generally includes headache, chills, myalgia, malaise, prostration, and gastrointestinal symptoms. Bubonic plague is characterized by acute regional lymphadenopathy that manifests as a bubo, most often in the inguinal, axillary, or cervical regions, depending upon where the infected flea inoculates the plague bacilli. These buboes, which are extremely painful to touch or movement, appear within 24 hours of the onset of systemic symptoms (McGovern & Friedlander, 1997). Septicemic plague can occur secondarily to bubonic plague or can develop without detectable lymphadenopathy. The case-fatality rate for bubonic plague is 50%–60%; septicemic plague is virtually invariably fatal (Chin, 2000).

The pneumonic form of plague is the most dangerous in terms of public health threat and is the form most likely to occur after the airborne release of a plague biological weapon (Inglesby, Dennis, Henderson, Bartlett, Ascher, Eitzen, et al., 2000). Primary pneumonic plague is characterized by a severe pneumonia, high fever, dyspnea, and hemoptysis, which occur within 1–3 days of the infective aerosol exposure from a biological weapon or another pneumonic plague patient (secondary spread). Secondary pneumonic plague, which may follow the bubonic or septicemic forms, results from hematogenous spread of the plague bacilli to the lungs. Without effective treatment, the case-fatality rate for pneumonic plague is essentially 100%.

Upon introduction into the human host, *Y. pestis* synthesizes a variety of virulence factors, including an anti-phagocytic capsule that allows the organism to resist phagocytosis and to replicate unimpeded (McGovern & Friedlander, 1997). The endotoxin of *Y. pestis* contributes to the development of septic shock in manners similar to those seen with other gram-negative organisms. As might be expected, complications of gram-negative sepsis could include disseminated intravascular coagulation, adult respiratory distress syndrome, and multiple organ system failure.

Inglesby and associates (2000), in their consensus work on the management of plague used as a biological weapon, suggest that the first indication of a covert attack with plague might be a sudden outbreak of illness presenting as severe pneumonia and sepsis. Since this would be primary pneumonic plague, buboes would rarely be seen. Autopsy findings would include areas of profound lobular exudation and bacillary aggregation (Dennis & Meier, 1997), since *Y. pestis* is believed to be the only gram-negative bacterium capable of causing fulminant pneumonia with blood-tinged sputum in an otherwise healthy individual.

Since either primary or secondary pneumonic plague patients are capable of creating infective aerosols, patients should be kept in droplet precautions for 72 hours after initiation of effective therapy (Garner, 1996). Plague is a reportable condition in nearly all 50 states; proven or suspect cases must be reported to state or local health authorities immediately (Rousch, Birkhead, Koo, Cobb, & Fleming, 1999).

There are little modern data that support clear recommendations for the best treatment of plague. Since the 1950s, intramuscular streptomycin has been used to treat plague (Perry & Featherston, 1997), but streptomycin is uncommonly found in the United States. Gentamicin has been used as an alternative to streptomycin as it is widely available and inexpensive (American Hospital Formulary Service, 2000). A critical review and development of consensus recommendations for therapies was conducted by Inglesby and colleagues (2000). They make two general recommendations based on the size of the population likely to require treatment. For treating a modest number of patients, parenteral administration of streptomycin or gentamicin is recommended. For a large casualty situation, where intravenous or intramuscular therapy is not logistically feasible, oral administration of doxycycline (or tetracycline) or ciprofloxicin is recommended. Presumptive treatment of persons in the exposed area with fever and cough should occur immediately. The special situations of treating children, immunosupressed persons, and pregnant women are also outlined in these recommendations. Asymptomatic close contacts of persons with pneumonic plague should receive a 7-day course of antibiotics as well.

The plague bacillus, in contrast to the anthrax bacillus, does not survive for extended periods of time outside of the host, nor does it form environmentally hardy spores. No special decontamination of environmental surfaces, more than normal hospital cleaning, is indicated.

OTHER CONSIDERATIONS

Depending on the scope of an intentional release of a pathogenic microbe, a potentially larger epidemic of psychological and psychiatric disorders will quickly follow the infectious disease threat. Holloway, Norwood, Fullerton, Engel, and Ursano (1997) point out that a significant number of psychological factors can be associated with the use of biological agents. These include horror, anger, panic, magical thinking about microbes, fear of invisible agents, fear of contagion, attribution of arousal symptoms to infection, and others. Clearly humans have deep-seated fear of infection and death. Unfortunately, many jurisdictions that have been developing response plans have focused solely on responding to the communicable disease epidemic. The fear, panic, and dread can spread, perhaps even faster than the microbial threat with the hyperbole of media coverage (Smith, Veenhuis, & MacCormack, 2000). The provision of mental health services must be a priority, concomitant with provision of medical services (DiGiovanni, 1999).

Much of the work toward understanding the impact of microbiological agents has been conducted in military settings. The populations exposed and studied have most often been predominantly young adult males in good physical condition. In the case of a release of a pathogenic microbe in the general population, the entire population spectrum of a city or region might be affected. This would include subpopulations with special vulnerabilities or needs, and these populations must be considered in preparedness planning. The American Academy of Pediatrics, Committees on Environmental Health and Infectious Diseases (2000), point out the special needs and concerns of the pediatric population with regard to exposure to chemical or biological terrorism.

The standard public health model of primary prevention is of limited utility to the health care community as it relates to bioterrorism. Prevention of a bioterrorism act falls mostly into the purview of law enforcement and criminal intelligence and outside the realm of most nurses, physicians, and health officials. Therefore, prevention of as many cases of disease in the face of an intentional release is a reasonable goal of bioterrorism response and preparedness planners. Kaufmann, Meltzer, and Schmid (1997) evaluated the economic impact of bioterrorist attacks using three different classic biological agents. The range was estimated at $477.7 million per 100,000 persons for their brucellosis scenario, to $26.2 billion per 100,000 persons exposed to the anthrax bacillus. Their study, using an insurance analogy, clearly indicated that post-attack prophylaxis and response is the single most important means of reducing the losses. Importantly, they suggest that the presence of a well-designed, implemented, and exercised response utilizing post-attack prophylaxis may act as a deterrent to those who would execute such an attack for maximum impact. Russell (1997) posits that the effectiveness of any post-attack intervention depends on a rapid response that requires prior planning, preparation, and training.

BIOTERRORISM PREPAREDNESS AND RESPONSE

Since a bioterrorist attack is likely to be a local, as opposed to a statewide, event, local hospitals, managed care organizations, clinics, and other health care delivery settings may be called upon to participate in response and response planning. Hospitals, which will be rapidly overwhelmed with ill and the "worried well" must prepare for medical care, security, decontamination when appropriate, and infection control issues.

Recommendations of a CDC Strategic Planning Workgroup on Biological and Chemical Terrorism Preparedness and Response (Centers for Disease Control and Prevention, 2000a) provide excellent background information and a sound foundation for development of a national response capacity, but do not provide direction at the local or facility level. Macintyre and associates (2000) point out that most health care facilities are poorly prepared to mount an effective response to the great influx of patients and their infections. The authors propose a concept of operation for civilian hospital settings that highlights prompt recognition, staff and facility protection, patient decontamination and triage, medical therapy, and external coordination with emergency response and public health agencies.

The Association of Professionals in Infection Control and Epidemiology, Inc. (APIC) (2000) has developed a bioterrorism readiness plan template for health care facilities that focuses on infection control and prophylaxis considerations in hospitals and other institutions. The plan fails, however, to detail the vital role infection control nurses play in the surveillance and reporting of communicable diseases. Timely detection and reporting of the first signals of an unusual (potentially intentionally-caused) outbreak is crucial to best possible response outcome (Institute of Medicine, 1999b).

Many of the nursing, medical, and public health aspects of bioterrorism preparedness and response are new to emergency response planners. Therefore, public health agencies are now being included in the planning process. This is a relatively new development and one that will benefit from the wisdom and guidance of health care professionals who will ultimately care for the sick and injured (including psychological injury). All health care settings should become involved in partnerships with local health agencies to ensure that the very best response plan is developed, exercised, and updated for their community. State health agencies are making preparations to assist local health authorities in detecting and responding to an intentionally-caused epidemic. In most cases, the office of the State Epidemiologist will serve as a contact for information for each state's plan. The CDC has a 24-hour emergency phone number (770-488-1700) for information and assistance, but all callers should first contact their local and state health departments for direct assistance. Local law enforcement agencies have a similar communications procedure that ensures that the Federal Bureau of Investigation is notified of a potential crime.

Nurses and other frontline health care providers have a variety of opportunities to participate in planning and preparing for a bioterrorist attack. It is commonly understood that a well executed plan will not guarantee that all morbidity and mortality will be prevented, but it is guaranteed that many more will die in the absence of such a plan.

REFERENCES

Abramova, F. A., Grinberg, L. M., Yampolskaya, O. V., & Walker, D. H. (1993). Pathology of inhalational anthrax in 42 cases from the Sverdlovsk outbreak of 1979. *Proceedings of the National Academy of Sciences of the United States of America, 90*, 2291–2294.

Alibek, K., & Handelman, S. (1999). *Biohazard.* New York: Random House.

American Academy of Pediatrics, Committee on Environmental Health and Committee on Infectious Diseases. (2000). Chemical-biological terrorism and its impact on children: A subject review. *Pediatrics, 105*, 662–670.

American Hospital Formulary Service. (2000) *AHFS drug information.* Bethesda, MD: American Society of Health System Pharmacists.

Association for Professionals in Infection Control and Epidemiology, Inc. (2000). *Bioterrorism readiness plan: A template for healthcare facilities* [On-line]. Available: http://www.apic.org/html/educ/readinow.html

Bauer, D. J., St. Vincent, L., Kempe, C. H., & Downie, A. W. (1963). Prophylactic treatment of smallpox contacts with N-methylisatin-thiosemicarbazone (compound 33T57, Marboran). *Lancet, 2*, 494–496.

Brachman, P. S. (1980). Inhalation anthrax. *Annals of the New York Academy of Sciences, 353*, 83–93.

Center for Nonproliferation Studies. (1999). Chronology of state use and biological and chemical weapons control. *Chemical & Biological Weapons Resource Page* [On-line]. Available: http://cns.miis.edu/research/cbw/pastuse.htm

Centers for Disease Control. (1988). Human cutaneous anthrax—North Carolina, 1987. *Morbidity and Mortality Weekly Report, 37*, 413–414.

Centers for Disease Control and Prevention. (1994a). Human plague—United States, 1993–1994. *Morbidity and Mortality Weekly Report, 43*, 242–246.

Centers for Disease Control and Prevention. (1994b). Update: Human plague—India, 1994. *Morbidity and Mortality Weekly Report, 43*, 761–762.

Centers for Disease Control and Prevention. (1996). Prevention of plague: Recommendations of the Advisory Committee on Immunization Practices (ACIP). *Morbidity and Mortality Weekly Report, 45*(RR-14), 1–15.

Centers for Disease Control and Prevention. (1999). Bioterrorism alleging use of anthrax and interim guidelines for management—United States, 1998. *Morbidity and Mortality Weekly Report, 48,* 69–74.

Centers for Disease Control and Prevention. (2000a). Biological and chemical terrorism: Strategic plan for preparedness and response. Recommendations of the CDC Strategic Planning Workgroup. *Morbidity and Mortality Weekly Report, 49*(RR-4), 5–6.

Centers for Disease Control and Prevention. (2000b). Surveillance for adverse events associated with anthrax vaccination—U.S. Department of Defense, 1998–2000. *Morbidity and Mortality Weekly Report, 49,* 341–345.

Centers for Disease Control and Prevention. (2000c). Use of anthrax vaccine in the United States. *Morbidity and Mortality Weekly Report, 49*(RR-15), 1–20.

Centers for Disease Control and Prevention. (2001a). Human anthrax associated with an epizootic among livestock—North Dakota, 2000. *Morbidity and Mortality Weekly Report, 50,* 677–680.

Centers for Disease Control and Prevention. (2001b). Update. Investigation of anthrax associated with intentional exposure and interior health guidelines, October 2001. *Morbidity and Mortality Weekly Report, 50,* 889–893.

Centers for Disease Control and Prevention. (2001c). Update: Investigation of bioterrorism-related anthrax—Connecticut 2001. *Morbidity and Mortality Weekly Report, 50,* 1077–1079.

Chin, J. (2000). Anthrax. In J. Chin (Ed.), *Control of communicable diseases manual* (pp. 20–21). Washington, DC: American Public Health Association.

Christopher, G. W., Cieslak, T. J., Pavlin, J. A., & Eitzen, E. M. (1999). Biological warfare: A historical perspective. In J. Lederberg (Ed.), *Biological weapons: Limiting the threat* (pp. 18–19). Cambridge, MA: MIT Press.

Cole, L. (1997). *The eleventh plague* (pp. 4–6). New York: W. H. Freeman and Co.

Dennis, D., & Meier, F. (1997). Plague. In C. R. Horsburgh & A. M. Nelson (Eds.), *Pathology of emerging infections* (pp. 21–47). Washington, DC: American Society of Microbiology Press.

DiGiovanni, C., Jr. (1999). Domestic terrorism with chemical or biological agents: Psychiatric aspects. *American Journal of Psychiatry, 156,* 1500–1505.

Dixon, T. C., Meselson, M., Guillemin, J., & Hanna, P. C. (1999). Medical progress: Anthrax. *New England Journal of Medicine, 341,* 815–826.

Dragon, D. C., & Rennie, R. P. (1995). The ecology of anthrax spores. *Canadian Veterinary Journal, 36,* 295–301.

Fainberg, A. (1997). Debating policy priorities and implications. In B. Roberts (Ed.), *Terrorism with chemical and biological weapons: Calibrating risks and responses* (pp. 75–94). Alexandria, VA: Chemical and Biological Arms Control Institute.

Fenner, F., Henderson, D. A., Arita, I., Jezel, Z., & Ladnyi, I. D. (1988). *Smallpox and its eradication* (p. 1460). Geneva, Switzerland: World Health Organization.

Franz, D. R., Jahrling, P. B., Friedlander, A. M., McClain, D. J., Hoover, D. L., Byrne, W. R., et al. (1997). Clinical recognition and management of patients exposed to biological warfare agents. *Journal of American Medical Association, 278*, 399–411.

Friedlander, A. M. (1997). Anthrax. In F. R. Sidell, E. T. Takafuji, & D. R. Franz (Eds.), *Medical aspects of chemical and biological warfare* (pp. 468–478). Washington, DC: Borden Institute.

Friedlander, A. M., Jr., & Longfield, R. N. (2000). Anthrax. In G. T. Strickland (Ed.), *Hunter's tropical medicine and emerging infectious diseases* (8th ed., pp. 384-388). Philadelphia: WB Saunders Co.

Garner, J. S. (1996). Guidelines for isolation precautions in hospitals: Hospital Infection Control Practices Advisory Committee. *Infection Control and Hospital Epidemiology, 17*, 53–80.

Hanna, P. C., Acosta, D., & Collier, R. J. (1993). On the role of macrophages in anthrax. *Proceedings of the National Academy of Sciences of the United States of America, 90*, 10198–10201.

Harris, S. H. (1997). *Factories of death*. New York: Routledge.

Henderson, D. A., Inglesby, T. V., Bartlett, J. G., Ascher, M. S., Eitzen, E., Jahrling, P. B., et al. (1999). Smallpox as a biological weapon: Medical and public health management. *Journal of the American Medical Association, 281*, 2127–2137.

Hinton, H. L. (1999). *Combating terrorism: Observations on biological terrorism and public health initiatives* (Testimony before the Committee on Veterans Affairs and the Subcommittee on Labor, Health and Human Services, Education and Related Agencies. Committee on Appropriations, U.S. Senate, GAO/T-NSAID-99-112, pp. 1–12). Washington, DC: U.S. Government Printing Office.

Holloway, H. C., Norwood, A. E., Fullerton, C. S., Engel, D., & Ursano, R. J. (1997). The threat of biological weapons: Prophylaxis and mitigation of psychological and social consequences. *Journal of the American Medical Association, 278*, 425–427.

Hughes, J. M. (1999). The emerging threat of bioterrorism. *Emerging Infectious Diseases, 5*, 494–495.

Inglesby, T. V., Henderson, D. A., Bartlett, J. G., Ascher, M. S., Eitzen, E., Jahrling, P. B., et al. (1999). Anthrax as a biological weapon: Medical and public health management. *Journal of the American Medical Association, 281*, 1735–1745.

Inglesby, T. V., Dennis, D. T., Henderson, D. A., Bartlett, J. G., Ascher, M. S., Eitzen, E., et al. (2000). Plague as a biological weapon: Medical and public health management. *Journal of the American Medical Association, 283*, 2281–2295.

Institute of Medicine. (1999a). *Assessment of future scientific needs for live variola virus* (pp. 20–86). Washington, DC: National Academy Press.

Institute of Medicine. (1999b). *Chemical and biological terrorism: Research and development to improve civilian medical response* (pp. 65–77). Washington, DC: National Academy Press.

Jernigan, J. A., Stephens, D. S., Ashford, D. A., Omenaca, C., Topiel, M. S., Galbraith, M., et al. (2001). Bioterrorism–related inhalational anthrax: The first 10 cases reported in the United States. *Emerging Infectious Diseases, 7*, 993–944.

Kaufmann, A. F., Meltzer, M. I., & Schmid, G. P. (1997). The economic impact of a bioterrorist attack: Are prevention and postattack intervention programs justifiable? *Emerging Infectious Diseases, 3*, 83–94.

LeDuc, J. W., & Jahrling, P. B. (2001). Strengthening national preparedness for smallpox: An update. *Emerging Infectious Diseases, 7*, 155–157.

Macintyre, A. G., Christopher, G. W., Eitzen, E., Gum, R., Weir, S., DeAtley, C., et al. (2000). Weapons of mass destruction events with contaminated casualties: Effective planning for health care facilities. *Journal of the American Medical Association, 283*, 242–249.

McClain, D. J. (1997). Smallpox. In F. R. Sidell, E. T. Takafuji, & D. R. Franz (Eds.), *Medical aspects of chemical and biological warfare* (pp. 543–548). Washington, DC: Borden Institute.

McDade, J. E., & Franz, D. (1998). Bioterrorism as a public health threat. *Emerging Infectious Diseases, 4*, 493–494.

McGovern, T. W., & Friedlander, A. M. (1997). Plague. In F. R. Sidell, E. T. Takafuji, & D. R. Franz (Eds.), *Medical aspects of chemical and biological warfare* (pp. 479–502). Washington, DC: Borden Institute.

Meselson, M., Guillemin, J., Hugh-Jones, M., Langmuir, A., Popova, I., Shelokov, A., & Yampolskaya, O. (1994). The Sverdlovsk anthrax outbreak of 1979. *Science, 266*, 1202–1208.

Mitra, A. C., Sarkar, J. K., & Mukherjee, M. K. (1974). Virus content of smallpox scabs. *Bulletin of the World Health Organization, 51*, 106–107.

Olsen, K. B. (1995). Overview: Recent incidents and responder implications. In *Proceedings of the seminar on responding to the consequences of chemical and biological terrorism* (No. 1996-416-003, pp. 2.36–2.93). Washington, DC: U.S. Government Printing Office.

O'Neill, J. P. (1995). Terrorism briefing. In *Proceedings of the seminar on responding to the consequences of chemical and biological terrorism* (No. 1996-416-003, pp. 1.20–1.23). Washington, DC: U.S. Government Printing Office.

Osterholm, M. T. (1999). Bioterrorism: Media hype or real potential nightmare? *American Journal of Infection Control, 27*, 461–462.

Osterholm, M. T., & Schwartz, J. (2000). *Living terrors* (pp. 113–117). New York: Delacorte Press.

Perrotta, D. M., Rawlings, J., & Eckman, M. (1998). The specter of chemical and biological terrorism. *Disease Prevention News, 58*(8), 1–6.

Perry, R. D., & Featherston, J. D. (1997). *Yersinia pestis*—etiologic agent of plague. *Clinical Microbiology Reviews, 10*, 35–66.

Rath, J., & Bürgel, J. L. (2001). Socioeconomic biological weapons. *Science, 293*, 425–426.

Ratsitorahina, M., Chanteau, S., Rahalison, L., Ratisofasoamanana, L., & Boisier, P. (2000). Epidemiological and diagnostic aspects of the outbreak of pneumonic plague in Madagascar. *Lancet, 355*, 111–113.

Roush, S., Birkhead, G., Koo, D., Cobb, A., & Fleming, D. (1999). Mandatory reporting of diseases and conditions by health care professionals and laboratories. *Journal of the American Medical Association, 282*, 164–170.

Sarkar, J. K., Mitra, A. C., Mukherjee, M. K., & De, S. K. (1973). Virus excretion in smallpox. 2. Excretion in the throat of household contacts. *Bulletin of the World Health Organization, 48*, 523–527.

Sellman, B. R., Mourez, M., & Collier, R. J. (2001). Dominant-negative mutants of a toxin subunit: An approach to therapy of anthrax. *Science, 292*, 695–697.

Sidell, F. R., Takafuji, E. T., & Franz, D. R. (Eds.). (1997). *Medical aspects of chemical and biological warfare*. Washington, DC: Borden Institute.

Simon, J. D. (1999). Biological terrorism: Preparing to meet the threat. In J. Lederberg (Ed.), *Biological weapons: Limiting the threat* (p. 238). Cambridge, MA: MIT Press.

Smith, C. G., Veenhuis, P. E., & MacCormack, J. N. (2000). Bioterrorism: A new threat with psychological and social sequelae. *North Carolina Medical Journal, 61*(3), 150–165.

Swartz, M. N. (2001). Recognition and management of anthrax—An update. *New England Journal of Medicine, 345*, 1621–1626.

Taylor, J. P., Dimmitt, D. C., Ezzell, J. W., & Whitford, H. (1993). Indigenous human cutaneous anthrax in Texas. *Southern Medical Journal, 86*(1), 1–4.

Török, T. J., Tauxe, R. V., Wise, R. P., Livengood, J. R., Sokolow, R., Mauvais, S., et al. (1997). A large community outbreak of salmonellosis caused by intentional contamination of restaurant salad bars. *Journal of American Medical Association, 278*, 389–398.

Tucker, J. B. (1999). Bioterrorism: Threats and responses. In J. Lederberg (Ed.), *Biological weapons: Limiting the threat* (pp. 283–285). Cambridge, MA: MIT Press.

United States General Accounting Office. (1999). *Combating Terrorism: Need for comprehensive threat and risk assessments of chemical and biological attacks* (GAO/NSAID-99-163). Washington, DC: U.S. Government Printing Office.

25

Behavioral and Cultural Aspects of Transmission and Infection

Barbara Jeanne Fahey

For many, but not all, emerging and reemerging infectious diseases, transmission is influenced by human behavior and/or cultural practices (Petney, 2001). Behavior may be thought of as the actions or reactions of persons under specified circumstances, while culture is "the totality of socially transmitted behavior patterns, arts, beliefs, institutions, and all other products of human work and thought characteristic of a community or population" (*The American Heritage Dictionary*, 1982). As a result of epidemiological and scientific research and nursing theory development, much is known about behavioral and cultural aspects of disease transmission and prevention, but much remains to be elucidated (Andrews & Boule, 1999; Giger & Davidhizer, 1999). The interplay, interrelations, and interdependence of behavior, culture, and disease transmission are complex. A transmissible emerging/reemerging infectious disease can arise at any given location and spread rapidly to other regions through travel and trade. The international emergence/resurgence of infectious diseases is the consequence of numerous factors that are discussed in chapter 1. The purpose of this chapter is to highlight areas of human behavior and culture that play important roles in emerging/reemerging disease transmission and to explore management strategies in the context of human behavior/culture. This chapter will focus on those topic areas most directly affected by behavioral or cultural practices, including sexual behavior, antibiotic utilization, hygienic practices, travel, nutritional behavior, breastfeeding, immunization behavior, threat of bioterrorism, and other selected behavioral/cultural considerations. Topic areas that will not be addressed in detail include availability of potable water, medical and microbiological technological advances, increasing sensitivity of detection systems, reallocation of funds away from public health and sanitation, deterioration of public health infrastructure, population growth, increased life expectancy, and shift to an older age composition of the world population.

SEXUAL BEHAVIORS

Sexual behaviors are integral to the perpetuation of sexually transmitted diseases (STDs). Because the sexual urges that influence sexual behaviors can be quite strong, modification of sexual practices is difficult. Sexual behavior is influenced by multiple interacting factors, including hormones, emotions, desire to procreate, culture/family tradition, personal belief system, religion, financial need or desire, and curiosity. While the practice of abstinence and/or the modification of sexual behavior can substantially reduce the toll of STDs, the morbidity and mortality attributable to sexual behavior are a continuing concern to health officials worldwide. The STD pandemic shows no signs of slowing. Building an international consensus about appropriate interventions to reduce STD risk and transmission is a daunting task, due in great measure to the diversity and idiosyncrasy of human behavioral and cultural traditions. Thus, the design, implementation, social acceptance, continuation, and acceptance of activities to reduce transmission of STDs are far from straightforward.

Sexual activity, voluntary and involuntary, is associated with transmission of numerous emerging/reemerging STDs, such as human immunodeficiency virus (HIV) (see chapter 12) (Durham & Lashley, 2000). The most common route for HIV transmission is sexual. In sub-Saharan Africa and other developing countries, HIV transmission occurs primarily through heterosexual contact. Sexual transmission of HIV is at epidemic levels in many areas of the world (Bartholet, 2000). The numbers of HIV infections are even more staggering. The Joint United Nations Programme on HIV/AIDS (2001) reported an estimated 36.1 million persons worldwide living with HIV/AIDS, the majority of these in developing nations. In 2000, 3 million persons died from the disease and 5.3 million became infected (Joint United Nations Programme on HIV/AIDS, 2001). In sub-Saharan Africa the World Health Organization has estimated that 5,000 people are infected with HIV each day (Gellman, 2000). Social instability may encourage sexual activity with multiple partners as migrant workers, refugees, and women resort to prostitution to feed and clothe themselves. Cultural practices can promote sex with multiple partners because in some parts of the world sexual relations with multiple sex partners is considered normal activity. Superstitions also may foster sexual relations with multiple partners; in some areas, intercourse with a virgin is believed to cure HIV infection (Bartholet, 2000). Other factors that influence the sexual transmission of HIV and other STDs include little or no condom use, low circumcision rates, low literacy rates, religious beliefs, and women's lack of control over the circumstances or safety of sex.

Strategies to address these behavioral and cultural issues are complex, difficult to design, hard to implement, and challenging to sustain. Effective education must be culturally sensitive, presented in the native language, readily available to the entire population in the targeted area, and must be adaptable to different ages. Efforts to improve the economic health of a targeted area must rely on initial and continued good will from investors and financiers. Work to improve social and political problems is dependent on the constructive interactions of entire communities; these constructive interactions can be hard to start and even harder to maintain. Accessibility to health care, medicine, and safe sex barrier supplies must be insured. Infrastructures to provide education and health care need to exist. Currently, many parts of the world have inadequate resources for education, are struggling to maintain the local economy, and have inadequate resources to assure access to health care, medicines, and contraceptives.

Despite formidable challenges, STD rate reduction via behavioral and cultural practice changes is possible. The decline in risk behavior in Thailand, particularly unprotected sex among young men, is one example (Kitsiripornchai, Markowitz, Ungchusak, Jenkins, Leucha, Limpitaks, et al., 1998). Maintaining safer sex patterns is possible. For example, the HIV infection rate in Senegal has remained less than 2% since the epidemic's inception. Introducing and sustaining safer sex patterns is possible—the infection rate in Uganda has been reduced by 50% during the 1990s (Bartholet, 2000). An example of a longer lasting intervention is the prevention strategy promoted in an AIDS clinic funded by the United Nations and the Kazakhstan government. The clinic offers a needle exchange program for drug addicts, free condoms, and seminars for children (Rao, 2000). Efforts to sustain decreased STD transmission after initial reduction is another consideration. For example, whereas HIV transmission was dramatically reduced among homosexual populations in San Francisco during the late 1980s and early 1990s, the trend reversed during the late 1990s, ostensibly associated with a younger generation that had not experienced firsthand the consequences of HIV infection and thus did not have strong motivation to practice "safer sex." In addition, extreme economic debt and political problems in developing countries impede economic development necessary to stem the STD epidemic. Behavioral approaches to lower STD rates include providing access to, education about, and validating proper use of safer sex practices. This approach is dependent upon multiple critical factors, such as adequate sustained financial resources, stable health program infrastructure, and ongoing support from political, religious, and public sources.

With all of these differences in behavioral and cultural practices, decreasing and sustaining a decrease in STD transmission will be dependent on the ability of each community to identify and engage the specific issues germane to its own individual culture or society that contribute to the continued transmission of STDs. Reducing and maintaining reduction of STD transmission is an international public health concern and should be a high priority for public health program funding and development.

ANTIBIOTIC USE

Antibiotics are becoming increasingly less effective as a tool to combat infectious diseases (see chapter 2). Decreasing effectiveness means increasing opportunity for the occurrence of new/reemerging diseases. Human behavior is culpable for much of the antibiotic resistance that has emerged and spread throughout the world. These behaviors include excessive use of antibiotics in agriculture and horticulture, lack of adherence to prescribed antibiotic regimens, inappropriate use of antibiotics by clinicians (especially in instances in which the antibiotics are not indicated), and demand for antibiotics by consumers (Cohen & Tartasky, 1997).

Until the early 1990s, the consequences of emerging drug resistance were largely dismissed because new drugs were introduced that countered developing resistance. For example, shortly after ampicillin-resistant gonococci emerged from Thailand and the Philippines (with international spread), new cephalosporins and beta-lactamase inhibitors were available (Brown, Warnnissorn, Biddle, Panikabutra, & Traisupa, 1982). But utilizing the newer antibiotic "quick fix" approach has delayed but not prevented the current situation of increasing resistance and fewer treatment options. The specter of organisms resistant to all antibiotic agents is all too probable and not too far in the future.

The common practice of using antibiotic agents in animal feed and agriculture products provides selective pressure for resistant strains that can be transmitted within the bacterial population of the involved animals and among others in the food chain. More than 40% of the antibiotics manufactured in the United States are administered to animals (Levy, 1998). The consequences of this wide-scale use are worrisome. For example, an interesting case report described the identification of ceftriaxone-resistant *Salmonella* infection from a 12-year-old boy who lived on a farm with herds of cattle (Fey, Safranek, Rupp, Dunne, Ribot, Iwen, et al., 2000). The child's *Salmonella enterica* serotype Typhimurium isolate was identical to one of the isolates from the cattle. Whereas the use of antibiotics in livestock has been epidemiologically linked with the emergence and dissemination of resistance in nontyphoidal salmonella strains, this investigation is unique in that it established a direct connection between the child's infection and related isolates from cattle (Van den Bogaard & Stobberingh, 1999).

Fortunately, corrective regulatory measures in animal husbandry have begun. The use of antibiotics to promote growth in animal feeds has been banned in some countries. For example, avoparcin, a widely used animal antibiotic mixed in feed to promote animal growth, was removed from the European market in 1999 (Kopecny, 1999). The biochemistry and molecular structure of avoparcin is very similar to vancomycin and a causal association between the use of avoparocin and increasing prevalence of vancomycin-resistant *Enterococcus* has been hypothesized. Hopefully, this action will serve as a catalyst for additional changes and will prolong the effective life of vancomycin as a treatment. In agriculture, antibiotics are applied to commercial fruit trees to control or prevent bacterial infections. Antibiotic residue on produce can promote development of resistance among normal gastrointestinal flora once the coated produce is ingested. In the event that resistant strains do develop, the strains are likely to colonize the gastrointestinal tract. Washing raw fruit and vegetables is a simple and probably effective technique to remove antibiotic residues.

Drug resistance has been a substantial problem with management of tuberculosis, a reemerging infectious disease (see chapter 16). The persistence of tuberculosis and the development of drug resistance is related to drug availability/distribution in developing countries as well as to the adherence (or lack thereof) to a possibly long-term single or multiple agent course of therapy (Small & Fujiwara, 2001). Issues of drug availability and distribution are ongoing—global health agencies and governing bodies struggle continuously with design and implementation of successful programs. Strategies to promote therapy adherence have included directly observed therapy plus other measures, but this mechanism is difficult to enforce on an international scale and in impoverished/isolated/developing regions of the world (Gupta, Kim, Espinal, Caudron, Pecoul, Farmer, et al., 2001).

Experience demonstrates that tuberculosis incidence and transmission can be reduced through behavioral and/or practice changes. During the late 1980s and early 1990s the U.S. reported an upsurge in the cases of tuberculosis and outbreaks of multidrug-resistant tuberculosis (Centers for Disease Control and Prevention, 1994). Initial and continued decreases in tuberculosis cases (both drug-sensitive and multidrug-resistant) occurred subsequent to aggressive implementation of country-wide controls that consisted of 1) administrative measures (early identification, isolation, and effective treatment of persons with active tuberculosis [e.g., directly observed therapy]); 2) engineering controls (to prevent spread and reduce concentration of tuberculosis droplet nuclei); and 3) personal protective equipment (e.g., appropriate masks for exposed health care workers) (Centers for Disease Control and Prevention, 1994).

The successful tuberculosis control program implemented in the United States may be difficult to replicate in all parts of the world. Fortunately, promising research is being conducted on alternative strategies designed to decrease tuberculosis rates. Because successful completion of 6–12 months of therapy is difficult, shorter antibiotic courses for asymptomatic tuberculosis infection are being explored. Recent research, such as an international randomized trial of short-course tuberculosis preventive therapy conducted by Gordin, Chaisson, Matts, Miller, De Lourdes Garcia, Hafner, and associates (2000) in HIV-infected persons, has suggested that a daily 2-month course of rifampin and pyrazinamide is similar in safety and efficacy to the standard 12-month isoniazid regimen. Shortened courses of therapy will likely facilitate adherence, which in turn will lead to fewer and smaller institutional and community tuberculosis outbreaks and a lowered incidence of multidrug-resistant tuberculosis (De Cock, Grant, & Porter, 1995; Whalen, Johnson, Okwera, Hom, Huebner, Mugyenyi, et al., 1997). For further discussion see chapter 16 and Small and Fujiwara (2001).

Excessive antibiotic use is associated with development of antibiotic resistance. In developed countries, a prescription is needed for many antibiotics. Whereas this screening filter should promote judicious antibiotic utilization, the mechanism guarantees neither proper ordering nor proper use (Levy, 1998). Many patients in U.S. hospitals receive antibiotics unnecessarily. Nearly 30 years ago, one study reported that on surgical units up to 48% of treated patients had no evidence of infection (Kunin, 1973). Similar patterns were noted in British hospitals almost 20 years ago (Geddes, 1982). Pediatricians report that parents usually expect their child to receive antibiotics, even when not clinically indicated (e.g., to treat upper respiratory viral infections) (Nyquist, Gonzales, Steiner, & Sande, 1998); however, antibiotics are not indicated for children with upper respiratory viral infections. Repeated use of antibiotics over time can predispose skin flora and gastrointestinal flora to develop antibiotic resistance. In developing countries, many antibiotics marketed by prescription in developed countries are available over the counter, increasing the likelihood of antibiotic misuse and the potential for resistance.

As with other dimensions of human behavior influencing antibiotic resistance, data demonstrate that the behavior of excessive antibiotic use can be modified. For example, during the late 1980s, Finnish public health officials noted an increase in erythromycin resistance among group A streptococcal isolates (Seppala, Klaukka, Vuopio-Varkila, Muotiala, Helenius, Lager, et al., 1997). In 1991, to stem the trend, national guidelines were issued that were intended to reduce the use of macrolides in the treatment of respiratory and skin infections. Within a year's time, macrolide use had decreased more than 40% and significant declines in erythromycin resistance among group A streptococcal isolates occurred in Finland. A more modest intervention occurred during a 1999 cholera outbreak in Madagascar. The

Ministry of Defense erected extensive roadblocks and required all travelers to take oral antibiotics; nonselective antibiotic administration to those without cholera increased selective pressure for antibiotic resistance. The Ministry of Defense subsequently modified the control program such that only travelers reporting diarrhea were given antibiotics (Markon, 2000).

Behaviors that predispose to the development of antibiotic resistance can be altered. Strategies that are likely to promote judicious antibiotic use include

- formation of coalitions (with professional and nonprofessional membership) to promote and coordinate antibiotic control,
- development of peer education programs for medical care providers,
- provision of timely feedback from databases to physicians,
- promotion of ready access (written and electronic) to information on antibiotics and their utilization,
- formation of partnerships with mass media and public health agencies for press releases and public service announcements, and
- collaboration with child care setting administrators (Centers for Disease Control and Prevention/National Center for Infectious Diseases, 1997).

HYGIENIC BEHAVIOR: COMMUNITY SETTING

Poor hygienic behaviors (including poor personal hygiene, poor food preparation techniques, and inadequate occupational/environmental hygiene) have been associated with emerging/reemerging disease transmission in the community and home. Inadequate hygienic practices have been associated with reemerging foodborne and waterborne transmission of such infections as cholera, *E. coli* O157:H7 (see chapters 4 and 9), viral gastroenteritis, zoonoses, and hemorrhagic fevers (see chapter 8) (Scott, 1999).

The importance of inadequate hygienic behaviors in the occurrence of reemerging infectious diseases is demonstrated in the African experience with cholera (see chapter 4). In Madagascar, only one in three people has access to clean water; only 3% have access to flush toilets; money is usually not available to purchase charcoal to boil water, a critical step in preventing cholera (Markon, 2000). Poor hygiene, contaminated water, or contaminated soil clinging to vegetables can be vectors for cholera transmission. Effective control measures include public health campaigns that recommend good hygiene, hand washing, boiling water, and sprinkling chlorine in shallow wells.

Inadequate hygienic practices have also been associated with transmission of Ebola hemorrhagic fever (EHF), an emerging disease first recognized in 1976 (Peters & LeDuc, 1999) (see chapter 8). Current theory is that the index patient of an outbreak becomes infected through contact with an infected animal. Other people then become exposed by direct contact with the blood and/or other potentially infectious fluids of the infected person. Thus, the virus readily spreads through families and friends of the infected person because close contact and accidental exposure to infectious fluids is likely to occur while feeding, holding, caring for, or otherwise assisting the infected person, and during postmortem body care (Kerstiëns & Matthys, 1999). EHF transmission can occur readily in the community in the absence/use of barrier equipment/hand washing. The exposure among health care workers who do not use personal protective equipment would thus be akin to household exposure with ensuing risk for EHF transmission. For example, in the Kikwit, Democratic Republic of the Congo EHF outbreak in 1995, before control measures were begun, 67 health care workers became infected with EHF; after interventions were started, only 3 health care workers developed EHF and no infections occurred among staff involved with body burial (Kerstiëns & Matthys, 1999). Upon initiation of control measures (provision of protective equipment, antiseptics and barrier-nursing technique training) EHF transmission to health care workers was reduced dramatically during EHF outbreaks (Guimard, Bwaka, Colebunders, Calain, Massamba, De Roo, et al., 1999). Difficulties encountered in maintenance of healthful hygienic practices include limited access to potable water; inadequate plumbing facilities; population migration to refugee camps; crowding; and disruption of goods and supplies due to civil unrest, war, or economic hardship. One innovative approach to promoting improved community hygiene is a recently launched website (http://www.ifh-homehygiene.org) where the International Scientific Forum on Home Hygiene has provided comprehensive guidelines for the prevention of infection in the domestic environment.

Hygienic practices are important to the overall health and health promotion for each individual in the home or community. Personal, family, and cultural practices all affect the type of hygienic practices that are used. Access to water, cleaning supplies, and waste disposal systems are also important components of hygienic practices. On a global scale, continuous education should be provided about the chain of infection (host to susceptible host via route of transmission) and the value of hygienic practices to reduce the risk for disease transmission. On an international level, strategies should be explored and implemented to assist areas of the world that do not have potable water and access to cleaning supplies.

HYGIENIC BEHAVIOR: HEALTH CARE SETTING

Hygienic behavior in the health care setting includes environmental cleaning, hand hygiene, and use of Standard Precautions. Environmental surfaces (i.e., floors, walls, furniture, beds, medical equipment) become contaminated from infected, transiently colonized, or chronically colonized patients, visitors, or health care personnel. A contaminated environment may become a reservoir for emerging infectious diseases, such as vancomycin-resistant enterococci (see chapter 19), and must be considered as a potential reservoir for disease transmission. Routine microbiological surveillance of the environment is of limited value, should not be routinely performed, and should only be considered in unique circumstances (e.g., to support epidemiological investigations or to promote quality control for biological indicator programs) (Vesley & Streifel, 1996). Continuous fomite disinfection, soil removal, and waste removal are necessary to reduce the likelihood of disease transmission from the health care environment. Although sanitizing or disinfecting agents can be used, less expensive nongermicidal cleaning agents are usually sufficient for routine cleaning and are less likely to cause chemical sensitivity reactions. The selection of cleaning products should be carefully considered and decisions should be congruent with public health recommendations (e.g., those of the Centers for Disease Control [1985]). Health care settings should have written procedures for environmental cleaning that emphasize practices to suppress dust, dirt, and aerosolization (e.g., vacuum cleaners should include exhaust filters). Spill cleanup procedures should specify use of protective barriers (gloves) to protect staff from exposure to the spill and use of disinfectants that inactivate bloodborne pathogens (e.g., a dilute hypochlorite sodium (bleach) solution). Availability of supplies is important. Disinfection/sterilization protocols should consider newer agents such as prions (see chapter 17).

Hand washing is the single most important means of preventing the spread of emerging/reemerging infectious diseases and infection in general. Good hand washing reduces carriage of transient flora and thus reduces risk for disease transmission. A causal association between hand hygiene and reduced infection transmission, morbidity, and mortality related to hospital-acquired infections is well established, beginning more than 150 years ago with the eloquent work of Semmelweis (Wiese, 1930). Quite ironically, health care personnel hand washing practices remain remarkably poor (Boyce, 1999). For reasons that are not fully understood, hand washing adherence varies by personal practice, by occupation, by clinical setting, and by perception of risk (to self and others). Health care personnel have reported that nonadherence is attributable to excessive workload and to skin irritation, sensitivity, and dryness caused by hand washing (Larson & Killien, 1982; Zimakoff, Kjelsberg, Larsen, & Holstein, 1992). Hand hygiene should be considered an integral component of quality care in all health care settings. Due to the need for in-depth understanding of the logistical barriers and behavioral issues, an ongoing multidisciplinary approach to attempt to improve hand washing adherence, including elements of adherence monitoring and frequent feedback to health care personnel is likely to be most successful (Boyce, 1999). A comprehensive review of the issues surrounding adherence to hand washing may be found in Pittet (2001).

Innovative strategies and interesting technologies to promote hand washing adherence are being explored and implemented, such as water-free hand washing agents with emollients; sinks with electronic sensors; dedicated hand washing machines; and combination hand washing agent/skin care product lines. Nonetheless, promoting adherence to simple hand washing techniques remains a challenge.

"Standard Precautions" is an infection control strategy designed to reduce the risk of transmission of bloodborne pathogens as well as pathogens from moist body substances. This concept and practice is firmly embraced in United States, but has not yet become established as an international infection control standard (Occupational Safety and Health Administration, 1991). The behavior patterns specified by Standard Precautions—administrative controls (e.g., annual training, participation in a hepatitis B vaccination program), engineering controls (e.g., access to sharps disposal containers), thoughtful use of barrier equipment (e.g., gloves most frequently)—are designed to reduce risk for disease transmission in the health care setting, from patient to staff, staff to patient, and patient to staff to patient. Eventual evolution of Standard Precautions to an international infection control standard should be encouraged to promote reduction of transmission of emerging/reemerging infectious diseases in all health care settings. Primary barriers to the universal adoption of Standard Precautions are inadequate education and lack of resources.

INJECTED AND RECREATIONAL DRUG USE

Injected and recreational drug use is behavior initiated, maintained and sustained by each individual person. The culture and behavior of persons who participate in injected and recreational drug use is extremely complex and beyond the scope of this chapter. Injected and recreational drug user behavior is known, however, to contribute to transmission of emerging/reemerging infectious diseases. Injected drug use is a recognized risk factor for HIV infection, accounting for about 25% of single risk group of U.S. cases of AIDS, and 32% when the category of injecting drug use (IDU) and "men who have sex with men" is added (Centers for Disease Control and Prevention, 2001). Despite ongoing alerts about the dangers for disease transmission via sharing used needles, and despite the implementation of needle exchange programs in various parts of the world, the sharing behavior persists and the reality of bloodborne disease transmission continues. Injected drug use and sharing of cocaine straws are also risk factors for transmission of such emerging infectious diseases as hepatitis C (see chapter 11) (Bonkovsky & Mehta, 2001). Interventions to modify risk behavior change among drug using populations are labor intensive and time intensive. Interventions include cross-training of substance abuse counselors, provision of substance abuse education among school-age children, access to trained health care personnel, and legal efforts to remove illegal drug supplies. In developing countries, use of injected drugs by nonmedical practitioners using equipment that is not sterilized, may be routine, expected treatment.

TRAVEL

The increased ease of travel is associated with increased risk for transmission of emerging/reemerging diseases (see chapter 22). Increased ease of travel by land, air, and water has provided a mechanism for rapid dissemination and transmission of infectious agents. Political changes in many parts of the world have eased previous restrictions on travel across borders. Air travel provides service to most global locations within a 24-hour period and thus expands the potential for rapid spread of diseases, examples of which have been discussed elsewhere in this book. Political unrest, resulting in the migration and immigration of large numbers of refugees, has resulted in the emergence of infectious diseases in areas where these diseases were previously unknown or rare. Research, investigation, and control measures for emerging/reemerging infectious disease transmission associated with travel behavior will remain important for the foreseeable future.

NUTRITIONAL BEHAVIOR

The adage "you are what you eat" applies to nutritional behavior and is associated with emerging/reemerging infectious disease transmission. Case reports of Creutzfeldt-Jakob disease have detailed patient histories that have included consumption of the brains of wild goats or squirrels (Kamin & Patten, 1984) (see chapter 17). More recently, variant Creutzfeldt-Jakob disease (vCJD) has been identified in the United Kingdom and plausibly linked to an epidemic of bovine spongiform encephalopathy (BSE) in cattle (Will, Ironside, Zeidler, Cousens, Estibiero, Alperovitch, et al., 1996). The outbreak is thought to have started when cattle were fed with meat-and-bonemeal made from offal (animal tissue discarded by slaughterhouses) whose origin included scrapie-infected sheep. The outbreak was then accelerated by feeding offal from infected cattle to other cattle. In 1988, Britain banned the feeding of ruminant-derived protein (milk excluded) to ruminants; a decrease in the annual incidence of BSE since the ban is compatible with outbreak etiology from meat and bonemeal (Alter, 2000). An estimated half million BSE-infected cows entered the human food chain before the offal ban; as a result of the estimated prolonged incubation period for vCJD (up to 30 years or longer), the expected vCJD epidemic should peak about the year 2009 (Brown, Will, Bradley, Asher, & Detwiler, 2001). Identification of a likely causal relation with occurrence of vCJD, with subsequent implementation of corrective policies, will lead we hope to timely identification/destruction of suspected BSE-infected animals and a decrease in the incidence of vCJD among the human population. There are particular infection control specifications for health care settings to consider for management of individuals suspected or diagnosed with vCJD or any transmissible spongiform encephalopathy.

Food and eating preferences/and or methods of food preparation also contribute to acquisition of such emerging infectious diseases as *Escherichia coli* O157:H7, cholera, and cyclosporiasis. In these cases, infection can be associated with the eating of undercooked food such as hamburgers (*E. coli*, see chapter 9), choosing out-of-season imported produce such as raspberries (cyclosporiasis, see chapter 6), or eating raw or undercooked shellfish from contaminated beds (cholera, see chapter 4).

Breastfeeding is recommended as an excellent source for nutrition for neonates and infants. The benefits of breastfeeding have been questioned with the unfolding of the HIV epidemic because HIV can be transmitted in breast milk. Transmission frequency was initially estimated to range from 14% (established maternal infection) to 29% (acute maternal infection) (Dunn, Newell, Ades, & Peckham, 1992; Van de Perre, Simonon, Msellati, Hitimana, Vaira, Bazubagira, et al., 1991). However, more recent research suggests absolute transmission rates to be 3.2–9.2 per 100 years of breastfeeding among infants 6 months or younger, with more than 40% of infant HIV infections acquired via breastfeeding occurring during the first months of life (Nduati, John, Mbori-Ngacha, Richardson, Overbaugh, Mwatha, et al., 2000).

The standard of care among industrialized countries is that infants of HIV-infected women should not be breastfed. Women in industrialized countries are likely to have access to potable water, ample supplies of infant formula, and access to medical resources to help insure that the formula is properly mixed and administered. A standard for HIV-infected women not to breastfeed makes sense when safe alternative nourishment is available to the infants. In parts of the world where malnutrition and infectious diseases are the primary causes of infant mortality, however, the World Health Organization Global Program on AIDS recommends breastfeeding, regardless of the mother's HIV status (Joint United Nations Program on HIV/AIDS [UNAIDS] and infant feeding, 1992). In these parts of the world, the drinking water may be laden with disease-causing bacteria; the mother may not have access to or may not be able to afford infant formula; and she may not have access to medical resources to insure that the formula is being properly prepared and administered. Whereas randomized clinical trials suggest that breast milk substitutes could prevent 44% of infant HIV infections, caution is critical. Before discouraging breastfeeding, public health authorities must ensure that mothers have access to clean water, adequate supplies of formula, and meticulous teaching in formula preparation and administration (Nduati et al., 2000). Each community needs to assess the resources available to HIV-infected mothers, to discuss resource availability with public health officials, and to proceed together with a breastfeeding recommendation that, given data relevant to the individual community, is most likely to promote infant health and reduce infant mortality.

IMMUNIZATION BEHAVIOR

With fewer and fewer diagnosed cases of vaccine-preventable diseases, an increasing number of people challenge the value of vaccination and do not participate themselves or enroll their children in vaccine programs. This behavior has created an increasing reservoir of persons susceptible to, at risk for contracting, and potentially able to be sources for continued transmission of vaccine-preventable diseases. Physicians and health agencies strongly recommend vaccination against diseases that can cause significant morbidity and mortality. The importance of receiving vaccinations has not changed, but immunization behavior—the culture and behavior of vaccine acceptance—has shifted in recent years. In the early 1970s, because of widespread concern in Britain, Japan, and Sweden about adverse effects of pertussis vaccination, fewer children were immunized (Rosenfeld, 2000). In Japan, pertussis cases rose from 400 in 1971–1974 to 13,000 between 1975–1979 (Rosenfeld, 2000). Russia experienced a similar increase in diagnosed cases of diphtheria: pediatric and booster vaccinations decreased around 1989 and the number of identified diphtheria cases rose from 900 in 1989 to 50,000 in 1994 (Rosenfeld, 2000).

Poor immunization program adherence (vaccine/booster rejection) is associated with reemergence of preventable diseases (e.g., pertussis and diphtheria). Education and continuing education on the personal and public health merits of vaccination may encourage ongoing cooperation with vaccine programs. However, factors other than behavior are involved with failure to immunize—vaccines such as those for hepatitis B and *Hemophilus influenzae* are often too costly in developing countries (Okie, 1999). Thus, achieving and sustaining adequate immunization behavior and immunization levels is a multifaceted international challenge.

BIOTERRORISM

The behavior of bioterrorism is a worrisome global concern (see chapter 24). Bioterrorists intentionally introduce agents with the anticipated outcome of morbidity and mortality. Persons engage in this behavior to further ideological, material, or spiritual objectives. They believe that achievement of their goal can be achieved more effectively by hurting people, killing people, and wreaking societal/cultural/personal havoc. The threat of deployment of biologic weapons on both civilian and military targets has many unknowns—the targets; the agents (e.g., anthrax, botulinum toxin, plague, smallpox); routes for delivery and distribution; and the ability of public health and health care systems to mount timely and appropriate response (Centers for Disease Control and Prevention, 2000). The intentional release of *Bacillus anthracis* resulting in 23 cases of both cutaneous and inhalational anthrax by November 28, 2001 (Centers for Disease Control and Prevention, 2001) spurred countries to accelerate efforts to develop programs that will counter bioterrorism. For example, the United States Department of Defense has established a mandatory anthrax vaccination program for military personnel, and organizations have published bioterrorism management procedures. Continued preparation for bioterrorism is ongoing and will likely include the development of management procedures for other potential infectious diseases that may be used in bioterrorism.

OTHER BEHAVIORAL/CULTURAL CONSIDERATIONS

Socioeconomic changes influence emerging disease transmission. The Mexican experience with efforts to control the major vector for dengue virus, *Aedes aegypti*, is a good example. The Pan American Health Organization conducted an effective elimination campaign in the 1950s–1960s (Pan American Health Organization, 1994). Mexico reported elimination of the mosquito species in 1963, but subsequent social and economic shifts allowed vector reinfestation. These changes included population emigration from rural to urban areas without adequate housing, water, or sewage and waste management systems; proliferation of nonrecyclable products that provided plentiful breeding locations for *Aedes aegypti*; and diminished public health infrastructure and resources (Gubler & Trent, 1993; Pan American Health Organization, 1994).

Civil unrest, ever present in various parts of the world (e.g., Chechnya, Kosovo, Sierra Leone, Somalia, Philippines) invites transmission of emerging/reemerging diseases. Resources and organization for public health programs are undermined. Nonadherence with recommended vaccination schedules increases the pool of susceptible persons and the likelihood of vaccine-preventable disease occurrence and transmission. Increased homelessness increases the risk for tuberculosis transmission. Lack of access to potable water and clean food increases the likelihood of foodborne and waterborne diseases. Interruption of regular market patterns disrupts access to contraceptives and promotes STD transmission.

Body art involves tattooing, piercing, and branding. Emerging/reemerging disease may occur when instruments are not sterilized, poor technique is used, and/or adequate wound care is not maintained (Fisman, 1999; Sperry, 1992). Body art practitioners are largely unlicensed, unregulated, and not subject to routine health inspections (Braithwaite, Stephens, Sterk, & Braithwaite, 1999). Body art procedures are associated with actual or potential transmission of tetanus, hepatitis B, hepatitis C, HIV, and other organisms at the time of the procedure and in the course of wound care (Loscalzo, Ryan, Loscalzo, Sarna, & Caday, 1995; Nishioka & Gyorkos, 2001; O'Malley, Smith, Braun, & Prevots, 1998; Pugatch, Mileno, & Rich, 1998; Tweeten & Rickman, 1998). An anecdotal report of a 45-day-old infant who developed fatal septicemia with a resistant strain of *Pseudomonas aeruginosa* after ritual cutting illustrates the risk for disease transmission introduced by body art behavior (Mathur & Sahoo, 1984). Body art and ritual cutting occur in many areas of the world.

Death rituals or "funerary practices" are richly diverse, being reflective of the broad international cultural variety enfolding death (Stephen, 1998). Mortuary staff and all persons who wash and drape bodies before burial/cremation are at risk for emerging/reemerging diseases such as hepatitis C, HIV, and Ebola hemorrhagic fever (see chapter 8) (Gatrad, 1994). Adherence to standard precautions in all funerary practices will lower risk for disease transmission but in many cases are difficult to incorporate because of cultural beliefs and practices.

Human body part consumption traditions (e.g., to attempt to cure illness) are well documented in Chinese and Western cultures (Chen & Chen, 1998; MacCulloch, 1925). Although cannibalism is uncommon and unusual, in instances in which it has been practiced, disease transmission has been documented. For example, ritualistic postmortem cannibalism practiced until the late 1950s by the Fore highlanders of New Guinea was directly related to the transmission of kuru, a fatal transmissible spongiform encephalopathy (see chapter 17) (Gajdusek, 1977). Disease transmission halted when the cultural ritual of postmortem cannibalism was discontinued.

SUMMARY

Management of emerging/reemerging infectious diseases will depend in large part on the integration of social sciences into the structure and functioning of national/international public health policy and programs. Infant mortality provides an indication of the overall health of populations. Improved availability of health care resources, expansion of basic education—especially for women, and nutrition supplementation programs, have been associated with reduction in infant mortality; progress toward these goals should be encouraged (Peña, Wall, & Persson, 2000). Prevention through education of high-risk behaviors and immunization remain the best defense. Acknowledgment of the influence of civil unrest, war, and economic crisis on emerging/reemerging infectious diseases is critical to facilitating early disease identification and management.

REFERENCES

Alter, M. (2000). How is Creutzfeldt-Jakob disease acquired? *Neuroepidemiology, 19*, 55–61.

The American heritage dictionary (2nd ed.). (1982). Boston: Houghton Mifflin.

Andrews, M. M., & Boule, J. S. (Eds.). (1999). *Transcultural concepts in nursing care* (3rd ed.). Philadelphia: Lippincott, Williams and Wilkins.

Bartholet, J. (2000, January 17). Africa's plague years. *Newsweek*, pp. 32–37.

Bonkovsky, H. L., & Mehta, S. (2001). Hepatitis C: A review and update. *Journal of the American Academy of Dermatology, 44*, 159–182.

Boyce, J. M. (1999). Is it time for action: Improving hand hygiene in hospitals. *Annals of Internal Medicine, 130*, 153–155.

Braithwaite, R. L., Stephens, T., Sterk, C., & Braithwaite, K. (1999). Risks associated with tattooing and body piercing. *Journal of Public Health Policy, 20*, 459–470.

Brown, S., Warnnissorn, T., Biddle, J., Panikabutra, K., & Traisupa, A. (1982). Antimicrobial resistance of *Neisseria gonorrhoea* in Bangkok: Is single-drug treatment passê? *Lancet, 2*, 1366–1368.

Brown, P., Will, R. G., Bradley, R., Asher, D. M., & Detwiler, L. (2001). Bovine spongiform encephalopathy and variant Creutzfeldt-Jakob disease: Background, evolution, and current concerns. *Emerging Infectious Diseases, 7*, 6–16.

Centers for Disease Control. (1985). *Guideline for handwashing and hospital environmental control, 1985*. Atlanta, GA: Author.

Centers for Disease Control and Prevention. (1994). Guidelines for preventing the transmission of *Mycobacterium tuberculosis* in health-care facilities. *Morbidity and Mortality Weekly Report, 43*(RR-13), 1–132.

Centers for Disease Control and Prevention/National Center for Infectious Diseases. (1997). *Careful antibiotic use to prevent resistance, 1*, 1–4. Atlanta, GA: Author.

Centers for Disease Control and Prevention. (2000). Biological and chemical terrorism: Strategic plan for preparedness and response. Recommendations of the CDC Strategic Planning Workgroup. *Morbidity and Mortality Weekly Report, 49*(RR-4), 5–6.

Centers for Disease Control and Prevention. (2001). Update: Investigation of bioterrorism-related inhalational anthrax—Connecticut, 2001. *Morbidity and Mortality Weekly Report, 50*, 1049–1051.

Chen, T., & Chen, S. Y. (1998, Spring). Medical cannibalism in China: The case of ko-ku. *Pharos*, 23–25.

Cohen, F. R., & Tartasky, D. (1997). Microbial resistance to drug therapy: A review. *American Journal of Infection Control, 25*, 51–64.

De Cock, K. M., Grant, A., & Porter, J. D. (1995). Preventive therapy for tuberculosis in HIV-infected persons. *Lancet, 345*, 833–836.

Dunn, D. T., Newell, M. L., Ades, A. E., & Peckham, C. S. (1992). Risk of human immunodeficiency virus type 1 transmission through breastfeeding. *Lancet, 340*, 585–588.

Durham, J. D., & Lashley, F. R. (Eds.). (2000). *The person with HIV/AIDS: Nursing perspectives* (3rd ed.). New York: Springer Publishing Co.

English, J. F. (1999). Overview of bioterrorism readiness plan: A template for health care facilities. *American Journal of Infection Control, 27*, 468–469.

Fey, P. D., Safranek, T. J., Rupp, M. E., Dunne, E. F., Ribot, E., Iwen, P. C., et al. (2000). Ceftriaxone-resistant salmonella infection acquired by a child from cattle. *New England Journal of Medicine, 342*, 1242–1249.

Fisman, D. (1999). Infectious complications of body piercing. *Clinical Infectious Diseases, 28*, 1340.

Gajdusek, D. C. (1977). Unconventional viruses and the origin and disappearance of kuru. *Science, 197*, 943–960.

Gatrad, A. (1994). Muslim customs surrounding death, bereavement, postmortem examinations, and organ transplants. *British Medical Journal, 309*, 521–523.

Geddes, A. M. (1982). The impact on clinical practice of antibiotic-resistant microorganisms. In C. H. Stuart-Harris & D. M. Harris (Eds.), *The control of antibiotic-resistant bacteria* (pp. 1–16). London: Academic Press.

Gellman, B. (2000, April 30). Clinton administration declares AIDS a national security threat. *The Washington Post*, pp. A1, A28–A29.

Giger, J. N., & Davidhizer, R. E. (Eds.). (1999). *Transcultural nursing assessment and intervention* (3rd ed.). St. Louis: Mosby.

Gordin, F., Chaisson, R. E., Matts, J. P., Miller, C., De Lourdes Garcia, M., Hafner, R., et al. (2000). Rifampin and pyrazinamide vs. isoniazid for prevention of tuberculosis in HIV-infected persons: An international randomized trial. *Journal of the American Medical Association, 283*, 1445–1450.

Gubler, D. J., & Trent, D. W. (1993). Emergence of epidemic dengue/dengue hemorrhagic fever as a public health problem in the Americas. *Infectious Agents and Disease, 2*, 383–393.

Guimard, Y., Bwaka, M. A., Colebunders, R., Calain, P., Massamba, M., De Roo, A., et al. (1999). Organization of patient care during the Ebola hemorrhagic fever epidemic in Kikit, Democratic Republic of the Congo, 1995. *Journal of Infectious Diseases, 179*(Suppl. 1), S268–S273.

Gupta, R., Kim, J. Y., Espinal, M. A., Caudron, J-M., Pecoul, B., Farmer, P. E., et al. (2001). Responding to market failures in tuberculosis control. *Science, 293*, 1049–1051.

Joint United Nations Programme on HIV/AIDS (UNAIDS) and infant feeding. (1992). *Weekly Epidemiologic Record, 67*, 177–179.

Joint United Nations Programme on HIV/AIDS (UNAIDS). (2001). *AIDS Epidemic Update* [On-line]. Available: http://www.unaids.org/index.html

Kamin, M., & Patten, B. M. (1984). Creutzfeldt-Jakob disease: Possible transmission to humans by consumption of wild animal brains. *American Journal of Medicine, 76*, 142–145.

Kerstiëns, B., & Matthys, F. (1999). Interventions to control virus transmission during an outbreak of Ebola hemorrhagic fever: Experience from Kikwit, Democratic Republic of the Congo, 1995. *Journal of Infectious Diseases, 179*(Suppl. 1), S263–S267.

Kitsiripornchai, S., Markowitz, E. E., Ungchusak, K., Jenkins, R. A., Leucha, W., Limpitaks, T., et al. (1998). Sexual behavior of young men in Thailand: Regional differences and evidence of behavior change. *Journal of Acquired Immune Deficiency Syndromes and Human Retrovirology, 18*, 282–288.

Kopecny, E. (1999, December 21). *Antibiotic in poultry feed discontinued-worldwide* [On-line]. Available: http://www.sare.org/htdocs/hypermail/html-home/41-html/0200.html

Kunin, C. M. (1973). Evaluation of antibiotic use: A comprehensive look at alternative approaches. *Reviews of Infectious Diseases, 3*, 745–753.

Larson, E., & Killien, M. (1982). Factors influencing handwashing behavior of patient care personnel. *American Journal of Infection Control, 10*, 93–99.

Levy, S. B. (1998). The challenge of antibiotic resistance. *Scientific American, 278*(3), 46–53.

Loscalzo, I., Ryan, J., Loscalzo, J., Sarna, A., & Cadag, S. (1995). Tetanus: A clinical diagnosis. *American Journal of Emergency Medicine, 13*, 488–490.

MacCulloch, J. (1925). Cannibalism. In J. Hastings (Ed.), *Encyclopedia of religion and ethics* (pp. 194–209). New York: Charles Scribner's Sons.

MacDonald, M., Crofts, N., & Kaldor, J. (1996). Transmission of hepatitis C virus: Rates, routes and cofactors. *Epidemiologic Reviews, 18*, 137–147.

Markon, C. (2000, March 20). *Cholera, diarrhea and dysentery update* [On-line]. Available: http://www.cnr.berkeley.edu/~slist/ns113/msg00096.html

Mathur, D., & Sahoo, A. (1984). *Pseudomonas* septicaemia following tribal tattoo marks. *Tropical and Geographical Medicine, 36*, 301–302.

Nduati, R., John, G., Mbori-Ngacha, D., Richardson, B., Overbaugh, J., Mwatha, A., et al. (2000). Effect of breastfeeding and formula feeding on transmission of HIV-1: A randomized clinical trial. *Journal of the American Medicine Association, 283*, 1167–1174.

Nyquist, A., Gonzales, R., Steiner, J. F., & Sande, M. A. (1998). Antibiotic prescribing for children with colds, upper respiratory tract infections, and bronchitis. *Journal of the American Medical Association, 279*, 875–877.

Occupational Safety and Health Administration. (1991). 29CFR Part 1910.1030: Occupational exposure to bloodborne pathogens. *Federal Register, 56*(235), 64004–65182.

Okie, S. (1999, August 10). Science races to stem TB's threat. *The Washington Post*, pp. A1, A4.

O'Malley, C., Smith, N., Braun, R., & Prevots, D. R. (1998). Tetanus associated with body piercing. *Clinical Infectious Diseases, 27*, 1343–1344.

Pan American Health Organization. (1994). Dengue and dengue hemorrhagic fever in the Americas: Guidelines for prevention and control. *Scientific Publications, 548*, 3–22.

Peña, R., Wall, S., & Persson, L. (2000). The effect of poverty, social inequity, and maternal health on infant mortality in Nicaragua, 1988–1993. *American Journal of Public Health, 90*, 64–69.

Peters, C., & LeDuc, J. W. (1999). An introduction to Ebola: The virus and the disease. *Journal of Infectious Diseases, 179*(Suppl. 1), ix–xvi.

Petney, T. N. (2001). Environmental, cultural and social changes and their influence on parasite infections. *International Journal for Parasitology, 31*, 919–932.

Pittet, D. (2001). Improving adherence to hand hygiene practice: A multidisciplinary approach. *Emerging Infectious Diseases, 7*, 234–240.

Pugatch, D., Mileno, M., & Rich, J. D. (1998). Possible transmission of human immunodeficiency virus type 1 from body piercing. *Clinical Infectious Diseases, 26*, 767–768.

Rao, S. (2000, January 04). Kazakh steel town struggles with AIDS. *Reuters* [On-line]. Available:

Rosenfeld, I. (2000, January 09). Don't worry about vaccinations. *The Washington Post Magazine*, pp. 10, 15.

Sampton, D. E., Parker, R., & Sistrom, M. G. (1999). "We is 'et' up with methamphetamine": Sex and needle-sharing in rural Virginia, 1997 (Abstract no. 433). *1999 National HIV Prevention Conference.*

Scott, E. (1999). Hygienic issues in the home. *American Journal of Infection Control, 27,* S22–S25.

Seppala, H., Klaukka, T., Vuopio-Varkila, J., Muotiala, A., Helenius, H., Lager, K., et al. (1997). The effect of changes in the consumption of macrolide antibiotics on erythromycin resistance in group A streptococci in Finland. *New England Journal of Medicine, 337,* 441–446.

Small, P. M., & Fujiwara, K. I. (2001). Management of tuberculosis in the United States. *New England Journal of Medicine, 345,* 189–200.

Sperry, K. (1992). Tattoos and tattooing. Part II: Gross pathology, histopathology, medical complications, and applications. *American Journal of Forensic Medicine and Pathology, 13*(1), 7–17.

Stephen, M. (1998). Consuming the dead: A Kleinian perspective on death rituals cross-culturally. *International Journal of Psychoanalysis, 79*(Pt. 6), 1173–1194.

Tweeten, S., & Rickman, L. S. (1998). Infectious complications of body piercing. *Clinical Infectious Diseases, 26,* 735–740.

Van den Bogaard, A. E., & Stobberingh, E. E. (1999). Antibiotic usage in animals: Impact on bacterial resistance and public health. *Drugs, 58,* 589–607.

Van de Perre, P., Simonon, A., Msellati, P., Hitimana, D. G., Vaira, D., Bazubagira, A., et al. (1991). Postnatal transmission of human immunodeficiency virus type 1 from mother to infant: A prospective cohort study in Kigali, Ramada. *New England Journal of Medicine, 325,* 593–598.

Vesley, D., & Streifel, A. J. (1996). Environmental services. In C. G. Mayhall (Ed.), *Hospital epidemiology and infection control* (pp. 818-823). Baltimore: Williams & Wilkins.

Whalen, C. C., Johnson, J. L., Okwera, A., Hom, D. L., Huebner, R., Mugyenyi, P., et al. (1997). A trial of three regimens to prevent tuberculosis in Ugandan adults infected with the human immunodeficiency virus. *New England Journal of Medicine, 337,* 801–808.

Wiese, E. R. (1930). Semmelweis. *Annals of Medical History, 2,* 80–88.

Will, R. G., Ironside, J. W., Zeidler, M., Cousens, S. N., Estibeiro, K., Alperovitch, A., et al. (1996). A new variant of Creutzfeldt-Jakob disease in the UK. *Lancet, 347,* 921–925.

Zimakoff, J., Kjelsberg, A. B., Larsen, S. O., & Holstein, B. (1992). A multicenter questionnaire investigation of attitudes toward hand hygiene, assessed by the staff in fifteen hospitals in Denmark and Norway. *American Journal of Infection Control, 20,* 58–64.

26

Into the Future

C. J. Peters

The public health and the research communities have made strides in responding to emerging infectious diseases, but much more needs to be done. These infections deserve our attention because of trends in our modern world that are placing important evolutionary pressures on microbes. Simultaneously we are providing greater opportunities for the infectious agents to emerge locally as well as to move around the world and set up housekeeping in new places.

The combination of changing ecology and travel and transport of organisms is nowhere seen more clearly than in antibacterial resistance (see chapter 2). The selective forces of widespread antibiotic use have led to the emergence and movement of populations of resistant bacteria carrying the genetic information to elude our therapeutic efforts. Sometimes, the distance traveled is only from one bed to another in the intensive care unit, but in other cases the movement has been worldwide. Even the pneumococcus is now widely resistant to penicillin (see chapter 18), denying us the use of the best antibiotic we have ever developed in treating this common and often life-threatening infectious agent. Simultaneously there is a huge genetic pool in bacteria that are not notable human pathogens but that are subject to selection in human and animal reservoirs and may subsequently transfer their genetic material to other bacteria of more direct importance.

The role of selection is more subtle but not less important in viral diseases. Some chronic or latent viruses such as herpes viruses or polyomaviruses have coevolved with humans and uncommonly cause serious disease in the normal host. Other viruses are transmitted in nature and infect humans as a "sideline." These may be important pathogens directly but they also form a pool of agents that can potentially adapt to inter-human transmission, much as viruses such as measles did centuries ago and HIV has done more recently (Fenner, 1970; Gao, Bailes, Robertson, Chen, Rodenburg, Michael, et al., 1999). Influenza A could be thought of as an avian virus that periodically generates mutants and reassortants that can adapt to human transmission (Hay, 2001). The flow of viruses between different species and within a single species is critically dependent on selection, ecology, and movement of infected hosts.

IMPORTANCE OF ECOLOGICAL CHANGE

What is the driving force in the emergence of zoonotic viral disease? We can divide the factors into three broad categories: viral mutation, ecological change, and travel or transport (Figure 26.1). In most cases the evidence points to changes in ecology; that is, ecology in the broad sense. For a rodent-borne virus, changes in the plant and animal surroundings or climate change such as might occur with deforestation or an El Niño/southern oscillation (ENSO) event could be the ecological force. For a virus such as HIV, changes in human sexual behavior or needle use could be the relevant ecological alterations. Many of the emerging pathogens are RNA viruses and these agents are continuously generating mutants because of the poor fidelity of the polymerase and the lack of the error-checking mechanism operating with DNA

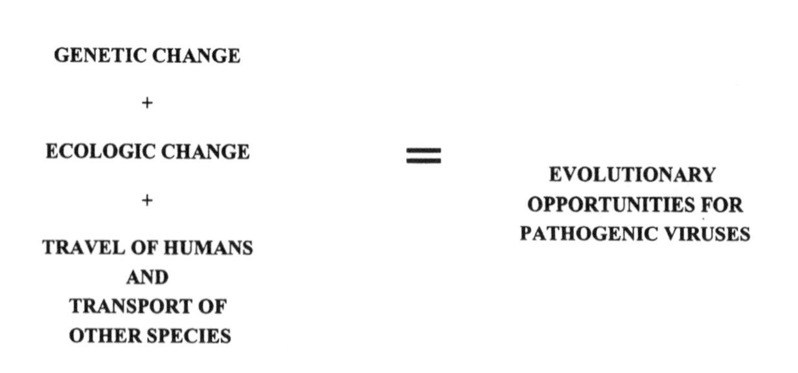

FIGURE 26.1 A schema for emerging infections.

replication. Interestingly, the role of viral mutants in driving the emergence of disease seems to be relatively small with the exception of influenza and a few other viruses. Mutations are adaptive and allow the viruses to function in changing situations.

IMPORTANCE OF TRAVEL AND TRANSPORT

Another obvious factor is travel by humans with consequent transport of viruses, vectors, and reservoirs. This became a major factor in the 1500s with the age of exploration. Ships began to traverse the oceans with increasing frequency and travel and exploration further breached intracontinental barriers. In the last quarter century we have multiplied the number of ships and further accentuated the process with rapid movement by airplanes.

To illustrate the importance of ecology and the mixing effect of travel and transport, let us consider emergences of hazardous virus diseases over the last 5 years such as hantaviruses, Ebola virus, Hendra virus, Nipah virus, Congo-Crimean hemorrhagic fever virus, smallpox, Rift Valley fever virus, and Marburg virus (see Appendix A, Tables A.1–A.3). The epidemics these diseases cause are often sufficiently dramatic to motivate a reasonable investigation of the inciting circumstances, and these episodes are one of the categories we should be concerned about in the future. They are usually zoonotic viruses transmitted in nature and often are highly hazardous in the laboratory. These viruses will be used to give a framework for examining emerging infections in general, but the lessons from this group apply broadly to most of the emerging pathogens, particularly the viruses.

HANTAVIRUS PULMONARY SYNDROME, SURPRISES FOR MEDICINE

In 1993 a mysterious epidemic of fatal respiratory disease occurred in the southwestern U.S. Investigations were at first stymied but soon discarded a toxin explanation and identified a hantavirus as the cause (Ksiazek, Peters, Rollin, Zaki, Nichol, Spiropoulou, et al., 1995; Nichol, Spiropoulou, Morzunov, Rollin, Ksiazek, Feldmann, et al., 1993). In spite of the fact that previously known hantaviruses caused hemorrhagic fever with renal syndrome, the mechanisms underlying the pathogenesis of the "mystery disease" were consonant with those of other hantavirus infections (Ksiazek et al., 1995; Zaki, Greer, Coffield, Goldsmith, Noted, Foucar, et al., 1995). In fact, with newer diagnostic approaches and awareness of the clinical syndrome, the American hantaviruses were soon found to be numerous and to generally cause "hantavirus pulmonary syndrome" or HPS (Peters, 1998). Several hundred cases have now been diagnosed in North, Central, and South America.

Local outbreaks were usually precipitated by changes in weather conditions. Longitudinal studies of rodent populations and rodent infection in the southwestern U.S. have shown a close relationship with rainfall and this has been driven by the climatic changes following ENSO events (Mills, Yates, Ksiazek, Peters, & Childs, 1999; Yates, Mills, Parmenter, Ksiazek, Calisher, Nichol, et al., 2001). There are no practical interventions to protect human populations in rural areas other than rodent-proofing of homes (see Appendix C, Table C.6).

One of the biggest surprises from the hantavirus story has been the finding that one of the American hantaviruses, Andes virus, has caused at least one Argentine epidemic with human-to-human transmission (Wells, Sosa, Estani, Yadon, Enria, Padula, Pini, et al., 1997). This is the only example of such spread and has not been seen with any other hantavirus, including Sin Nombre virus in the U.S. (Wells, Young, Williams, Armstrong, Busico, Khan, et al., 1997).

NIPAH VIRUS, MONOCULTURES, AND SPECIES JUMPING

Both Hendra and Nipah viruses were discovered during relatively recent epidemics (Chua, Bellini, Rota, Harcourt, Temin, Lam, et al., 2000; Murray, Eaton, Hooper, Wang, Williamson, & Young, 1998). They belong to the scientifically venerable virus family Paramyxoviridae but are sufficiently different from known members that they have been assigned to a new genus in that family. Both viruses apparently have their usual life in megachiropterans, also known as fruit-eating bats or flying foxes. In the case of Hendra virus, a limited number of horses and humans have been infected and the cause of emergence is unknown. Undoubtedly the movement of flying foxes into suburban sites (possibly related to habitat destruction) facilitated the equine infections, and the unusual disease in a prominent horse trainer caring for sick racing horses led to increased interest and could well have been important in the discovery.

In the case of Nipah virus, the proximity of flying foxes to a pig-raising industry that had been modernized to provide a large number of animals in close proximity seemed to be an important factor. Movement of pigs between farms was felt to be a major factor in spread within Malaysia, and export of pigs to Singapore resulted in disease among abattoir workers there. Virus infection was found in humans (who suffered encephalitis with a high case fatality and sometimes severe residua), horses, dogs, and cats. Genetic analyses of the viruses are underway but have not yet shown a difference between the virus in its natural reservoir and the virus in its new host so far; in fact, if differences were found they would most probably be adaptive rather than the origin of the epidemics.

Nipah virus is a very dangerous agent with the capability of spreading directly from pig to pig and in addition infecting several other species. This ability to cross species is unusual, particularly for a paramyxovirus. Presumably the availability of a monoculture of pigs was the event that led to its ability to adapt from its original flying fox host, and the movement of these animals enhanced its spread within Malaysia and elsewhere. The slaughter of more than a million pigs was needed to control the virus, a feat that would have been much more difficult to accomplish expeditiously in a country such as the U.S. where more environmental and other regulations are in place. Fortunately the prompt containment prevented the progress of the disease from peninsular Malaysia to the Asian mainland where pigs are a very important part of the economy and the food supply.

FILOVIRUSES AND INTERHUMAN TRANSMISSION

The filoviruses are undoubtedly viruses with a reservoir in nature, but scientists have been unable to find the source of either of the two major viruses, Ebola virus and Marburg virus (see chapter 8). Both have emerged sporadically from their natural cycles and been brought into contact with multiple humans through the intermediary of nonhuman primates or nosocomial spread (Peters & LeDuc, 1999). One operative mechanism is movement of the primates to Europe or the U.S. for use in vaccine production and/or biomedical research. Another is the poor hygienic standards in African hospitals; proper barrier nursing has been shown to stop Ebola transmission in Zaire in 1995 (Khan, Tshioko, Heymann, Le Guenno, Nabeth, Kerstiëns, et al., 1999). This experience has been replicated in epidemics in Gabon and South Africa.

The South African experience is particularly relevant to the U.S. (Richards, Murphy, Jobson, Mer, Zinman, Taylor, et al., 2000). A sick physician from Gabon was admitted to a well-equipped hospital but the diagnosis was not suspected. He underwent extensive workup and was cared for using routine precautions. One of the nurses who was involved in a cut-down procedure became critically ill, and in an attempt to make a diagnosis, samples were sent for testing for Crimean Congo hemorrhagic fever, an important pathogen in South Africa. The virus laboratory routinely sought all known viral hemorrhagic fever agents in their examinations and diagnosed the nurse with Ebola. Retrospectively the index case was identified and confirmed by blood serology and virus isolation from semen. The occurrence of only one secondary case even though no special Ebola-related precautions were taken suggests the pattern we would likely see in the U.S. if Ebola virus were introduced: very limited spread in hospital staff and intimate contacts (Dowell, Mukunu, Ksiazek, Khan, Rollin, Peters, et al., 1999). Of course, if a known Ebola patient were admitted, any hospital would take special precautions, but an attitude of panic would not be justified (Peters, Jahrling, & Khan, 1996).

Thus the danger of Ebola virus does not lie in its ability to cause spreading epidemics that would defy control. It remains an important problem because its reservoir is unknown and thus we have no way to understand the factors underlying its transition into humans. The epidemics that occur when Ebola or Marburg viruses are introduced into the human population are stalking horses for inadequate hygiene in hospitals, reuse of needles and syringes without sterilization contributing to hepatitis and HIV transmission, and inadequate surveillance. The potential future danger is that failure to terminate chains of transmission could set the stage for genetic adaptation of the virus to interhuman spread.

RIFT VALLEY FEVER AND VECTOR-BORNE DISEASES

Rift Valley fever virus is a mosquito-borne pathogen of domestic animals and humans in sub-Saharan Africa (Peters, 1997). It first showed its ability to spread in 1977 when it caused a major epidemic in Egypt. After dying out there, it recurred in the 1990s. More recently it has caused a major epidemic in eastern Africa after the inciting ENSO event in 1997–1998 (Linthicum, Anyamba, Tucker, Kelley, Myers, & Peters, 1999). The waning of that epidemic was followed by an introduction of the virus into the western area of the Arabian peninsula (Centers for Disease Control and Prevention, 2000). The extensive animal and human epidemic claimed more than 120 human lives and established once again the ability of this virus to move to new environments (Shope, Peters, & Davies, 1982).

It is of interest to examine some of the worst offenders among the mosquito-borne viruses for factors that predispose to geographical movement. In the cases of urban yellow fever, dengue, and chikingunya viruses, the vector utilized in its transported mode is *Aedes aegypti*, a mosquito that is capable of living with humans whenever they allow standing water to exist in containers, tires, and other receptacles. In these cycles, humans are the relevant vertebrate host (Peters & Dalrymple, 1990). West Nile virus came to North America and found a home with avian vertebrate hosts, and the ubiquitous *Culex pipiens* mosquito transmits the virus (Despommier, 2001). The American togavirus Venezuelan equine encephalitis virus seems to be evolving to use equines introduced in post-Columbian times as its vertebrate amplifier and to be transmitted by a variety of relatively common mosquito vectors (Weaver, 1998). Rift Valley fever has also acquired "new" vertebrate amplifying hosts with the introduction and reintroduction of sheep and cattle to Africa. It also has a very broad range of potential mosquito vectors, specifically including common North American mosquitoes (House, Turell, & Mebus, 1992). This would seem to be a versatile and dangerous virus simply awaiting a stochastic event to cause major problems outside Africa.

SMALLPOX AND THE RETURN OF OLD FOES

It is ironic that the eradication of a virus could be the cause for even greater anxiety than when it was causing extensive human disease. No one would prefer to have smallpox present in nature, but interruption of its obligatory inter-human transmission chain in 1977 led to a cessation of vaccination that has left humans at risk of extensive epidemics should the virus be reintroduced. The revelations that the virus has been used to produce a biological weapon by the former Soviet Union, the conclusions that other countries may possess smallpox, and the rise of concern with bioterrorism lead to the conclusion that defenses against smallpox are needed. A susceptible population, inadequate vaccine stocks, rapid and extensive travel, and loss of medical expertise simply make the remote possibility of a reintroduction unacceptable. Of all the viruses discussed, this is the only one with a proven track record of epidemic inter-human spread and its roughly 30% mortality leaves little doubt as to the human and social impact of a smallpox epidemic.

In the context of smallpox, it is worth remembering other high hazard viruses could be agents of bioterrorism or biological warfare (see chapter 24). Will they be used, and will they show us new faces of some of the viral hemorrhagic fevers and other lethal viruses (Peters, 2000)?

FORECAST FOR THE FUTURE

The last decade provides many examples of changes in infectious disease patterns. Some emergences are directly related to the increasing pool of immunosuppressed or otherwise compromised hosts in the human population that provide a substrate for the infecting agent. Other infectious diseases do not represent any change of incidence but rather are a consequence of our improved ability to recognize or test for the condition. At first glance the latter would not seem to be an "emergence" but this situation meets the definition of the Institute of Medicine for an emerging infectious disease (Lederberg, Shope, & Oaks, 1992). The inclusion of this category as emerging infections is justified because we must go through the same process of evaluation, public health response, education, and research as for other diseases that represent true increases in incidence. HPS provides an excellent example.

The most important challenges for the future are agents that attack the normal host. We have made the case that ecological change provides the selective forces to which viruses and their vectors/reservoirs adapt. Furthermore, the rapidly increasing pace of travel and transport increases the occasions for genetically flexible RNA viruses to exploit opportunities arising through ecological shifts (Figure 26.1) (Peters, 2001). Some of the factors that are quite generally related to the increasing pace of infectious disease emergence in humans are exemplified in Table 26.1, briefly considering high hazard virus disease emergence over the last 5 years.

The combined impact of ecological change and travel is multiplied; disturbed environments have long been recognized to be the most receptive to introductions of exotic flora and fauna (Elton, 1958; Vitousek, D'Antonio, Loope, & Westbrooks, 1996). If we look at the total impact of humans on the earth through these processes, we find an alarming degree of change (Table 26.2). From space, satellites show us that more than half the earth's land surface has been modified by human behavior (Vitousek, Mooney, Lubchenco, & Melillo, 1997).

TABLE 26.1 Some Generally Applicable Factors in Emergence

- New diagnostic methods or recognition of a new syndrome can uncover a common disease not previously appreciated (HPS).
- "New" agents are still being discovered. Some are doing what they have always done (HPS) but others are changing host range and posing completely new threats (Nipah virus).
- Most of the viruses are not readily spread from person to person with the exception of the old pathogen, smallpox. Some may be a threat to increase their interhuman capability (filoviruses) and some have been truly surprising (Andes hantavirus).
- In the case of zoonotic diseases, great fluctuations in incidence can occur depending on climatic conditions; ENSO provides one of the driving forces (HPS, Rift Valley fever).
- Local disturbances in land use or agricultural practices may lead to changes in virus, vector, or reservoir circulation (Rift Valley fever, hantaviruses, Nipah virus).
- Changes in "human ecology" can favor the emergence of diseases (Ebola and Marburg viruses).
- Local and intercontinental movement of viruses is possible and may die out (filoviruses) or may cause protracted transmission (Rift Valley fever).
- Advances in one country can be major setbacks in another (disposable needles and filoviruses).
- Eradication of a disease brings its own problems, including accumulation of susceptibles, deterioration of vaccine stocks, and changing vaccine standards (smallpox).
- Vectors and reservoirs can be subject to distant introduction.
- Study of epidemics yields important information.
- Prediction is an important goal but not yet accurate.

TABLE 26.2 Human Impact on Earth's Ecology

- Half of land surface transformed by human action
- Extinction rates of animal species increased 100–1000 times
  One fourth of bird species extinct
  Many fishing areas depleted with many actual and threatened extinctions
- Biological invasions are common
  Nonnative plants comprise 20% of continental and 50% of island species
  West Nile is latest recognized viral invasion to North America
  Foot and mouth disease invades U.K. and Europe in 2001
- More than one half all surface freshwater used by humans
  98% of U.S. rivers have at least one major dam
  Two thirds of all Earth's rivers have at least one dam
  Projected shortages of clean water for two thirds of Earth's inhabitants in next quarter century
  WHO identifies more than 1 billion humans without clean water today
- Impact on climate and weather
  Global warming is certain
  How much is anthropogenic?
  Weekly cycle of rainfall off North American coast demonstrates human impact on weather
- More nitrogen fixed by humans than all other sources
  Major impact on S, Hg, Pb and other elements
  DDT, PCB, and other toxic, slowly degraded compounds made by humans accumulating in environment and in living organisms

Adapted from: Leakey & Lewin, 1995; Holland & Peterson, 1995; Vitousek et al., 1997.

We are driving extinction of animals and plants at a rate far greater than ever seen before (Leakey & Lewin, 1995). Water, an essential resource, is being usurped extensively by humans; and it is projected that it will become a limiting resource in quantity and quality within a decade or two. These changes are clearly documented, without entering controversial areas such as anthropogenic contributions to global warming or "hot-button" issues such as old growth forests and the rain forest. The extensive use of our planet's bounty leaves less and less room for any mistakes and fewer avenues of remediation. Increasingly, the old adage about "dilution is the solution to pollution" is no longer valid. In 2001, the U.S. has come face to face with power shortages on the west coast; increasing hydroelectric power from the northwestern states to alleviate this problem would result in further ecological modifications, and additional pressure on endangered species.

The lack of flexible alternatives will become increasingly problematic as world population forces more dependence on modern intensive agriculture. Intensive cultivation of plants and animals will lead to situations in which a single genetically homogenous species will be grown in a limited area, making a perfect target for emerging diseases. This situation has been recognized since the Irish potato famine and amply documented subsequently.

The modification of centuries old practices of rice growing and irrigation in the island ecosystem of Bali provides an instructive example (Lansing, 1991). In an attempt to increase the production of rice, "green" rice strains and intensive water-fertilizer regimens were introduced. The changes in planting and irrigation practices led to eruptions of pests and the need for intensive pesticide use. Water supplies became inadequate and the distribution of water was skewed. Crops underwent cycles of infection by fungi and viruses requiring repeated introductions of resistant rice strains. This type of problem may be soluble and lead to increased food production in the long run, but it is sure to introduce vulnerabilities to agricultural diseases. The 2001 outbreak of foot and mouth disease in England and its rapid spread only serves to emphasize the impact of agricultural diseases in today's mobile, intensive food production industry.

If we are going to successfully deal with the increasing amount of change and the accelerating rate of change, we need both local action and technology. Technology (Table 26.3) has given us powerful tools in the struggle, but many of these approaches are today used in a reductionist fashion. For example, molecular biology today often focuses on the individual organism or gene. We need to emphasize, however, the power of integrative approaches in which we use molecu-

TABLE 26.3 Scientific Tools Helpful in Dealing With Infectious Diseases

- Molecular biology, immunology
- Genomics, proteomics
- Advances in study of veterinary, wildlife, and human diseases
- Remote sensing

lar biology to follow the movement of genes and the structure of complex ecological systems. Genomics so far has been about one genome from a species and not a population of genomes interacting with populations of other species' genomes and an environment. As noted in the Bali example, we also have to bear in mind some of the unintended consequences of technology.

The local action needed to recognize emerging infections is fairly well understood (Table 26.4) (Peters, 2001). Indeed, these activities are primarily those of a good health care system and a well-supported public health infrastructure. This is perhaps unfortunate, because it might be easier to mobilize the global community for some sort of specialized technological project than to attempt to improve activities that we already know are in various degrees of trouble.

TABLE 26.4 Recognition of Emerging Human Diseases Is Critically Dependent on Local Health Care Services

- Competent and alert health care providers
- Pathologists and autopsies
- Routine clinical diagnostic laboratories to identify the usual disease offenders
- Public health institutions to collate information and compare it to background surveillance data
- Public health microbiology laboratory backup
- Access to reference capability (clinicians, pathologists, microbiology laboratory, and other expertise) for unusual or complex problems

TABLE 26.5 Elements for Dealing With Emergence That Are Absent From the World Stage

- Adequate public health and curative health infrastructure in most countries in the world
- Will to improve public and curative health infrastructure in all countries in the world
- Enough resources for adequate surveillance
- Research designed to elucidate more of the principles underlying emergence
- The ability to make practical vaccines for human use
- Smooth regulatory atmosphere to facilitate responses to threats

In spite of the positive features in our struggle against infectious diseases, there are some real obstacles. We show no sign of taking important steps to stabilize the world's ecological change or the population growth that is a major driving force for ecological change. Bioterrorism and biological warfare are wild cards; will they be used more extensively than merely anthrax spores placed in a few letters? Now that the barrier has been broken and someone with the obvious capability of preparing a dry powder with the very dangerous particle size and aerosol properties of the October 2001 attack is involved we can most assuredly expect further attempts with anthrax. The former Soviet Union prepared literally tons of infectious agents such as tularemia, plague, Machupo virus, Rift Valley Fever virus, and Marburg virus. Massive dissemination of these agents could lead to new patterns of infectious disease distribution. We are faced with critical deficits in a number of areas (Table 26.5), and their reversal is not likely. I think those of us working in the arena of emerging infections are going to be in business for a long time.

REFERENCES

Centers for Disease Control and Prevention. (2000). Update: Outbreak of Rift Valley fever—Saudi Arabia, August–November 2000. *Morbidity and Mortality Weekly Report, 49*, 982–985.

Chua, K. B., Bellini, W. J., Rota, P. A., Harcourt, B. H., Temin, A., Lam, S. K., et al. (2000). Nipah virus: A recently emergent deadly paramyxovirus. *Science, 288*, 1432–1435.

Despommier, D. (2001). *West Nile story*. New York: Apple Trees Productions.

Dowell, S. F., Mukunu, R., Ksiazek, T. G., Khan, A. S., Rollin, P. E., Peters, C. J., & the EHF Study Group. (1999). Transmission of Ebola hemorrhagic fever: A study of risk factors in family members, Kikwit, Democratic Republic of the Congo, 1995. *Journal of Infectious Diseases, 179*(Supp. 1), S87–S91.

Elton, C. S. (1958). *The ecology of invasions by animals and plants*. London: Methuen & Co., Ltd.

Fenner, F. (1970). In S. V. Boyden (Ed.), *The impact of civilization on the biology of man*. Canberra: Australian National University Press.

Gao, F., Bailes, E., Robertson, D. L., Chen, Y., Rodenburg, C. M., Michael, S. F., et al. (1999). Origin of HIV-1 in the chimpanzee *Pan troglodytes troglodytes*. *Nature, 397*, 436–441.

Hay, A. J. (2001). Potential of influenza A viruses to cause pandemics. In W. L. Irving, J. W. McCauley, D. J. Rowlands, & G. L. Smith (Eds.), *New challenges to health: The threat of virus infection, 60th Symposium of the Society for General Microbiology* (pp. 89–104). Cambridge: Cambridge University Press.

Holland, H. D., & Petersen, U. (1995). *Living dangerously: The earth, its resources, and the environment*. Princeton, NJ: Princeton University Press.

House, J. A., Turell, M. J., & Mebus, C. A. (1992). Rift Valley fever: Present status and risk to the Western Hemisphere. *Annals of the New York Academy of Sciences, 653*, 233–242.

Khan, A. S., Tshioko, F. K., Heymann, D. L., Le Guenno, B., Nabeth, P., Kerstiëns, B., et al. (1999). The reemergence of Ebola hemorrhagic fever, Democratic Republic of the Congo, 1995. *Journal of Infectious Diseases, 179*(Suppl. 1), S76–S86.

Ksiazek, T. G., Peters, C. J., Rollin, P. E., Zaki, S., Nichol, S., Spiropoulou, C., et al. (1995). Identification of a new North American hantavirus that causes acute pulmonary insufficiency. *American Journal of Tropical Medicine and Hygiene, 52*, 117–123.

Lansing, J. S. (1991). *Priests and programmers. Technologies of power in the engineered landscape of Bali*. Princeton, NJ: Princeton University Press.

Leakey, R., & Lewin, R. (1995). *The sixth extinction*. New York: Anchor/Doubleday.

Lederberg, J., Shope, R. E., & Oaks, S. (1992). *Emerging microbial threats*. Washington, DC: U.S. National Academy of Sciences Press.

Linthicum, K. J., Anyamba, A., Tucker, C. J., Kelley, P. W., Myers, M. F., & Peters, C. J. (1999). Climate and satellite indicators to forecast Rift Valley fever epidemics in Kenya. *Science, 285*, 397–400.

Mills, J. N., Yates, T. L., Ksiazek, T. G., Peters, C. J., & Childs, J. E. (1999). Long-term studies of hantavirus reservoir populations in the southwestern United States: Rationale, potential, and methods. *Emerging Infectious Diseases, 5*, 95–101.

Murray, K., Eaton, B., Hooper, P., Wang, L., Williamson, M., & Young, P. (1998). Flying foxes, horses, and humans: A zoonosis caused by a new member of the *Paramyxoviridae*. In W. M. Scheld, D. Armstrong, & J. M. Hughes (Eds.), *Emerging infections 1* (pp. 43–58). Washington, DC: ASM Press.

Nichol, S. T., Spiropoulou, C. F., Morzunov, S., Rollin, P. E., Ksiazek, T. G., Feldmann, H., et al. (1993). Genetic identification of a hantavirus associated with an outbreak of acute respiratory illness. *Science, 262*, 914–917.

Peters, C. J. (1997). Emergence of Rift Valley fever. In J. F. Saluzzo & B. Dodet (Eds.), *Factors in the emergence of arbovirus diseases* (pp. 253–264). Paris: Elsevier.

Peters, C. J. (1998). Hantavirus pulmonary syndrome in the Americas. In W. M. Scheld, W. A. Craig, & J. M. Hughes (Eds.), *Emerging infections 2* (pp. 17–64). Washington, DC: ASM Press.

Peters, C. J. (2000). Are hemorrhagic fever viruses practical agents for biological terrorism? In W. M. Scheld, W. A. Craig, & J. M. Hughes (Eds.), *Emerging infections 4* (pp. 203–211). Washington, DC: ASM Press.

Peters, C. J. (2001). The viruses in our past, the viruses in our future. In G. L. Smith, W. L. Irving, J. W. McCauley, & D. J. Rowlands (Eds.), *New challenges to health: The threat of virus infection, 60th Symposium of the Society for General Microbiology* (pp. 1–32). Cambridge: Cambridge University Press.

Peters, C. J., & Dalrymple, J. M. (1990). Alphaviruses. In B. N. Fields & D. M. Knipe (Eds.), *Virology* (pp. 713–761). New York: Raven Press.

Peters, C. J., Jahrling, P. B., & Khan, A. S. (1996). Management of patients infected with high-hazard viruses: Scientific basis for infection control. *Archives of Virology* (Suppl. 11), 1–28.

Peters, C. J., & LeDuc, J. W. (1999). An introduction to Ebola: The virus and the disease. *Journal of Infectious Diseases, 179*(Suppl. 1), ix–xvi.

Richards, G. A., Murphy, S., Jobson, R., Mer, M., Zinman, C., Taylor, R., et al. (2000). Unexpected Ebola virus in a tertiary setting: Clinical and epidemiologic aspects. *Critical Care Medicine, 28,* 240–244.

Shope, R. E., Peters, C. J., & Davies, F. G. (1982). The spread of Rift Valley fever and approaches to its control. *Bulletin of the World Health Organization, 60,* 299–304.

Vitousek, P. M., D'Antonio, C. M., Loope, L. L., & Westbrooks, R. (1996). Biological invasions as global environmental change. *American Scientist, 8,* 468–478.

Vitousek, P. M., Mooney, H. A., Lubchenco, J., & Melillo, J. M. (1997). Human domination of Earth's ecosystems. *Science, 277,* 494–499.

Weaver, S. C. (1998). Recurrent emergence of Venezuelan equine encephalomyelitis. In W. M. Scheld, D. Armstrong, & J. M. Hughes (Eds.), *Emerging Infections 1* (pp. 27–42). Washington, DC: ASM Press.

Wells, R. M., Sosa Estani, S., Yadon, Z. E., Enria, D., Padula, P., Pini, N., et al. (1997). An unusual hantavirus outbreak in southern Argentina: Person-to-person transmission? *Emerging Infectious Diseases,* 3, 171–174.

Wells, R. M., Young, J., Williams, R. J., Armstrong, L. R., Busico, K., Khan, A. S., et al. (1997). Hantavirus transmission in the United States. *Emerging Infectious Diseases,* 3, 361–365.

Yates, T., Mills, J., Parmenter, C., Ksiazek, T., Calisher, C., Nichol, S., et al. (in press). Biocomplexity and Sin Nombre virus: The ecology of an outbreak. *Nature.*

Zaki, S. R., Greer, P. W., Coffield, L. M., Goldsmith, C. S., Noted, K. B., Foucar, K., et al. (1995). Hantavirus pulmonary syndrome: Pathogenesis of an emerging infectious disease. *American Journal of Pathology, 146,* 552–579.

Appendices

Appendix A

Emerging/Reemerging Diseases by Organism

Felissa R. Lashley

TABLE A.1 Examples of Emerging/Reemerging Bacteria

Bacteria	Major Disease(s)	Comments
Bartonella grahamii	Neuroretinitis	Described in Europe. Major reservoir is bank voles.
Bartonella clarridgeae	Cat scratch disease	Only recently identified as a human pathogen. Described in 1995. Found in cats. Can cause cat scratch disease.
Bartonella elizabethae	Endocarditis, bacteremia	Identified as a new species in 1993. Formerly called *Rochalimaea*. See chapter 3.
Bartonella henselae	Bacillary angiomatosis (BA), cat scratch disease, bacteremia, endocarditis, peliosis	Causes cat scratch disease. BA first described in persons with AIDS in 1987. Also causes relapsing fever and endocarditis. The cat is a major reservoir. Children and persons with HIV disease are most susceptible to cat scratch disease. See chapter 3.
Bartonella quintana	Bacillary angiomatosis (BA), trench fever, endocarditis, peliosis, bacteremia	BA occurs almost exclusively in immunocompromised persons. BA lesions may be multifocal and highly vascular. Peliosis usually occurs in the immunosuppressed. See chapter 3.

(continued)

TABLE A.1 *(continued)*

Bacteria	Major Disease(s)	Comments
Borrelia burgdorferi	Lyme disease	Recognized in 1978 in Lyme, CT. Transmitted to humans via deer ticks. Can have severe chronic sequelae. Characterized by a skin lesion known as erythema migrans that appears in about 60% at the site of the tick bite. Other symptoms may include rash, malaise, headache, chills, fever, backache arthralgia, and myalgia. Later effects may include arthritis and neurological and cardiac manifestations. See chapter 14.
Burkholderia (formerly *Pseudomonas*) *pseudomallei*	Melioidosis	Endemic in Thailand, Guam, and now present in India and the Caribbean. Present in Australia and Malasia. Considered a tropical disease. Most persons develop inapparent infection that may be latent, appearing after many years when the person is immunosuppressed. May cause parotid abscess in children, or acute septicemia or a neurologic syndrome, or suppuration in the liver or other organs in adults. Persons with cystic fibrosis who travel may be especially susceptible. Considered by some to be reemerging because of geographic spread and antimicrobial resistance, especially to aminoglycosides and most β-lactams.
Campylobacter jejuni	Enteritis	A zoonotic infection. Became recognized as a human pathogen in the 1970s. Symptoms include fever, diarrhea (watery or bloody), and abdominal pain. Trigger for Guillain-Barré syndrome.

TABLE A.1 *(continued)*

Bacteria	Major Disease(s)	Comments
Chlamydia pneumoniae	Association with coronary heart disease, pharyngitis, bronchitis, sinusitis, and pneumonia	Considered emerging in context of its association with coronary heart disease. In 1983 was recognized in connection with pneumonia, pharyngitis, and other infections. See chapter 21.
Clostridium novyl	Soft tissue inflammation and infection	Outbreak in April, 2000, of unexplained illness and deaths in injecting drug users in Great Britain thought due to *C. novyl*. High mortality rate.
Cornyebacterium diptheriae	Diphtheria	Reemerging in places where public heath systems are in disarray such as the former Soviet Union states. Vaccine preventable.
Ehrlichia chaffeensis	Human monocytic ehrlichiosis	Recognized in 1987. Rickettsiae. Transmitted by ticks and also transfusion, rarely. Illness ranges in severity from mild to severe. Fever, headache, chills, myalgia, malaise with nausea, vomiting, anorexia. Rash occurs in 20%–35%. Multiorgan failure can occur. See chapter 14.
*Ehrlichia equi/ Ehrlichia phagocytophila-*like agent	Human granulocytic ehrlichiosis	Identified during 1992–1993 outbreak in midwest. Is a rickettsiae. Tick-borne. Can rarely be transmitted by transfusion. Fever, chills, myalgia headache, malaise. Rash not usual. Ranges in severity. See chapter 14.
Ehrlichia ewingii	Ehrlichiosis	Identified in patients from Missouri beginning in 1996. Tick-borne rickettsiae. Presentation includes fever, headache, and thrombocytopenia. Clinical disease can be clinically identical to that of *E. chaffeensis* or the agent of HGE. See chapter 14.

(continued)

TABLE A.1 *(continued)*

Bacteria	Major Disease(s)	Comments
Ehrlichia sennetsu	Illness similar to mononucleosis	First reported in 1985. Found in Japan and Malaysia.
Enterococcus faecalis	Vancomycin-resistant nosocomial surgical infections	See chapter 19. G-I tract and skin are reservoirs. Accounts for about 15%–18% of vancomycin-resistant enterocci (VRE) infections.
Enterococcus faecium	Vancomycin-resistant nosocomial surgical infections	See chapter 19. Same reservoirs as above. Accounts for 80%–85% of VRE infections.
Escherichia coli O157:H7	Diarrheal illness, hemolytic uremic syndrome	See chapter 9. First recognized in outbreak in the early 1980s. A foodborne illness associated with several vehicles including alfalfa sprouts, ground beef, unpasteurized apple juice, and others. Can be waterborne.
Helicobacter pylori	Peptic ulcer disease, gastritis, mucosa-associated lymphoid tissue gastric lymphoma, gastric adenocarcinoma	Was isolated in 1982 and given its present name in 1989. Has been designated as a class I carcinogen by WHO. May also be responsible for recurrent childhood abdominal pain. See chapter 21.
Legionella pneumophila	Legionnaires' disease (LD), Pontiac fever	LD recognized after infection occurred in attendees at an American Legion convention in Philadelphia in July, 1976. Causes pneumonia. See chapter 13.

TABLE A.1 *(continued)*

Bacteria	Major Disease(s)	Comments
Leptospira spp. Includes *L. interrogans*, *L. borgpeterseni*, *L. weillei* and others	Leptospirosis	A zoonotic disease of worldwide distribution. Results from exposure to infected animal urine directly or indirectly through contaminated soil or water. Can penetrate skin or mucous membranes. More usual in children and young adult men related to occupational exposure. Is considered reemerging due to outbreaks in Nicaragua (1995), and in U.S. travelers to Costa Rica (1996) from contaminated river water during white water rafting. Two types of illness—one with mild febrile illness without jaundice, and one with jaundice, fever, chills, headache, rash, myalgia, conjunctivitis, prostration. Icteric form may have hepatic dysfunction, renal insufficiency, hemorrhage. Can develop complications (including pulmonary or conjunctival gastrointestinal) and CNS involvement. See chapter 22.
Listeria monocytogenes	Listeriosis	A gram-positive bacteria only recently considered as causing gastrointestinal disease, diarrhea, nausea, vomiting, and abdominal cramps often with fever. Most cases of listeriosis occur in immunocompromised persons, the elderly, or pregnant women. Typical illness manifestations are flu-like symptoms, sepsis, or central nervous system illness. Frequently contaminated foods include deli meats, soft cheeses. See chapter 3.

(continued)

TABLE A.1 ***(continued)***

Bacteria	Major Disease(s)	Comments
Mycobacterium avium complex	Pulmonary and disseminated disease in persons with HIV disease	Ubiquitous soil and water bacteria considered emerging because of the increase in persons with HIV disease. May also affect the GI tract causing diarrhea, malabsorption, and abdominal pain. Disseminated disease usually seen in persons with CD4 counts less than 50 mm^3.
Mycobacterium celatum	Pulmonary and disseminated disease in persons with HIV disease	Usually found in immunosuppressed persons such as those with HIV disease.
Mycobacterium genavense	Disseminated disease in patients with HIV disease	Described first in 1990. Accounts for about 13% of disseminated mycobacterial infections in Switzerland. Manifestations include diarrhea, pain, weight loss, fever, anemia, pancytopenia, and hepatosplenomegaly.
Mycobacterium haemophilum	Cutaneous, pulmonary, and disseminated disease; causes arthritis, osteomyelitis	Usually found in immunosuppressed persons such as those with HIV disease. Described in 1978. Cause of a syndrome consisting of a dermatitis and necrotizing painful skin lesions, in immunocompetent and immunosuppressed persons who also may have joint infections. Reservoir is unknown. Considered emerging by virtue of increasing infection rates and increase in geographic distribution.
Mycobacterium kansasii	Pulmonary disease, disseminated disease	Usually found in persons with HIV disease, and is considered emerging in that context.

TABLE A.1 *(continued)*

Bacteria	Major Disease(s)	Comments
Mycobacterium marinum	Skin lesions	Causes skin nodules or small ulcers on extremities taking years to heal. May result in some scarring. May disseminate in the immunosuppressed. Transmitted through contaminated water including aquariums. May result following skin abrasions. An EID by virtue of increasing rates of infection.
Mycobacterium ulcerans	Buruli ulcer	Reservoir is unknown. Primarily in children. Necrotic skin ulcers. Infections may be linked to environmental disturbances, such as flooding in Uganda and from the use of recycled sewage water to irrigate a golf course in Australia. Scarring during healing. Frequently results in deformities including contracture. Becoming third most prevalent mycobacterial disease.
Mycoplasma penetrans	Antiphospholipid syndrome	Has been more frequently described in persons with HIV infection but affects others as well. Characterized by hemocytopenic and vaso-occlusive manifestations, pulmonary and neurologic manifestations including stroke, myelitis.
Rhodococcus equi	Pneumonia most common	First human case reported in 1967 in a person receiving steroids for hepatitis. Most cases occur in persons with AIDS and CD4 counts less than 200 mm^3. Is considered emerging because of the increase in cases. Extrapulmonary infections can occur, particularly brain and renal abscesses, and osteomyelitis.

(continued)

TABLE A.1 *(continued)*

Bacteria	Major Disease(s)	Comments
Staphylococcus aureus (Toxin-producing strains)	Toxic shock syndrome	In 1978, toxic shock syndrome in healthy young women (especially 15–19 yrs.) was identified. After a peak in 1980, cases have markedly declined. The illness was associated with the menstrual cycle and rise of super-absorbent tampons and vaginal infection followed by toxin production leading to the syndrome. Nonmenstrually associated cases can occur in both sexes. See chapter 3.
Streptococcus pyogenes	Fasciitis, toxic shock syndrome	Emergence of invasive group A streptococcal infections in the mid-1980s. See chapter 3.
Vibrio cholerae	Cholera	Cholera is an old disease causing severe diarrheal illness, but the seventh cholera pandemic began in Indonesia in 1961 caused by the *V. cholerae* O1 serogroup, El Tor biotype. The organism is curved, gram-negative. In 1992, *V. cholerae* O139 was identified in India. Epidemic cholera appeared in Latin America in 1991 after nearly 100 years of absence. Characterized by "rice water" diarrheal stools. See chapter 4.
Vibrio parahaemolyticus	Gastroenteritis	Rare outbreaks before 1997. In 1998, the first outbreak of serotype O3: K6 occurred in the U.S. and 416 persons developed gastroenteritis from eating oysters from Galveston Bay in Texas.

TABLE A.1 *(continued)*

Bacteria	Major Disease(s)	Comments
Vibrio vulnificus	See comments	Emergence reported in 1979. Infections usually result from consumption of shellfish, especially raw oysters from the Gulf of Mexico. An increase is seen in the summer. Infection can result in septicemia with bulbous skin lesions, shock, and rapid death. Persons with iron overload such as hemochromatosis are especially vulnerable.

Sources: Buller, Arens, Hmiel, Paddock, Sumner, & Rikihisa, 1999; Centers for Disease Control and Prevention, 2000; Dance, 2000; Dobos, Quinn, Ashford, Horsbaugh, & King, 1999; French, Benator, & Gordin, 1997; Guerrant, Walker, & Weller, 1999; Hseuh, Teng, Lee, Yu, Yang, Ho, & Luh, 2001; IARC Working Group on the Evaluation of Carcinogenic Risks to Humans, 1994; Koehler, 1998; Lehane & Rawlin, 2000; Levett, 2001; Maguiña & Gotuzzo, 2000; Pechère, Opravil, Wald, Chave, Bessesen, Sievers, et al., 1995; Pretorius & Kelly, 2000; Steere, 2001; Strickland, 2000; Yáñez, Cedillo, Neyrolles, Alonso, Prévost, Rojas, et al., 1999; Zaki & Spiegel, 1998.

TABLE A.2 Selected Emerging/Reemerging Fungal Pathogens[1]

Organism	Major Disease(s)	Comments
Aspergillus spp. Includes *Aspergillus fumigatus*, *Aspergillus flavis*, *Aspergillus niger*	Aspergillosis	Are common ubiquitous, filamentous fungi found in soil and decaying organic matter. Usually affects immunosuppressed persons especially if neutropenic or on corticosteroid therapy. Portal of entry is usually respiratory tract. The most common cause of nosocomial fungal pneumonia. Symptoms include pleuritic chest pain, fever, dyspnea, and cough. May disseminate as well as cause severe pulmonary disease.
Blastomyces dermatitidis	Blastomycosis	Is endemic in parts of North America (around the Great Lakes, Mississippi, Ohio, and St. Lawrence Rivers). May cause acute pneumonia, skin or bone lesions, or CNS disease. Dissemination can occur but is not common.
Candida spp. Includes *C. albicans*, *C. tropicalis*, *C. kruseii*, *C. glabrata*, *C. lusitanieae*	Candidiasis	Is a yeast. Formerly considered of minor importance in relation to mucosal surfaces. Increasing in frequency as a nosocomial infection. Increased awareness of pathogenicity of non-*albicans* species. Increase in both superficial and systemic *Candida* infections especially in those who are immunosuppressed or have medical devices. Can affect oropharynx, eye, esophagus, vagina, anorectal area, and can disseminate.

TABLE A.2 *(continued)*

Organism	Major Disease(s)	Comments
Coccidioides immitis	Coccidioidomycosis	A dimorphic fungal infection endemic in the southwestern U.S. and parts of Mexico and Central and South America. Increased coccidioidomycosis cases have been seen in California and Arizona since the early 1990s, apparently related to cycles of aridity and rainfall along with construction-related soil turnover. Acquired by inhalation usually. Disproportionately affects elderly and HIV-infected individuals. Primary infection is asymptomatic in about half. In immunocompetent, acute infection is usually flu-like, confined to the lung with chest pain and cough. Can lead to meningitis, chronic pulmonary disease, skin lesions, lymph node, or urogenital infection. May affect persons with indwelling medical devices. Can also cause disease in a variety of organs (especially after dissemination) such as the gastrointestinal tract, respiratory tract, bones, muscles, joints, heart, urinary tract, eye, and central nervous system, especially as meningitis or encephalitis.

(continued)

TABLE A.2 *(continued)*

Organism	Major Disease(s)	Comments
Cryptococcus neoformans	Cryptococcal disease	Is an encapsulated yeast found in soil especially if contaminated with pigeon or chicken droppings causing disease in both immunocompetent and immunosuppressed. Overall incidence has increased greatly due to the numbers of HIV-infected persons and transplant recipients. Usually enters through respiratory tract causing pulmonary disease. May disseminate to extrapulmonary sites. Often causes meningitis, and less commonly can cause disease in nearly any tissue, especially joints, oral cavity, skin lesions, pericardium, myocardium, and genitourinary tract. Various varieties and serotypes are known with specific predilections.
Fusarium spp. Includes *Fusarium solani*, *Fusarium moniliforme*	Fusariosis	Are common filamentous fungi inhabiting soil. Acquire infection usually by inhalation, direct inoculation, or through ingestion of toxin. Are considered representative of emerging hyaline molds. Their toxins are potentially lethal and are monitored in crops. Immunosuppressed persons with neutropenia are most vulnerable. Cause respiratory, skin lesions, paronychia, disseminated infection, and chronic liver infection. Portals of entry may be through catheters, lungs, sinuses, and other areas.

TABLE A.2 *(continued)*

Organism	Major Disease(s)	Comments
Histoplasma capsulatum	Histoplasmosis	Endemic in fertile valleys of North America in the central and eastern U.S. but distribution is worldwide. Is a dimorphic fungus found in soil, especially that which has been contaminated by fowl or bats. Causes self-limited pulmonary infection in immunocompetent. Disseminated disease may occur, especially in immunosuppressed. Chronic illness such as granuloma or cavitary disease may occur.
Penicillium marneffei	Penicillinosis	Most prevalent among HIV-infected persons. In southeast Asia is considered an AIDS-indicator disease. Also found in HIV-negative people who traveled in endemic areas such as Thailand, China, Hong Kong, Vietnam, Indonesia, Singapore, and Myanmar (Burma). Signs/symptoms include cough, hepatosplenomegaly, skin lesions (papules, generalized papular rash, nodules), fever, weight loss, anemia, leukocytosis. May disseminate. First reported human infection in 1959, then no reports until 1984.
Pneumocystis carinii	Pneumocystosis, pneumonia	Classified as a fungus (from a protozon parasite) relatively recently. Usually seen in immunosuppressed persons and was originally the most frequent opportunistic infection seen in persons with HIV infection. Increased in incidence with HIV epidemic. Most common infection is seen in lungs causing pneumonia. Other sites are lymph nodes, adrenal glands, liver, eye, ear, thyroid, kidney, spleen, gastrointestinal sites, skin, mediastinum, and disseminated disease.

(continued)

TABLE A.2 *(continued)*

Organism	Major Disease(s)	Comments
Sporothrix schenckii	Sporotrichosis	A dimorphic fungus found in soil, sphagnum moss, and hay. Usually localized to skin, subcutaneous tissue, lymphocutaneous disease, especially in immunocompromised. May disseminate. Other forms include pulmonary, meningeal, and osteoarticular.
Trichosporon beigelii	See comments	A yeast infection that usually is invasive in the immunosuppressed, especially those with neutropenia. Usually enters through the respiratory or gastrointestinal tract or vascular catheters. May disseminate, causing cutaneous lesions, chorioretinitis, renal failure, cellulitis, meningitis, endocarditis, hepatic disease, and peritonitis. High mortality rate.

[1]Most are emerging due to a greater prevalence of persons with altered host immunity.
Sources: Cooper & McGinnis, 1997; Kauffman, Hajjeh, Chapman, for the Mycoses Study Group, 2000; Mandell, Bennett, & Dolin, 2000; Minari, Hachem, & Raad, 2001; Robinson, 1999; Sirisanthana, 2001; Strickland, 2000; Walsh, 1998.

TABLE A.3 Selected Emerging/Reemerging Parasites

Parasite	Disease	Comments
Babesia microti and spp (WA1, CA1, MO1)	Babesiosis	Usually a tick-borne disease. Some cases can result from blood transfusion. Manifestations can include fever, chills, malaise, headache, myalgia, abdominal pain, mild hepatosplenomegaly, and depression. Complications can include renal failure, adult respiratory distress syndrome, myocardial infarction. Can range from asymptomatic to severe disease especially in the elderly or immunocompromised. See chapter 14.
Brachiola vesicularum	Microsporidiosis	Described in 1998. Can cause myositis especially in those with HIV infection.
Cryptosporidum parvum	Cryptosporidiosis	Causes diarrhea and gastrointestinal illness. Usually results from contaminated water ingestion, but can be foodborne. Contamination of water supplies or crops can result from leaking septic tanks or runoff from manure in fields after heavy rain. Largest outbreak of about 403,000 was in Milwaukee in 1993. See chapter 5.
Cyclospora cayetanensis	Cyclosporiasis	A coccidian protozoan first recognized to infect humans in Papua New Guinea. Manifestations include diarrhea, bloating, abdominal pain, fatigue, fever, and weight loss. Outbreaks have been recognized in the U.S. since the late 1990s. Guatemalan raspberries, mesclun lettuce, and basil have been identified as vehicles in various outbreaks. See chapter 6.

(continued)

TABLE A.3 *(continued)*

Parasite	Disease	Comments
Echinococcus multilocularis	Alveolar hydatid disease	A heminth. In Canada, U.S.-Canadian border, central Europe, and Siberia. Imported red foxes from these areas to southeast U.S. may be infected. Potential for establishing endemic foci there. Maintained in foxes, but wolves, coyotes, cats, and dogs are also final hosts. Intermediate hosts include mice, voles, and lemmings.
Encephalitozoon cuniculi	Microsporidiosis	Hepatitis, disseminated disease. Renal insufficiency and cough may follow infection. In the immunocompetent, seizures have been described.
Encephalitozoon hellum	Usually disseminated infection	Described in humans in 1991. May cause keratoconjunctivitis in persons with AIDS.
Encephalitozoon intestinalis	Enteritis, disseminated infection	Not usually seen in non-HIV-infected persons. First identified in persons with AIDS in 1993. Causes chronic diarrhea. Formerly called *Septata intestinalis*. May cause cholangitis in persons with AIDS. See chapter 3.
Enterocytozoon bienusi	Enteritis, biliary tract disease	First identified in a person with HIV in 1985. Usually limited to gastrointestinal tract. Can cause diarrhea and cholangitis. Possibility of potential of waterborne transmission. May cause cholangitis in persons with AIDS. Rarely causes respiratory infection. Can infect immunocompetent persons. See chapter 3.

TABLE A.3 *(continued)*

Parasite	Disease	Comments
Gnathostomosis spinigerum and other species	See comments	This nematode has had a high prevalence in southeast Asia and is now emerging in South America and Mexico, especially Acapulco. Humans acquire infection from eating raw or undercooked fish containing larvae in their muscles especially in the form of sashimi or ceviche. In humans, swelling occurs in skin, subcutaneous tissue, and certain organs, which is caused by larvae migration. Within 24–48 hours of ingestion may see fever, malaise, nausea, vomiting, diarrhea, and pain.
Leishmania spp, especially *L. donovani*	Leishmaniasis	Usually transmitted by sandflies. Endemic in many areas. Has expanded in range and increased in frequency with deforestation in Latin America. Has increased in fox and pet dog population. Coffee growing facilitates development of parasites in vectors. Outbreak in southern Sudan due to ecological changes favoring sandflies and waves of nonimmune immigrants.
Metorchis conjunctus	Liver disease	A helminth considered to have emerged in 1993. The long-term oncogenic potential is unknown. An outbreak occurred in Montreal from eating contaminated sashimi at a picnic.
Nosema connori	See comments	A microsporidia first associated with disease in 1973. Can cause disseminated disease in non-HIV-infected persons.
Nosema ocularum	Keratitis	A microsporidia. Can cause keratitis in non-HIV-infected persons.

(continued)

TABLE A.3 *(continued)*

Parasite	Disease	Comments
Pleistophora spp	Myositis	A microsporidia. Can cause myositis in persons with and without AIDS. Little known about epidemiology.
Taenia solium	Neurocystericosis	Becoming the most important parasitic nervous system infection and a cause of epilepsy. Endemic in South America, Africa, and most of Asia. Seen more frequently in Europe, North America, and Australia because of immigration of infected persons and tourism. Increasing numbers of cases have been seen in the U.S. since the 1970s, and the majority are in persons from Mexico or Central America. In one instance in the early 1990s a cluster of cases among orthodox Jews in the U.S. were traced to infected domestic workers from Central America.
Trachipleistophora hominis	Microsporidiosis	Associated with myositis, keratoconjunctivitis, disseminated disease, and sinusitis usually in those with AIDS. Identified in 1996.
Trypanosoma cruzi	Chagas' disease (American trypanosomiasis)	Acute disease is relatively rare in the U.S., with most cases occurring in Texas. However, the number of people with chronic infections is about 100,000 due to immigration, thus posing a potential risk to the blood supply where there is a high concentration of immigrants from endemic areas.
Vittaforma corneae	See comments	A microsporidia first associated with disease in 1973. Can cause disseminated disease in persons with HIV disease. Can cause keratitis in the immunocompetent and urinary tract infection.

Sources: Didier, 1998; Framm & Soave, 1997; Franzen & Müller, 2001; Guerrant, Walker, & Weller, 1999; MacLean, 1998; Rojas-Molina, Pedraza-Sanchez, Torres-Bibiano, Meza-Martinez, & Escobar-Gutierrez, 1999; Strickland, 2000; White, 2000.

TABLE A.4 Selected Emerging/Reemerging Viruses

Virus	Major Disease Association	Comments
Australian bat lyssavirus	Encephalitis	Virus identified in 1996 in a black flying fox (a bat species) in Australia. Carried by bats. Causes a rabies-like disease. First known human case was in a woman in 1996 who died.
Barmah Forest virus	See comments	Confined to Australia currently. Isolated from mosquitoes in southeast Australia in 1974. Reported as infecting humans in 1986. Symptoms include arthralgia, myalgia, fever, rash, lethargy that can last 6 months. Outbreak in 1993–1994.
Enterovirus 71 (EV71)	Encephalomyelitis	Isolated as cause of encephalitis in 1969. In 1997 and 1998 caused neurovirulent outbreaks in Asia. Other outbreaks occurred later.
Hantaviruses		
Andes virus	Hantavirus pulmonary syndrome (HPS)	Found in Argentina and Chile. Primary reservoir is *Oligoryzomys longicaudatus* rodent. First seen in 1993.
Bayou virus	HPS	Found in southeastern U.S. Reservoir is *Oryzomys palustris* (the rice rat). Renal disease and myositis prominent. Cases have occurred in Louisiana and Texas.
Black Creek Canal virus	HPS	Reservoir is *Sigmodon hispidus* (cotton rat). Found in southeastern U.S. First identified in 1993 in Florida. Renal failure also seen. Myositis can be prominent.

(continued)

TABLE A.4 *(continued)*

Virus	Major Disease Association	Comments
Choclo virus	HPS	Reported from Panama. Outbreak in 1999–2000. Reservoir is *Oligoryzomys fulvescenes* rodent.
Hantaan virus	Hemorrhagic fever with renal syndrome (HFRS)	A bunyavirus. Most cases in Korea, China, and Japan. Abrupt onset with fever, chills, flushed face and torso, weakness, headache, myalgia, nausea, and vomiting. Hypotension or shock occurs on about day 5 followed by oliguria. Some patients get hemorrhagic manifestations such as epistaxis and subconjunctival hemorrhage. May have fluid, electrolyte, and central nervous system abnormalities. A diuretic phase then occurs about 2 weeks after onset and convalescence may be associated with polyuria. Mortality is 5%–15%.
HV39694 virus	HPS	Found in Argentina. Primary reservoir is unknown.
Juqutiba virus	HPS	Found in Brazil. Primary reservoir is unknown. First recognized in 1993.
Laguna Negra virus	HPS	Found in Paraguay and Bolivia. Primary reservoir is *Calomys laucha*. First seen in 1995.
Lechiguanas virus	HPS	Found in Argentina. First noted in 1988.
Monongahela virus	HPS	Found in eastern U.S. Primary reservoir is rodent, *Peromyscus maniculatus*.

TABLE A.4 *(continued)*

Virus	Major Disease Association	Comments
New York virus	HPS	Found in eastern U.S. Primary reservoir is *Peromyscus leucopus* (white footed mouse).
Oran virus	HPS	Found in Argentina. Primary reservoir is *Oligoryzomys longicaudatus*. First seen in 1984.
Puumala virus	Nephropathia epidemica/HFRS	Symptoms include fever, abdominal pain, renal dysfunction. Major reservoir is bank vole. Endemic in northern two thirds of Sweden. May be associated with Guillain-Barré syndrome. Mildest of the old-world hantaviruses under HFRS rubric.
Sin Nombre virus	HPS	See chapter 10. Recognized in 1993 after a cluster of persons with acute respiratory syndrome occurred in the southwestern U.S. Mice are reservoirs.
Hemorrhagic fever viruses		
Crimean-Congo hemorrhagic fever virus	Crimean-Congo hemorrhagic fever virus	Bunyavirus. Hard ticks are vectors and reservoir. Isolated in 1967.
Junin virus	Argentine hemorrhagic fever	Main reservoir is corn mouse. Arenavirus. Agent isolated in 1958.
Ebola virus	Ebola hemorrhagic fever	See chapter 8. Identified in 1976 with outbreaks in Zaire. Reservoir unknown. A filovirus.
Guanarito virus	Venezuelan hemorrhagic fever	Main host is cane mouse. Incubation period is 1–2 weeks. Recognized in 1989. An arenavirus.

(continued)

TABLE A.4 *(continued)*

Virus	Major Disease Association	Comments
Lassa virus	Lassa hemorrhagic fever	Virus first isolated from a patient in west Africa in 1969. An arenavirus. Transmitted to humans via a common rodent, contact with infected human secretions, and through contaminated needles in hospitals. Fever, weakness, malaise, joint pain, headache, sore throat, cough. Bleeding occurs in about 20%. Incubation period about 18 days. Ribavirin used in treatment. See chapter 8.
Machupo virus	Bolivian hemorrhagic fever	Large outbreak in 1964. Exposure through bush mice via food, water, direct contact. Fever, myalgia, petechiae, thrombocytopenia. Most often seen in agricultural workers in spring and summer.
Marburg virus	Marburg hemorrhagic fever	A filovirus first isolated in 1967 during an outbreak occurring among laboratory workers, medical personnel, and their families. Other outbreaks have been described in Zimbabwe and Kenya. See chapter 8.
Sabiá virus	Brazilian hemorrhagic fever	Isolated from a human case in 1990. An arenavirus. Little known to date.
Hendra virus (HEV) (formerly called equine morbillivirus)	Encephalitis, respiratory disease	First recognized in Australia in 1995. Reservoir is a type of fruit bat. See chapter 3. Humans apparently infected from contact with horses who had been infected by the bats.

TABLE A.4 *(continued)*

Virus	Major Disease Association	Comments
Hepatitis C virus	Hepatitis C	A flavivirus known to exist since the early 1970s but identified in 1988. Incubation period is 15–150 days. Can cause chronic hepatitis leading to cirrhosis. Many who develop disease are asymptomatic. The disease progresses slowly and insidiously and many do not know they are infected. See chapter 11.
Hepatitis D virus	See comments	Discovered in 1977, and recognized as causing infection in 1981 in Venezuela. The hepatitis delta virus is a RNA virus and infection with it usually depends on co-infection with hepatitis B. Can cause chronic hepatitis. Transmission is bloodborne and percutaneous with permucosal routes possible. Incubation period is 15–150 days.
Hepatitis E virus	Hepatitis E	A calicivirus detected in a patient with non A non B hepatitis in 1983. May not be new but was not differentiated from hepatitis A and B by previous techniques. Virus characterized in 1990. Believed to be responsible for large epidemics in developing countries, especially in Asia. Fecal-oral route is predominant transmission. Water contaminated by fecal matter is believed to be a primary source of infection.

(continued)

TABLE A.4 *(continued)*

Virus	Major Disease Association	Comments
Hepatitis G virus (GBV-C/HGV)	Suspected of causing some cases of hepatitis	A bloodborne RNA flavivirus with worldwide distribution but varying prevalence. Its role in causing hepatitis is uncertain but it is more prevalent in persons with hepatitis than the general population. Discovered in 1995.
Human herpesvirus 6 (HHV-6)	Exanthem subitum (roseola); see comments	Isolated in 1986 from persons with HIV and lymphoproliferative disorders. Believed to cause central nervous system complications in liver transplant recipients. Was a predictor of invasive fungal infections and was associated with late mortality. Infects most children by 2 years of age.
Human herpesvirus 7 (HHV-7)	Exanthem subitum (roseola)	Causes roseola and has been implicated in central nervous system complications but other disease associations unknown. Infects most children by 3 years of age.
Human herpesvirus 8 (HHV-8)	Kaposi's sarcoma (KS)	See chapter 8. Identified first in 1994. Found in KS lesions of HIV-infected person. Associated also with interstitial pneumonitis, encephalitis, hepatitis, and febrile illness.
Human immunodeficiency virus 1 (HIV-1)	HIV disease/AIDS	A retrovirus first identified in a group of homosexual men in 1981. Results in severe immunodeficiency and alterations leading to various opportunistic infections and neoplasms. See chapter 12.

TABLE A.4 *(continued)*

Virus	Major Disease Association	Comments
Human immunodeficiency virus 2 (HIV-2)	HIV disease/AIDS	Identified in 1985. Is largely confined to west Africa. Appears to cause milder disease than HIV-1, and to be somewhat less easily transmitted. See chapter 12.
Human papilloma virus	Genital warts, anal warts, cervical neoplasia; see comments	Was not realized as an etiologic agent of these conditions until 1980s. Closely associated with cervical intraepithelial neoplasia. Also causes anal and genital warts. Many types; HPV 16 is most important oncogenic type.
Human-T-lymphotropic virus-I (HTLV-I)	HTLV-I-associated myelopathy/tropical spastic paraparesis and adult T-cell leukemia/lymphoma (ATL)	Discovered in 1980, after ATL was characterized. A human retrovirus. See chapter 21. Has also been linked with uveitis and arthritis. Has worldwide distribution and is endemic in certain locales.
Human-T-lymphotropic virus-II (HTLV-II)	Adult hairy cell leukemia	A human retrovirus. See chapter 21.
LaCrosse encephalitis virus	California-LaCrosse encephalitis	*Aedes* mosquitos are reservoir and host. First isolated in 1964. Occurs primarily in children.

(continued)

TABLE A.4 *(continued)*

Virus	Major Disease Association	Comments
Nipah virus	Encephalitis	A paramyxovirus. Can cause encephalitis. Symptoms include fever, headache, dizziness, vomiting, reduced level of consciousness, seizures, focal neurologic signs such as nystagmus, absent or reduced reflexes, tachycardia, abnormal pupils, hypertension, segmental myoclonus, ptosis, thrombocytopenia, coma. In 1998 over 200 residents of a pig farming community in Malaysia were infected. Human-to-human transmission not known. High fatality rate of about 39%. Incubation period 1–3 weeks. Abbattoir workers in Singapore experienced an outbreak in 1999. Bats may be a reservoir. Related to Hendra virus.
Norwalk virus	Gastroenteritis	First associated in 1972 with material obtained from a 1968 outbreak of gastroenteritis in Norwalk, OH. Causes abrupt onset diarrhea, nausea, and vomiting with occasional additional symptoms. A strain of small round structured virus (SRSV) called calciviruses. Transmitted by fecally contaminated food and water, aerosolization, and person-to-person contact. Incubation period is 24–48 hours. Usually mild.

TABLE A.4 *(continued)*

Virus	Major Disease Association	Comments
O'nyong-nyong virus	O'nyong-nyong fever	A mosquito-borne alphavirus in the Togaviridae family, initially isolated during an epidemic in Uganda in 1959 affecting more than 2 million people. Another major outbreak occurred in 1996–1997. In the latter outbreak, the virus showed a genetic difference from the earlier outbreak. Signs/ symptoms include arthralgia, generalized skin rash, lymphadenopathy, fever. Usually nonfatal.
Oropouche virus	Oropouche fever	The virus was first isolated in 1955 in Trinidad from a febrile forest worker. The vector is the biting midge and/or mosquitos. Characterized by fever, headache, ocular pain, myalgia, and arthralgia.
Rift Valley fever virus	Rift Valley fever	While a few early human cases were recognized, the first large human epidemic was in Egypt in 1977–1978 involving about 200,000 cases and about 600 deaths. In humans signs/ symptoms range from flu-like syndrome to hemorrhagic fever, encephalitis, and/or retinitis. East African epidemic took place in 1997–1998 involving Kenya and Somalia. Is usually a zoonosis affecting sheep and cattle. Transmitted by mosquitos, aerosol, and contact.

(continued)

TABLE A.4 *(continued)*

Virus	Major Disease Association	Comments
Rocio virus	Encephalitis	A flavivirus detected during an encephalitis outbreak in Brazil in 1975–1976. Transmitted by mosquitos.
Rotavirus	Diarrheal illness	Rotavirus belonging to the *Reoviridiae* family and identified in 1973 in children with diarrhea in Australia. Worldwide distribution. Infection can be asymptomatic or cause mild to severe diarrheal disease. Incubation usually less than 48 hours with abrupt onset of vomiting, watery diarrhea, with or without low grade fever. Most cases resolve but in developing countries may be cause of mortality in children under 2 years.
SEN-V	May be associated with non-A-E hepatitis	Transmitted via transfusion but has not yet been proven to be associated with hepatitis.
Small round structured viruses	Gastrointestinal disease	Example is Norwalk strain. Visualized in 1972 in material from a gastroenteritis outbreak in a school in Norwalk, OH in 1968. Short incubation period. Classified as calicivirus. Usually mild disease.

TABLE A.4 *(continued)*

Virus	Major Disease Association	Comments
TT Virus (TTV)	Unknown at present	Small DNA virus identified in Japan in 1997, and named for patient, TT. May be transmissible by oral-fecal route and transfusion (not established). Possibly transfusion-hepatitis transmitted.
Venezuelan equine encephalitis virus (VEE)	Encephalitis	VEE virus characterized in 1930s. No outbreaks reported from 1973–1992. Large outbreak in 1995 in Venezuela and Colombia affecting humans and horses. Transmitted to humans via mosquitos. Usually mild infection with headache, chills, fever, myalgia, nausea, and vomiting.
West Nile virus	West Nile fever	Mosquito-borne flavivirus. Most infections are mild but can cause encephalitis. Outbreak in New York City in 1999. See chapter 20.
Whitewater Arroyo virus	Hemorrhagic fever	An arenavirus carried by wood rats and probably transmitted through exposure to rat urine, often by aerosol. First found in 1996 in western U.S. Associated with human deaths in 1999 and 2000.

Sources: Ali et al., 2001; Allain et al., 2000; Chew et al., 2000; Dewhurst, Skrincosky, & van Loon, 1997; De Souza Lopes, Coimbra, de Abrer Sacchetta, & Calisher, 1978; Durham & Lashley, 2000; Guerranta, Walker, & Weller, 1999; Laver & Walker, 2001; Mackenzie et al., 2001; Strickland, 2000; Vincent et al., 2000.

REFERENCES

Ali, R., Mounts, A. W., Parashar, U. D., Sahani, M., Lye, M. S., Isa, M. M., et al. (2001). Nipah virus infection among military personnel involved in pig culling during an outbreak of encephalitis in Malaysia, 1998–1999. *Emerging Infectious Diseases, 7,* 759–761.

Allain, J. P. (2000). Emerging viruses in blood transfusion. *Vox Sanguinis, 78*(Suppl. 2), 243–248.

Buller, R. S., Arens, M., Hmiel, S. P., Paddock, C. D., Sumner, J. W., & Rikihisa, Y. (1999). *Ehrlichia ewingii,* a newly recognized agent of human ehrlichiosis. *New England Journal of Medicine, 341,* 148–155.

Centers for Disease Control and Prevention. (2000). Update: *Clostridium novyi* and unexplained illness among injecting-drug users—Scotland, Ireland and England, April–June 2000. *Morbidity and Mortality Weekly Report, 49,* 201–205.

Chew, M. H. L., Arguin, P. M., Shay, D. K., Goh, K., Rollin, P. E., Shieh, W., et al. (2000). Risk factors for Nipah virus infection among abattoir workers in Singapore. *Journal of Infectious Diseases, 181,* 1760–1763.

Cooper, C. R., & McGinnis, M. R. (1997). Pathology of *Penicillium marneffei. Archives of Pathology and Laboratory Medicine, 121,* 798–804.

Dance, D. A. (2000). Melioidosis as an emerging global problem. *Acta Tropica, 5,* 115–119.

De Souza Lopes, O., Coimbra, T. L., de Abreu Sacchetta, L., & Calisher, C. H. (1978). Emergence of a new arbovirus disease in Brazil, I. Isolation and characterization of the etiologic agent, Rocio virus. *American Journal of Epidemiology, 107,* 444–449.

Dewhurst, S., Skrincosky, D., & van Loon, N. (1997, November 5). Human herpesvirus 6 (HHV-6). *Expert Reviews in Molecular Medicine* [On-line]. Available: http://www.ermm.cbcu.cam.ac.uk/sdr/txt001sdr.htm

Didier, E. (1998). Microsporidiosis. *Clinical Infectious Diseases, 27,* 1–8.

Dobos, K. M., Quinn, F. D., Ashford, D. A., Horsbaugh, C. R., & King, H. C. (1999). Emergence of a unique group of necrotizing mycobacterial diseases. *Emerging Infectious Diseases, 5,* 367–378.

Durham, J. D., & Lashley, F. R. (Eds.). (2000). *The person with HIV/AIDS: Nursing perspectives* (3rd ed.). New York: Springer Publishing Co.

Field, H., Young, P., Yob, J. M., Mills, J., Hall, L., & Mackenzie, J. (2001). The natural history of Hendra and Nipah viruses. *Microbes and Infection, 3,* 307–314.

Framm, S. R., & Soave, R. (1997). Agents of diarrhea. *Medical Clinics of North America, 81,* 427–447.

Franzen, C., & Müller, A. (2001). Microsporidiosis: Human diseases and diagnosis. *Microbes and Infection, 3,* 389–400.

French, A. L., Benator, D. A., & Gordin, F. M. (1997). Nontuberculous mycobacterial infections. *Medical Clinics of North America, 81,* 361–379.

Guerrant, R. L., Walker, D. H., & Weller, P. F. (Eds.). (1999). *Tropical infectious diseases.* Philadelphia: Churchill Livingstone.

Hsueh, P-R., Teng, L-J., Lee, L-N., Yu, C-J., Yang, P-C., Ho, S-W., & Luh, K-T. (2001). Melioidosis: An emerging infection in Taiwan? *Emerging Infectious Diseases, 7,* 428–433.

IARC Working Group on the Evaluation of Carcinogenic Risks to Humans. (1994). *Schistosomes, liver flukes and Helicobacter pylori: Views and expert opinions of an IARC Working Group on the Evaluation of Carcinogenic Risks in Humans* (Monograph 61). Lyon, France: International Agency for Research on Cancer.

Juranek, D. D. (2000). Cryptosporidiosis. In G. T. Strickland (Ed.), *Hunter's tropical medicine and emerging infectious diseases* (pp. 594–600). Philadelphia: WB Saunders Co.

Kauffman, C. A., Hajjeh, R., & Chapman, S. W., for the Mycoses Study Group. (2000). Practice guidelines for the management of patients with *Sporotrichosis. Clinical Infectious Diseases, 30,* 684–687.

Koehler, J. E. (1998). *Bartonella*: An emerging human pathogen. In W. M. Scheld, D. Armstrong, & J. M. Hughes (Eds.), *Emerging infections 1* (pp. 147–163). Washington, DC: ASM Press.

Lehane, L., & Rawlin, G. T. (2000). Topically acquired bacterial zoonoses from fish: A review. *Medical Journal of Australia, 173,* 256–259.

Levett, P. N. (2001). Leptospirosis. *Clinical Microbiology Reviews, 14,* 296–326.

Lauer, G. M., & Walker, B. D. (2001). Hepatitis C virus infection. *New England Journal of Medicine, 345,* 41–52.

Lindsay, M. D. A., Johansen, C. A., Broom, A. K., Smith, D. W., & Mackenzie, J. S. (1995). Emergence of Barmah Forest virus in Western Australia. *Emerging Infectious Diseases, 1,* 22–26.

Lyssavirus, Bat—Australia. (1999, August 13). *ProMED Digest, 99*(195), unpaginated.

Mackenzie, J. S., Chua, K. B., Daniels, P. W., Eaton, B. T., Field, H. E., Hall, R. A., et al. (2001). Emerging viral diseases of southeast Asia and the western Pacific. *Emerging Infectious Diseases, 7*(No. 3, Suppl.), 497–504.

MacLean, J. D. (1998). The north american liver fluke, *Metorchis conjunctus.* In W. M. Scheld, W. A. Craig, & J. M. Hughes (Eds.), *Emerging Infections 2* (pp. 243–256). Washington, DC: ASM Press.

Maguiña, C., & Gotuzzo, E. (2000). Bartonellosis. New and old. *Infectious Disease Clinics of North America, 14,* 1–22.

Mandell, G. L., Bennett, J. E., & Dolin, R. (Eds.). (2000). *Mandell, Douglas, and Bennett's principles and practice of infectious diseases* (5th ed.). Philadelphia: Churchill Livingstone.

McJunkin, J. E., Khan, R. R., & Tsai, T. F. (1998). California—La Crosse encephalitis. *Infectious Disease Clinics of North America, 12,* 83–91.

Minari, A., Hachem, R., & Raad, I. (2001). *Candida lusitaniae*: A cause of breakthrough fungemia in cancer patients. *Clinical Infectious Diseases, 32,* 186–190.

NIPAH Virus—Malasia: Official report. (1999, June 6). *ProMED Digest, 99*(134), unpaginated.

Pechère, M., Opravil, M., Wald, A., Chave, J. P., Bessesen, M., Sievers, A., et al. (1995). Clinical and epidemiologic features of infection with *Mycobacterium genavense.* Swiss HIV Cohort Study. *Archives of Internal Medicine, 155,* 400–404.

Pretorius, A-M., & Kelly, P. J. (2000). An update on human bartonelloses. *Central African Journal of Medicine, 46,* 194–200.

Robinson, L. A. (1999). Aspergillus and other fungi. *Chest Surgery Clinics of North America, 9,* 193–225.
Rojas-Molina, N., Pedraza-Sanchez, S., Torres-Bibiano, B., Meza-Martinez, H., & Escobar-Gutierrez, A. (1999). Gnathostomosis, an emerging foodborne zoonotic disease in Acapulco, Mexico. *Emerging Infectious Diseases, 5,* 264–266.
Sirisanthana, T. (2001). *Penicillium marneffei* infection in patients with AIDS. *Emerging Infectious Diseases,* 7(No. 3 Suppl.), 561.
Steere, A. C. (2001). Lyme disease. *New England Journal of Medicine, 345,* 115–124.
Stevens, D. L. (2001). Invasive streptococcal infections. *Journal of Infection and Chemotherapy,* 7, 69–80.
Strickland, G. T. (Ed.). (2000). *Hunter's tropical medicine and emerging infectious diseases* (8th ed.). Philadelphia: WB Saunders Co.
Terkeltaub, R. A. (2000). Lyme disease 2000. Emerging zoonoses complicate patient work-up and treatment. *Geriatrics, 44*(7), 34–47.
Thompson, G. K. (1999). Veterinary surgeon's guide to Australian bat lyssavirus. *American Veterinary Journal,* 77, 710–712.
Vincent, M. J., Quiroz, E., Gracia, F., Sanchez, A. J., Ksiazek, T. G., Kitsutani, P. T., et al. (2000). Hantavirus pulmonary syndrome in Panama: Identification of novel hantaviruses and their likely reservoirs. *Virology,* 277, 14–19.
Walsh, T. J. (1998). Emerging fungal pathogens: Evolving challenges to immunocompromised patients. In W. M. Scheld, D. Armstrong, & J. M. Hughes (Eds.), *Emerging infections 1* (pp. 221–232). Washington, DC: ASM Press.
White, A. C., Jr. (2000). Neurocysticercosis: Updates on epidemiology, pathogenesis, diagnosis and management. *Annual Review of Medicine, 51,* 187–206.
Yañez, A., Cedillo, L., Neyrolles, O., Alonso, E., Prévost, M. C., Rojas, J., et al. (1999). *Mycoplasma penetrans* bacteremia and primary antiphospholipid syndrome. *Emerging Infectious Diseases,* 5, 164–167.
Zaki, S. R., & Spiegel, R. A. (1998). Leptospirosis. In A. M. Nelson & C. R. Horsburgh, Jr. (Eds.), *Pathology of emerging infections II* (pp. 73–92). Washington, DC: American Society for Microbiology.

Appendix B

Emerging/Reemerging Diseases by Modes of Transmission

Felissa R. Lashley

TABLE B.1 Selected Emerging/Reemerging Foodborne and Waterborne Pathogens

Organism	Comments
Parasitic	
Cryptosporidium parvum	A waterborne emerging pathogen implicated in major outbreaks involving both contaminated drinking and recreational water. Causes diarrhea and gastrointestinal illness. See chapter 5.
Cyclospora cayetanensis	Responsible for large multistate and Canadian outbreaks in 1997 and 1998 due to contaminated Guatemalan raspberries, mesclun lettuce and basil. Causes gastrointestinal illness. See chapter 6.
Gnathostomosis spinigerum and other species	This nematode has had a high prevalence in Southeast Asia and is now emerging in South America and Mexico, especially Acapulco. Humans acquire infection from eating raw or undercooked fish containing larvae in their muscles, especially in the form of sashimi or ceviche. In humans, swelling caused by larvae migration occurs in skin, subcutaneous tissue, and certain organs.

(continued)

TABLE B.1 *(continued)*

Organism	Comments
Metorchis conjunctus	A helminth considered to have emerged in 1993. The long-term oncogenic potential is unknown. An outbreak occurred in Montreal from eating contaminated sashimi at a picnic.
Bacterial	
Campylobacter jejuni	A zoonotic infection. Became recognized as a human pathogen in the 1970s. Symptoms include fever, diarrhea (watery or bloody), and abdominal pain. Trigger for Guillain-Barré syndrome. See chapter 3.
Listeria monocytogenes	A gram-positive bacteria only recently considered as causing gastrointestinal disease, diarrhea, nausea, vomiting, and abdominal cramps, often with fever. Most cases of listeriosis occur in immunocompromised persons, the elderly, or pregnant women. Typical illness manifestations are flu-like symptoms, sepsis, or central nervous system illness. Frequently contaminated foods include deli meats, soft cheeses. See chapter 3.
Salmonella Enteriditis	A 41-state outbreak occurred in 1995 from ice cream prepared from a premix hauled in tanker trucks previously hauling raw eggs. Raw or undercooked eggs or poultry are frequent vehicles for infection. Causes gastroenteritis. See chapter 3.
Vibrio cholerae	Cholera is an old disease causing severe diarrheal illness, but the seventh cholera pandemic began in Indonesia in 1961 caused by the *V. cholerae* O1 serogroup, El Tor biotype. The organism is curved, gram-negative. In 1992, *V. cholerae* O139 was identified in India. Epidemic cholera appeared in Latin America in 1991 after nearly 100 years of absence. Characterized by "rice water" diarrheal stools. See chapter 4.

TABLE B.1 *(continued)*

Organism	Comments
Vibrio parahaemolyticus	Rare outbreaks before 1997. In 1998, the first outbreak of serotype O3: K6 occurred in the U.S. In this 416 persons developed gastroenteritis from eating oysters from Galveston Bay in Texas.
Vibrio vulnificus	Emergence reported in 1979. Infections usually result from consumption of shellfish, especially raw oysters from the Gulf of Mexico. An increase is seen in the summer. Infection can result in septicemia with bulbous skin lesions, shock, and rapid death. Persons with iron overload such as hemochromatosis are especially vulnerable.
Yersinia enterocolitica	Increasingly recognized as a source of gastroentenitis, sometimes with rectal bleeding and ileal perforation. Symptoms often suggest mesenteric adenitis or appendicitis. Serogroup O:3 is becoming more frequent. Hogs are an important reservoir, and eating pork is a risk factor for infection. Infants have acquired yersiniosis after transfer of the organism from the hands of caretakers who previously prepared chitterlings (pork intestines).
Viral	
Hepatitis A virus	While not an EID, a new vehicle for infection was identified. Frozen strawberries contaminated at a processing company in California and served in USDA-sponsored school lunch programs in several states in 1997 resulted in cases of hepatitis A in children in 2 states. Infection is by fecal-oral route.

(continued)

TABLE B.1 *(continued)*

Organism	Comments
Norwalk-like viruses	Gastroenteritis, for example, from eating contaminated raw oysters resulted from oyster gatherers who used toilets without holding tanks on their boats. Reports of outbreaks also from contaminated delicatessen meats, fresh produce items, and frozen raspberries. Belong to the small round structured viruses. Norwalk virus first visualized in 1972.

Sources: Atmar & Estes, 2001; Centers for Disease Control and Prevention, 2001a, 2001b; Franzen & Müller, 2001; MacLean, 1998; Prier & Solnick, 2000; Rojas-Molina, Pedraza-Sanchez, Torres-Bibiano, Meza-Martinez, & Escobar-Gutierrez, 1999; Strickland, 2000; Weber & Rutala, 2001.

TABLE B.2 Selected Transfusion Transmissible Emerging/ Reemerging Infectious Agents

Agent	Disease	Comments
Viruses		
Hepatitis C virus	Hepatitis C	A flavivirus known to exist since the early 1970s but identified in 1988. Incubation period is 15–150 days. Can cause chronic hepatitis leading to cirrhosis. Many who develop disease are asymptomatic. The disease progresses slowly and insidiously and many do not know they are infected. See chapter 11.
Hepatitis G virus (GBV-C/HGV)	See comments	May cause some commonly acquired hepatitis but role remains uncertain. At this time not believed to cause severe liver disease.
Human immunodeficiency virus (HIV)	HIV disease/AIDS	A retrovirus first identified in a group of homosexual men in 1981 for type 1 and in 1985 in west Africa for type 2. Results in severe immunodeficiency and alterations leading to various opportunistic infections and neoplasms. See chapter 12.
Human T-lymphotropic virus-I (HTLV-I)	Adult T-cell leukemia/ lymphoma and HTLV-I-associated myelopathy/tropical spastic paresis	See text in chapter 21. Identified in 1980. Has also been linked with uveitis and arthritis. Has worldwide distribution and is endemic in certain locales.
HTLV-II	Adult hairy cell leukemia	See text in chapter 21. Isolated in 1982. A retrovirus that may also play a role in myelopathies. Endemic in certain Native American and Indian populations in Panama, Brazil, and central Africa.

(continued)

TABLE B.2 *(continued)*

Agent	Disease	Comments
Parvovirus B19	Erythema infectiosum	Identified in 1975. Transmissible only during short period of viremia. Difficult to screen for. Causes self-limited disease associated with mild rash or arthropathy. More chronic or severe manifestation in immunocompromised; severe aplastic crises in persons with anemia; fetal infections can cause fetal hydrops, fetal death. Has induced aplastic anemia in some transfusion recipients, and symptoms in persons with hemophilia who received contaminated clotting factor.
TT Virus	Unknown	May be associated with hepatitis.
Parasites		
Babesia microti and *Babesia* spp	Babesiosis	About 26 transfusion-transmitted cases reported in U.S. as of 1998 from diverse U.S. geographical areas including the northeast and the state of Washington. May be tick-borne. Symptoms include fever, chills, sweating, malaise, weakness, headache, and myalgia, as well as mild hepatosplenomegaly. See chapter 14.

TABLE B.2 *(continued)*

Agent	Disease	Comments
Leishmania donovani	Leishmaniasis	Usually transmitted by sandflies. Endemic in many areas. Has expanded in range and increased in frequency with deforestation in Latin America. Has increased in fox and pet dog population. Coffee growing facilitates development of parasites in vectors. Outbreak in southern Sudan due to ecological changes favoring sandflies and waves of nonimmune immigrants.
P. vivax, *P. falciparum*, *P. malariae* and others	Malaria	Prevention of transfusion-transmitted malaria depends on donor travel history—1 year deferral for those who traveled to area with endemic malaria and 3 years for those who lived in endemic area or have a history of malaria is used. About three cases of transfusion-transmitted malaria per year in U.S. See chapter 15.
Trypanosoma cruzi	Chagas' disease	Overall risk in U.S. is 1 per 42,000 units of donated blood. Acute infection leads to chronic lifelong disease. Six cases reported in U.S. from transfusions as of 1999.

(continued)

TABLE B.2 *(continued)*

Agent	Disease	Comments
Bacteria		
Borrelia burgdorferi	Lyme disease	Recognized in 1978 in Lyme, CT. Transmitted to humans via deer ticks. Can have severe chronic sequelae. Characterized by a skin lesion known as erythema migrans that appears in about 60% at the site of the tick bite. Other symptoms may include rash, malaise, headache, chills, fever, backache, arthralgia, and myalgia. Later effects may include arthritis and neurological and cardiac manifestations. See chapter 14.
Ehrlichia chaffeensis	Human monocytic ehrlichiosis (HME)	First identified in 1987 in Arkansas. Symptoms include fever, headache, chills, myalgia, arthralgia, and malaise, nausea, vomiting, diarrhea, and weight loss may develop later. A rash may develop in up to 30%. Complications can include renal symptoms, a toxic shock-like syndrome and multiorgan failure. The fatality rate may be as high as 5%. See chapter 14.
Ehrlichia equi or *Ehrlichia phagocytophila*	Human granulocytic ehrlichiosis	Similar to HME. Rash is less likely to occur. The case fatality rate may be as high as 10%. First recognized in 1992–1993. See chapter 14.

TABLE B.2 *(continued)*

Agent	Disease	Comments
Other		
Abnormal Prions	Creutzfeldt-Jakob disease	Iatrogenic disease has resulted from corneal transplant, EEG electrodes, and duramater grafts. No confirmed reports from blood or blood-related transfusion products but theoretical possibility exists. Agent causes fatal spongiform encephalopathy. See chapter 17.
Abnormal Prions	vCreutzfeldt-Jakob disease	Theoretical risk only at this time. Agent causes fatal spongiform encephalopathy. See chapter 17.

Sources: Allain, 1998; Allain, 2000; Bowden, 2001; Brown, 2000; Dodd, 1998, 2000; Durham & Lashley, 2000; Klein, 2000; Moor, Dubbelman, VanSteveninck, & Brand, 1999; Mungai, Tegtmeier, Chamberland, & Parise, 2001; Poovorawan, Tangkijvanich, Theamboonlers, & Hirsch, 2001.

TABLE B.3 Selected Emerging/Reemerging Vector-Borne Diseases

Disease	Organism	Vector	Clinical Manifestation(s)	Comments
Bacterial				
African tick-bite fever	*Rickettsia africae*	*Amblyomma* ticks	Headache, fever, eschar at bite site, regional lymphadenopathy.	Isolated in Zimbabwe in 1990. Also seen in Tanzania, South Africa, and Guadeloupe.
Astrakhan fever	Bacteria closely related to *Rickettsia conorii*	Tick	Eruptive febrile illness occurring in summers.	First observed in 1983; 1989 identification. Reservoir includes dogs. Found near Caspian Sea.
California flea rickettsiosis	*Rickettsia felis*	Flea	Fever, headache, with or without rash. Description is not yet fully known.	Seen in California, Texas, France, and Brazil.
Flinders Island spotted fever	*Rickettsia honei*	Tick	Rash, fever, enlarged lymph nodes. Eschar may be present.	Agent identified in 1992 in Tasmania. May be related to Queensland tick typhus.
Human ehrlichiosis	*Ehrlichia ewingii*	Ticks (including Lone Star tick)	Fever, chills, headaches, leukopenia, myalgia.	Described in Missouri in 1999. See chapter 14. Reservoir includes dogs.

TABLE B.3 *(continued)*

Disease	Organism	Vector	Clinical Manifestation(s)	Comments
Human granulocytic ehrlichiosis	Agent closely related to *Ehrlichia equi* or *Ehrlichia phagocytophila*	Ticks	Fever, chills, myalgia headache, malaise. Rash not usual. Ranges in severity. Case fatality rate can be 10%. See chapter 14.	See chapter 14. Described in 1992–1993.
Human monocytic ehrlichiosis	*Ehrlichia chaffeensis*	Ticks (Lone Star ticks and American dog ticks)	Fever, headache, chills, myalgia, malaise with nausea, vomiting, anorexia. Rash occurs in 20%–30%. Case fatality rate can be 5%. Multiorgan failure can occur.	See chapter 14. Described in 1987. Reservoir includes white-tailed deer.
Israeli spotted fever/ Israeli tick typhus	*Rickettsia conorii* variants	Ticks	Mild spotted fever.	Described in 1974. Occurs in Israel and near Caspian sea.
Japanese or Oriental spotted fever	*Rickettsia japonica*	Ticks	Rash, fever, chills. May be black necrotic lesion at bite site.	Recognized in Japan in 1984. Agent isolated in 1986. Reservoir includes mice and other rodents.

(continued)

TABLE B.3 *(continued)*

Disease	Organism	Vector	Clinical Manifestation(s)	Comments
Lyme disease	*Borrelia burgdorferi*	Ticks	Rash, fever, chills, malaise, myalgias. May evolve into chronic illness with neurological symptoms and arthritis.	See chapter 14. Reservoirs include deer, mice, and birds.
Marseilles tick-bite fever	*Rickettsia mongoloti monae*	Ticks	A spotted fever with rash, fever, and headache.	Identified in Mongolia and Marseilles, France. First found in 1996. Reservoirs include migratory birds.
Parasitic				
Babesiosis	*Babesia microti*	Ticks	Manifestations can include fever, chills, malaise, headache, myalgia, abdominal pain, mild hepatosplenomegaly, and depression. Complications can include renal failure, adult respiratory distress syndrome, myocardial	See chapter 14.

TABLE B.3 *(continued)*

Disease	Organism	Vector	Clinical Manifestation(s)	Comments
			infarction. Can range from asymptomatic to severe disease, especially in the elderly or the immunocompromised.	
Leishmaniasis	*Leishmania donovani*	Sand fleas	Malaise, fever, chills.	Causes illness in one-half million yearly. Possibly emerging in U.S. through pet dogs brought back from endemic areas abroad by military families, and now found in fox hounds in U.S.
Malaria	*Plasmodium vivax*, *Plasmodium falciparum*, *Plasmodium ovale*, *Plasmodium malariae*	Mosquitos (*Anopheles* spp)	Chills, fever, anemia. Severity depends on species. See chapter 15.	Drug resistance is becoming problematic. Locally acquired cases have been described in the U.S. in the mid 1980s and 1990s.

Sources: Buller, Arens, Hmiel, Paddock, Sumner, & Rikihisa, 1999; Enserink, 2000; Goddard, 1999; Nichols, 2000; Parola & Raoult, 2001; Raoult & Olson, 1999; Raoult, Fournier, et al., 2001; Raoult, La Sala, et al., 2001; Steere, 2001; Strickland, 2000.

REFERENCES

Allain, J. P. (1998). Emerging viruses in blood transfusion. *Vox Sanguinis, 74,* 125–129.

Allain, J. P. (2000). Emerging viruses in blood transfusion. *Vox Sanguinis, 78*(Suppl. 2), 243–248.

Atmar, R. L., & Estes, M. K. (2001). Diagnosis of noncultivatable gastroenteritis viruses, the human caliciviruses. *Clinical Microbiology Reviews, 14,* 15–37.

Bowden, S. (2001). New hepatitis viruses: contenders and pretenders. *Journal of Gastroenterology and Hepatology, 16,* 124–131.

Brown, P. (2000). The risk of blood-borne Creutzfeldt-Jakob disease. *Developments in Biological Standardization, 102,* 53–59.

Buller, R. S., Arens, M., Hmiel, S. P., Paddock, C. D., Sumner, J. W., & Rikihisa, Y. (1999). *Ehrlichia ewingii,* a newly recognized agent of human ehrlichiosis. *New England Journal of Medicine, 341,* 148–155.

Centers for Disease Control and Prevention. (2001a). Diagnosis and management of foodborne illnesses: A primer for physicians. *Morbidity & Mortality Weekly Report, 50,* 1–69.

Centers for Disease Control and Prevention. (2001b). "Norwalk-like viruses." Public health consequences and outbreak management. *Morbidity and Mortality Weekly Report, 50*(No. RR-9), 1–20.

Dodd, R. Y. (1998). Transmission of parasites by blood transfusion. *Vox Sanguinis, 74,* 161–163.

Dodd, R. Y. (2000). Transmission of parasites and bacteria by blood components. *Vox Sanguinis, 78*(Suppl. 2), 239–242.

Durham, J. D., & Lashley, F. R. (Eds.). (2000). *The person with HIV/AIDS: Nursing perspectives.* New York: Springer Publishing.

Enserink, M. (2000). Has leishmaniasis become endemic in the U.S.? *Science, 290,* 1181, 1183.

Franzen, C., & Müller, A. (2001). Microsporidiosis: Human diseases and diagnosis. *Microbes and Infection, 3,* 389–400.

Goddard, J. (1999). Arthropods, tongue worms, leeches, and arthropod-borne diseases. In R. L. Guerrant, D. H. Walker, & P. F. Weller (Eds.), *Tropical infectious diseases: Principles, pathogens, & practice* (pp. 1325–1342). Philadelphia: Churchill Livinstone.

Guerrant, R. L., Walker, D. H., & Weller, P. F. (Eds.). (1999). *Tropical infectious diseases.* Philadelphia: Churchill Livingstone.

Klein, H. G. (2000). Will blood transfusion ever be safe enough? *Journal of the American Medical Association, 284,* 238–240.

Lauer, G. M., & Walker, B. D. (2001). Hepatitis C virus infection. *New England Journal of Medicine, 345,* 41–52.

MacLean, J. D. (1998). The North American liver fluke, *Metorchis conjunctus.* In W. M. Scheld, W. A. Craig, & J. M. Hughes (Eds.), *Emerging infections II* (pp. 243–256). Washington, DC: ASM Press.

Moor, A. C., Dubbelman, T. M., VanSteveninck, J., & Brand, A. (1999). Transfusion-transmitted diseases: Risks, prevention and perspectives. *European Journal of Haematology, 62,* 1–18.

Mungai, M., Tegtmeier, G., Chamberland, M., & Parise, M. (2001). Transfusion-transmitted malaria in the United States from 1963 through 1999. *New England Journal of Medicine, 344*, 1973–1978.

Nichols, G. L. (2000). Food-borne protozoa. *British Medical Bulletin, 56*(1), 209–235.

Parola, P., & Raoult, D. (2001). Ticks and tickborne bacterial diseases in humans: An emerging infectious threat. *Clinical Infectious Diseases, 32*, 897–928.

Poovorawan, Y., Tangkijvanich, P., Theamboonlers, A., & Hirsch, P. (2001). Transfusion transmissible virus TTV and its putative role in the etiology of liver disease. *Hepatogastroenterology, 48*, 256–260.

Prier, R., & Solnick, J. V. (2000). Foodborne and waterborne infectious diseases. *Postgraduate Medicine, 107*, 245–255.

Raoult, D., Fournier, P. E., Fenollar, F., Jensenius, M., Prioe, T., de Pina, J. J., et al. (2001). *Rickettsia africae*, a tick-borne pathogen in travelers to sub-Saharan Africa. *New England Journal of Medicine, 344*, 1504–1510.

Raoult, D., La Scola, B., Enea, M., Fournier, P-E., Roux, V., Fenollar, F., et al. (2001). A flea-associated rickettsia pathogenic for humans. *Emerging Infectious Diseases, 7*, 73–81.

Rauolt, D., & Olson, J. G. (1999). Emerging rickettsioses. In W. M. Scheld, W. A. Craig, & J. M. Hughes (Eds.), *Emerging infections 3* (pp. 17–35). Washington, DC: ASM Press.

Rojas-Molina, N., Pedraza-Sanchez, S., Torres-Bibiano, B., Meza-Martinez, H., & Escobar-Gutierrez, A. (1999). Gnathostomosis, an emerging foodborne zoonotic disease in Acapulco, Mexico. *Emerging Infectious Diseases, 5*, 264–266.

Steere, A. C. (2001). Lyme disease. *New England Journal of Medicine, 345*, 115–124.

Strickland, G. T. (Ed.). (2000). *Hunter's tropical medicine and emerging infectious diseases* (8th ed.). Philadelphia: WB Saunders Co.

Weber, D. J., & Rutala, W. A. (2001). The emerging nosocomial pathogens *Cryptosporidium, Escherichia coli* O157:H7, *Helicobacter pylori*, and hepatitis C: Epidemiology, environmental survival, efficacy of disinfection, and control measures. *Infection Control and Hospital Epidemiology, 22*, 306–315.

Appendix C

Prevention of Emerging Infectious Diseases

Felissa R. Lashley

TABLE C.1 Prevention of Foodborne Illness[1]

- Avoid raw or undercooked meat and poultry. Use a thermometer to measure the internal temperature of meat. Meats should be cooked to an internal temperature of at least 160° F, and poultry to 170° F for turkey breast and 180° F for others. Fish should be opaque and firm; shellfish in shells should be cooked till the shells open.
- Eggs should be cooked until the yolk is firm. Avoid raw or undercooked eggs or foods containing raw or lightly cooked eggs, including certain salad dressings, cookie and cake batters, sauces, and beverages such as unpasteurized eggnog. If you use recipes in which eggs remain raw or only partially cooked, use pasteurized eggs.
- Avoid raw or undercooked fish or shellfish, including oysters, clams, mussels, and scallops. Properly cooked fish should be opaque and flake easily with a fork.
- Avoid raw or unpasteurized milk or cheeses.
- Avoid unpasteurized fruit or vegetable juices.
- When cooking in a microwave oven, make sure there are no cold spots where pathogens can survive.
- Bring sauces, soups, and gravy to a boil when reheating. Heat other leftovers thoroughly to at least 165° F.
- Avoid cross-contaminating foods by washing hands, utensils, counter tops, and cutting boards with hot soapy water after they have been in contact with food items and before going on to prepare the next food. If possible, use a different cutting board for raw meat, poultry, and seafood products.

(continued)

TABLE C.1 *(continued)*

- Rinse poultry before cooking.
- Wash hands with hot, soapy water before preparing and after handling food each time and after using the bathroom or touching a pet or changing a diaper.
- Put cooked meat on a clean platter, rather than back on one that held the raw meat. Use separate plates for cooked food and raw foods.
- Refrigerate leftovers promptly—do not leave at room temperature. Refrigerate or freeze perishables, prepared foods, and leftovers within 2 hours or sooner.
- Divide large amounts of leftovers into shallow containers for quick cooling in the refrigerator. Don't pack the refrigerator. Cool air must circulate to keep food safe.
- Avoid leaving cut produce at room temperature for many hours.
- Never defrost food at room temperature. Thaw food in the refrigerator, under cold running water, or in the microwave oven.
- Marinate foods in the refrigerator.
- Separate raw meat, poultry, and seafood from other foods in your grocery shopping cart and in your refrigerator.
- Rinse fresh fruits and vegetables in running tap water to remove visible dirt and grime. Do not use soap or detergents. If necessary, use a small vegetable brush to remove surface dirt. Also wash packaged salad mixes even if marked prewashed.
- Be careful not to contaminate foods while slicing them up on the cutting board.
- Avoid preparing food for others if you yourself have a diarrheal illness.
- Avoid eating food prepared from nonlicensed street vendors, particularly in developing countries.
- When eating out, eat in establishments with high ratings from the health department.
- In developing countries, avoid eating cut fresh fruits and vegetables, salads, and non-peelable fruit and vegetables. Hot foods should be served piping hot.
- Avoid eating food and organ parts from certain high-risk animals including rodents, bushmeat, squirrels, and game animals.

Special Added Prevention for Immunocompromised Persons

- Avoid soft cheeses, such as feta, brie, Camembert, blue-veined, and Mexican-style cheese.
- Avoid raw sprouts (alfalfa, clover, and radish).
- Reheat to hot some foods that are bought precooked, because they can become contaminated with pathogens after they have been processed and packaged. These foods include: hot dogs, luncheon meats (cold cuts), fermented and dry sausage, and other deli-style meat and poultry products.

- Additional preventive measures may be found in Centers for Disease Control and Prevention, 1999.

[1]Other preventive measures involving the ways in which foods are grown, harvested, stored, prepared, served, packaged, and transported are not covered here.

Sources: Centers for Disease Control and Prevention, 1999, 2001a; Strickland, 2000; USPHS/IDSA, 1999, 2001.

TABLE C.2 Measures to Prevent Waterborne Infection

- Safe storage of treated water.
- In developing countries, avoid drinking tap water or using ice made from tap water.
- Proper treatment of potable water.
- Keep cattle and other such animals away from surface water such as rivers or ponds that serve community drinking systems.
- Locate human waste disposal systems such as latrines in areas where they will not contaminate the water supply by either underground seepage or runoff.
- Wash all fruits and vegetables thoroughly in safe water.
- Proper hand washing.
- Avoid drinking water directly from lakes, rivers, ponds, or streams.
- In developing countries avoid swallowing water while showering; use safe water for brushing teeth.
- Waterborne infection might also result from swallowing water during recreational activities. Avoid swimming in water that is likely to be contaminated with human or animal waste and avoid swallowing water during swimming.
- Always wash hands thoroughly
  after any contact with animals,
  after any contact with soil (e.g., gardening),
  after changing diapers,
  before eating or preparing food.
- Address cultural practices with the community that include washing with, playing in, or using for drinking, water in which untreated human or animal waste is disposed of or where funeral rites such as washing and preparing the body are carried out.
- Environmental and policy issues such as proper flood control, proper water treatment and maintenance and replacement of water treatment, storage and distribution systems, control of animal runoff to surface water and wells, and proper waste elimination from shipping vessels must be addressed at the appropriate levels.

Additional Measures for Immunocompromised Persons

- Specific education about risks and prevention.
- Avoid exposure to young animals such as calves and lambs, for instance on farms or at petting zoos.
- Avoid travel in developing countries or use protective measures.
- Avoid sexual practices that may result in exposure to feces.
- Avoid swimming in lakes, rivers, streams, ponds, public swimming pools, or recreational water parks.
- Avoid working with diaper-aged children.

TABLE C.2 *(continued)*

- Avoid contact with feces of all animals, particularly young farm animals such as calves.
- Consume only water that has been purified by boiling for 1 minute, or by treatment with certain filters. The CDC AIDS Hotline (1-800-342-2437) has information on filters that remove *Crytosporidium* from water.

Sources: Barwick, Levy, Craun, Beach, & Calderon, 2000; Centers for Disease Control and Prevention, 1999; Ford, 1999; Guerrant, Walker, & Weller, 1999; Juranek, 2000; Strickland, 2000; USPHS/IDSA, 1999, 2001; Working Group on Waterborne Cryptosporidiosis, 1997.

Note: For prevention of waterborne infections in health-care settings also see Emmerson (2001).

TABLE C.3 Prevention of Recreational Waterborne Infection*

- Provide adequate bathroom facilities including diaper-changing areas at recreational areas.
- Limit the number of swimmers per unit area.
- Patron and operator education.
- Improvement of filtration methods, disinfection methods, and pool design.
- Change recreational water industry practices (e.g., provide specific pools with dedicated filtration systems for children so the water is not mixed with adult pools, limit access of young children to adult pools, and operate filtration systems at higher turnover rates).
- Those experiencing diarrhea should refrain from swimming and continue to do so for weeks after the resolution of their diarrhea.
- Swimmers, boaters, rafters, and water skiers should avoid swallowing recreational water.
- Encourage persons not to enter the water if they have diarrhea. People can spread germs in the water even without having an "accident."
- Hands should be washed thoroughly after using the toilet or changing diapers, and the rectal area should be cleaned thoroughly after a bowel movement.
- Lifeguards should be notified of fecal matter in the water or persons changing diapers on tables and chairs in pool/beach area.
- Parents should be encouraged to take children to the toilet often for bathroom breaks.
- Diapers should be changed in a bathroom, not near the pool or shore.
- Children should be washed thoroughly (especially his or her bottom) with soap and water before swimming. Everyone has invisible amounts of fecal matter on his or her bottom that ends up in the water.
- Include in education programs that swim diapers or pants may not keep fecal matter from leaking into the water. These products are not leakproof.

Note: Technical information on filtration and disinfection may be obtained from the Environmental Protection Agency. Immunocompromised persons may need special precautions. Also see Table C.2.

Sources: Barwick et al., 2000; USPHS/IDSA, 1999, 2001; Working Group on Waterborne Cryptosporidiosis, 1997.

*Information about preventing recreational waterborne illness is available online at http://www.cdc.gov/healthyswimming

TABLE C.4 Measures to Prevent Tick-Borne Infectious Diseases

- Avoid tick-infested areas when possible.
- Walk in middle of trails, avoiding side vegetation.
- Wear appropriate barrier clothing.
- Carefully remove any attached ticks promptly and properly.
- Wear long pants.
- Tuck pant legs into socks.
- Tuck shirt into pants.
- Wear hat.
- Use appropriate tick repellants correctly.
- Treat clothing with permethrin repellant.
- Apply DEET insect repellant to exposed skin.
- Do body checks for ticks at least once a day and more often if necessary.
- Wear light-colored clothing so ticks are visible in contrast.
- Check clothing once a day for ticks.
- If hair is long, pull back.
- Clear brush and leaf litter from around houses—keep grassy areas mowed.
- Limit food available to rodents from house areas, such as keeping bird feeders distant from houses.
- Keep wildlife such as deer away from houses and gardens.

Sources: Guerrant, Walker, & Weller (1999); Parola & Raoult (2001); Strickland (2000); Terkeltaub (2000).

TABLE C.5 Preventing Mosquito Bites

- Sleep in an air-conditioned, well-screened area whenever possible.
- Keep unscreened windows closed.
- Use a mosquito net saturated with permethrin (Elamite; Nix) if screens or pyrethrin insecticides are not available (nets available at camping supply retailers).
- Use permethrin spray on clothes to repel mosquitoes (e.g., tick repellants, Duranon, Permanonel).
- Use an aerosol "knock-down" spray in the rooms, including shower areas.
- Always wear dark-colored, long sleeved clothing and long pants, especially at night.
- Spray an insecticide or repellent on clothing, as mosquitoes may bite through thin clothing.
- Apply an insect repellent that contains either N, N-diethyl-m-toluamide (DEET), or dimethyl phthalate to exposed areas such as wrists and ankles.
- Be watchful for mosquitoes, especially in the evening. Stay inside if possible.
- Avoid using perfume or any other kind of scented cosmetic.
- Use household insecticides for flying insects in a hotel room.
- When possible, travel during low transmission seasons.
- Seek accommodation in facilities at higher elevations, if possible.
- For outdoor lounging, use burning coils or candles formulated with mosquito repellants.
- Try to stay in air-conditioned or well-screened quarters.
- Change water in birdbaths regularly.
- Tightly cover stored water in receptacles.
- Eliminate potential mosquito breeding sites such as old tires, tree holes, and open containers that collect water.
- Promptly and appropriately dispose of refuse.
- Aggressively campaign for education on the above items.

Note: Vitamin B and ultrasound devices do not prevent mosquito bites. Environmental methods of mosquito control are not covered here.

Adapted from: Baird & Hoffman, 1999; Centers for Disease Control and Prevention, 2001b; Newton & White, 1999.

TABLE C.6 Prevention of Rodent-Borne Infection

Around the Home

Wash dishes and clean floors and counters.
Discard leftover pet food and empty water bowls at night inside and outside the home.
Store food and garbage in containers with tight lids inside and outside the home.
Clear brush and grass from foundations.
Seal holes and cracks or use metal flashing around base of buildings.
Conduct ongoing trapping if plague is a problem.
Spread flea powder in area being careful to follow directions to protect humans and domestic animals.
Elevate hay, wood piles, and garbage cans.
Locate them 100 feet from the house.
Remove junk or things that provide shelter to rodents.
Store animal feed in containers with lids.

When Cleaning Rodent-Infested Areas

Air out the area before entering.
Wear rubber gloves.
Do not stir up or breathe in dust.
Soak contaminated areas with disinfectant (e.g., Lysol, bleach solution).
Dispose of dead animals properly—do not handle with bare hands, and bury, burn, or use double plastic bag for trash.
Disinfect and dispose of used gloves.

When Camping or Hiking

Air out abandoned or unused cabins.
Inspect cabins for rodent infestation—if present do not use if possible.
Check potential outdoor sleeping areas for rodent droppings and burrows.
Do not disturb rodent burrows or dens.
Do not sleep near woodpiles or garbage areas.
Avoid sleeping on bare ground—use mats or elevated cots.
Store all food in rodent-proof containers and promptly discard, bury, or burn garbage.
Do not handle wild rodents even if friendly (like chipmunks, ground squirrels, etc.).

Sources: Centers for Disease Control and Prevention, 1995; Mertz, Hjelle, & Bryan, 1997.

REFERENCES

Baird, J. K., & Hoffman, S. L. (1999). Prevention of malaria in travelers. *Medical Clinics of North America, 83,* 923–944.

Barwick, R. S., Levy, D. A., Craun, G. F., Beach, M. J., & Calderon, R. L. (2000). Surveillance for waterborne-disease outbreaks—United States, 1997-1998. *Morbidity and Mortality Weekly Report, 49*(SS4), 1-35.

Centers for Disease Control and Prevention. (1995). *Preventing hantavirus pulmonary syndrome.* Pamphlet, unpaginated.

Centers for Disease Control and Prevention. (2001a). Diagnosis and management of foodborne illnesses: A primer for physicians. *Morbidity & Mortality Weekly Report, 50,* 1–69.

Centers for Disease Control and Prevention. (2001b). Underdiagnosis of dengue—Laredo, Texas, 1999. *Morbidity & Mortality Weekly Report, 50,* 57–59.

Emmerson, A. M. (2001). Emerging waterborne infections in health-care settings. *Emerging Infectious Diseases, 7,* 272–276.

Ford, T. E. (1999). Microbiological safety of drinking water: United States and global perspectives. *Environmental Health Perspectives, 107*(Suppl. 1), 191–206.

Guerrant, R. L., Walker, D. H., & Weller, P. F. (Eds.). (1999). *Tropical infectious diseases.* Philadelphia: Churchill Livingstone.

Juranek, D. D. (2000). Cryptosporidiosis. In G. T. Strickland (Ed.), *Hunter's tropical medicine and emerging infectious diseases* (pp. 594–600). Philadelphia: WB Saunders Co.

Mertz, G. J., Hjelle, B. L., & Bryan, R. T. (1997). Hantavirus infection. *Advances in Internal Medicine, 42,* 369–421.

Newton, P., & White, N. (1999). Malaria: New developments in treatment and prevention. *Annual Review of Medicine, 50,* 179–192.

Parola, P., & Raoult, D. (2001). Ticks and tickborne bacterial diseases in humans: An emerging infectious threat. *Clinical Infectious Diseases, 32,* 897–928.

Strickland, G. T. (Ed.). (2000). *Hunter's tropical medicine and emerging infectious diseases* (8th ed.). Philadelphia: WB Saunders Co.

Terkeltaub, R. A. (2000). Lyme disease 2000. Emerging zoonoses complicate patient work-up and treatment. *Geriatrics, 55*(7), 34–47.

USPHS/IDSA. (1999). Appendix. Recommendations to help patients avoid exposure to opportunistic pathogens. *Morbidity and Mortality Weekly Report, 48*(RR-10), 61–66.

USPHS/IDSA Prevention of Opportunistic Infections Working Group. (November 28, 2001). Final. 2001 USPHS/IDSA guidelines for the prevention of opportunistic infections in persons infected with human immunodeficiency virus [Online]. Available: http://www.hivatis.org/trtgdlns.html

Working Group on Waterborne Cryptosporidiosis. (1997). Cryptosporidium *and water: A public health handbook.* Atlanta, GA: Author.

Appendix D

Selected Resources

Jerry Durham and Felissa Lashley

Note: The resources listed include Web sites, organizations, government agencies, universities, and publications. Information on the majority of these topics can also be obtained through the Centers for Disease Control and Prevention, (CDC) http://www.cdc.gov and the World Health Organization (WHO), http://www.who.int/home_page, and National Institute of Allergy and Infectious Diseases (NIAID), National Institutes of Health, http://www.niaid.nih.gov. Thus, these particular resources are not repeated under each listed topic.

SELECTED RESOURCES FOR SPECIFIC DISEASES/TOPICS

Acquired Immunodeficiency Syndrome (AIDS)
See Human Immunodeficiency Virus

Antimicrobial Resistance

- CDC Antimicrobial Resistance Action Plan. [On-line]. Available: http://www.cdc.gov/drugresistance/actionplan/index.htm
- Food and Drug Administration (FDA). [On-line]. Available: http://www.fda.gov/cvm/antimicrobial/antimicrobial.html
- FDA, Center for Veterinary Medicine, National Antimicrobial Monitoring System [On-line]. Available: http://www.fda.gov/cvm/index/narms/narms_pg.html

Babesia

- *Babesia* project. [On-line]. Available: http://www.vetmed.ucdavis.edu/vbdp/babesia.htm

Bovine Spongiform Encephalopathy (also see nondiseases)

- FDA Center For Veterinary Medicine. [On-line]. Available: http://www.fda.gov/cvm/index/bse/bsetoc.html
- US Department of Agriculture (USDA). [On-line]. Available: http://www.aphis.usda.gov/oa/bse/
- Department of Environment, Food and Rural Affairs, United Kingdom. [On-line]. Available: http://www.maff.gov.uk/animalh/bse/index.html

Cholera

- World Health Organization Report on Global Surveillance of Epidemic-prone Infectious Diseases. [On-line]. Available: http://www.who.int/emc-documents/surveillance/docs/whocdscsrisr2001.html/cholera/cholera

Creutzfeldt-Jakob Disease (also see Prion diseases)

- UK Creutzfeldt-Jakob Disease Surveillance Unit. [On-line]. Available: http://www.cjd.ed.ac.uk/

Cryptosporidiosis

- Parasitology link: [On-line]. Available: www.ksu.edu/parasitology/links. This site provides links to many parasitology-related journals and societies as well as to specific parasites such as *Cryptosporidia.*

Cyclospora cayatenensis (Also see parasites)

- *Cyclospora.* [On-line]. Available: http://www.ksu.edu/parasitology/cyclospora/cyclospora.html FDA, Foodborne Pathogenic Microorganisms and Natural Toxins Handbook [On-line]. Available: http://vm.cfsan.fda.gov/~mow/cyclosp.html

Ebola

- University of Wisconsin Institute for Molecular Virology [On-line]. Available: http://www.bocklabs.wisc.edu/outbreak.html
- World Health Organization, Communicable Disease Surveillance and Response [On-line]. Available: http://www.who.int/emc/diseases/ebola/#Ebola

Escherichia coli

- FDA, Center for Food Safety and Applied Nutrition. [On-line]. Available: http://vm.cfsan.fda.gov/~mow/chap15.html
- Food Safety News on the Net. [On-line]. Available: http://www.mednews.net/bacteria/

Foodborne diseases

- Centers for Disease Control and Prevention site provides an abundance of information on food safety. [On-line]. Available: http://www.cdc.gov/foodsafety
- Food safety and Foodborne illness information [On-line]. Available: http://www.cfsan.fda.gov/~mow/intro.html
- Food safety research information office [On-line]. Available http://www.nal.usda.gov/fsrio/
- Gateway to government food safety information. [On-line]. Available: http://www.foodsafety.gov

Hantavirus

- American Lung Association. [On-line]. Available: http://www.lungusa.org/diseases/hantavirus_factsheet.html.
- CDC, National Center for Infectious Diseases. [On-line]. Available: http://www.cdc.gov/ncidod/diseases/hanta/hps/index.htm
- Tropical Diseases Web Ring. [On-line]. Available: http://www.hantavirus.net/

Helicobacter pylori

- European *Helicobacter pylori* Study Group. [On-line]. Available: http://www.helicobacter.org

Hepatitis C

- Hepatitis Foundation International. [On-line]. Available: http://www.hepfi.org/
- National Digestive Diseases Information Clearinghouse. [On-line]. Available: http://www.niddk.nih.gov/Health/Digest/Pubs/Chrnhepc/Chrnhepc.htm
- N ational Hepatitis C Coalition. [On-line]. Available: http://nationalhepatitis-c.org/

Human Immunodeficiency Virus (HIV)

- AIDS Education Global Information System (AEGIS). [On-line]. Available: http://www.aegis.com/
- AIDS Research Information Center. [On-line]. Available: http://www.critpath.org/aric/
- AIDS Treatment Information Service. [On-line]. Available: http://www.hivatis.org
- CDC, National Prevention Information Network. [On-line]. Available: http://www.cdcnpin.org/
- CDC National AIDS Clearinghouse. [On-line]. Available: http://www.maghrebnet.net.ma/alcs/links/cdcnac_aspensys_com.html
- International Association of AIDS Physicians. Covers international conferences and updates in HIV/AIDS therapy and policy. [On-line]. Available: http://www.iapac.org
- National Institute of Allergy and Infectious Diseases, Division of Acquired Immunodeficiency Syndrome, NIH [On-line]. Available: http://www.niaid.nih.gov/daids/default.htm
- National Library of Medicine, Specialized Information Services. [On-line]. Available: http://sis.nlm.nih.gov/HIV/HIVMain.html

Immunocompromised Persons

- Immune Deficiency Foundation. [On-line]. Available: http://www.primaryimmune.org/
- Jeffrey Modell Foundation. [On-line]. Available: http://www.jmfworld.com/
- National Institute of Allergy and Infectious Diseases. [On-line]. Available: http://www.niaid.nih.gov/Publications/pid/contents.htm

- New York State Department of Health Immunization Guidelines for Health Care Providers. [On-line]. Available: http://www.health.state.ny.us/nysdoh/immun/guide/table4d.htm

Lassa Virus

- CDC, Lassa Fever Online Slide Set. [On-line]. Available: http://www.cdc.gov/ncidod/dvrd/spb/mnpages/dispages/lassaf.htm

Legionellosis

- Legionnaire's Disease Links. [On-line]. Available: http://www.q-net.net.au/~legion/Legionnaire's_Disease_Links.htm
- Maryland Department of Health and Mental Hygiene. [On-line]. Available: http://www.dhmh.state.md.us/html/legionella.htm
- Occupational Safety and Health Administration. [On-line]. Available: http://www.osha-slc.gov/SLTC/legionnairesdisease/index.html

Lyme Disease

- CDC, Division of Vector-Borne Infectious Diseases. [On-line]. Available: http://www.cdc.gov/ncidod/dvbid/lymeinfo.htm
- International Lyme and Associated Diseases Society. [On-line]. Available: http://www.ilads.org/
- Links on Lyme Disease. [On-line]. Available: http://www.geocities.com/HotSprings/Oasis/6455/lyme-links.html
- Lyme Disease Resource Center. [On-line]. Available: http://www.lymedisease.org/
- New Jersey Department of Health. [On-line]. Available: http://www.state.nj.us/health/cd/f_lyme.htm

Malaria

- Malaria Foundation International. [On-line]. Available: http://www.malaria.org/
- Malaria Genome Project. [On-line]. Available: http://www.sanger.ac.uk/Projects/P_falciparum/
- Malaria Links. [On-line]. Available: http://www.geocities.com/aaadeel/malaria.html

- Multilateral Initiative on Malaria (MIM). [On-line]. Available: http://www.wellcome.ac.uk/en/1/biosfginttrpmim.html
- Special Programme for Research and Training in Tropical Diseases. [On-line]. Available: http://www.who.int/tdr/diseases/malaria/

Parasites

- Parasitology link: [On-line]. Available: www.ksu.edu/parasitology/links. This site provides links to many parasitology-related journals and societies as well as to specific parasites such as *Cryptosporidia.*

Plague

- World Health Organization, Communicable Disease and Surveillance Response. http://www.who.int/emc/diseases/plague/

Prion Diseases

- British Medical Journal's BSE-CJD Homepage. [On-line]. Available: http://www.bmj.com/cgi/collection/mad_cow
- CJD Foundation. [On-line]. Available: http://cjdfoundation.org/
- CliniWeb Internation, Prion Diseases. [On-line]. Available: http://www.ohsu.edu/cliniweb/C10/C10.228.228.800.html
- FDA, Center for Veterinary Medicine. [On-line]. Available: http://www.fda.gov/cvm/index/bse/bsetoc.html
- National Institute of Neurological Disorders and Stroke. [On-line]. Available: http://www.ninds.nih.gov/
- National Organization for Rare Disorders. [On-line]. Available: http://www.rarediseases.org/
- The Official Mad Cow Disease Home Page. [On-line]. Available: http://www.cyber-dyne.com/~tom/mad_cow_disease.html
- Prionics AG, University of Zurich. [On-line]. Available: http://www.prionics.ch/review_e.html
- The UK Creutzfeldt-Jakob Disease Surveillance Unit, Western General Hospital, Edinburgh. [On-line]. Available: http://www.cjd.ed.ac.uk/

Streptococcus pneumoniae

- National Foundation for Infectious Diseases. [On-line]. Available: http://www.nfid.org/library/pneumococcal/

Travel/Recreation-Associated Diseases

- CDC, Division of Parasitic Diseases: Swimming Pools/Recreational Waters. [On-line]. Available: http://www.cdc.gov/healthyswimming.htm
- CDC, National Center for Infectious Diseases: Travelers' Health. [On-line]. Available: http://www.cdc.gov/travel/index.htm
- International Society of Travel Medicine. [On-line]. Available: http://www.istm.org/
- Medical College of Wisconsin: Travel Medicine. [On-line]. Available: http://healthlink.mcw.edu/content/topic/Travel_Medicine
- The International Travel Medicine Clinic. [On-line]. Available: http://www.hsc.unt.edu/
- Travel Health Online. [On-line]. Available: http://www.tripprep.com/
- United States Department of State. [On-line]. Available: http://www.travel.state.gov/travel_warnings.html
- World Health Organization, International Travel and Health. [On-line]. Available: http://www.who.int/ith/english/
- Travelers Health Information site provides health information on specific destinations. Includes useful resources such as the CDC book *Health Information for International Travel* (the "Yellow Book"), the "Blue Sheet," and links to other related sites. [On-line]. Available: http://www.cdc.gov/travel/index.html

Tuberculosis

- Johns Hopkins Center for Tuberculosis Research. [On-line]. Available: http://www.hopkins-tb.org/
- Stanford Center for Tuberculosis Research. [On-line]. Available: http://molepi.stanford.edu/index.html tb.net. [On-line]. Available: http://www.tb.net.np/
- World Health Organization Global Tuberculosis Programme. [On-line]. Available: http://www.who.int/gtb/publications/gmdrt/

Vancomycin-Resistant Enterococci

- CDC, Division of Healthcare Quality Promotion. [On-line]. Available: http://www.cdc.gov/ncidod/hip/Aresist/vre.htm

West Nile Virus

- American Mosquito Control Association. [On-line]. Available: http//www.mosquito.org
- Cornell University. [On-line]. Available: http//:www.cfe.cornell.edu/risk/WNV
- National Atlas. [On-line]. Available: http//:www.nationalatlas.gov/virusmap.html
- National Pesticide Telecommunications Network. [On-line]. Available: http//:www.ace.orst.edu/info/nptn/wnv/
- New York State Department of Health. [On-line]. Available: http://www.health.state.ny.us/nysdoh/westnile/index.html
- United States Department of Agriculture. [On-line]. Available: http://www.aphis.usda.gov/oa/wnv/
- United States Geological Survey. [On-line]. Available: http://www.usgs.gov/west_nile_virus.html

SELECTED GENERAL RESOURCES INCLUDING GROUPS AND ORGANIZATIONS FOCUSING ON EMERGING INFECTIOUS DISEASES

"All the Virology on the WWW" from Garry Lab at Tulane: is a collection of virology-related Web. [On-line]. Available: http://www.tulane.edu/~dmsander/garryfavweb.html

An infectious disease resource developed by the **American Medical Association** (AMA) to provide physicians and interested consumers with scientifically accurate information on current and relevant issues in infectious disease. [On-line]. Available: http://www.ama-assn.org/ama/pub/category/1797.html

American Society for Microbiology is the oldest and largest single life science membership organization in the world. Its mission is to promote the microbiological sciences and their applications for the common good. They publish various professional journals and books. [Online]. Available: http://www.asmusa.org.

Association of State and Territorial Directors of Health Promotion and Public Health Education Home Page: information on various specific EID's. [On-line]. Available: http://www.astdhpphe.org/

Center for Complex Infectious Diseases: The primary mission of CCID is to determine the nature, origin, disease associations, modes of transmission, methods of diagnosis and responses to therapy of complex infectious diseases, and to disseminate such information. CCID is currently specializing in the detection and characterization of viruses which have undergone a "stealth" adaptation to avoid elimination by the immune system. [On-line]. Available: http://www.ccid.org/

The **Centers for Disease Control and Prevention** (CDC) is an agency of the Department of Health and Human Services that promotes health and quality of life by preventing and controlling disease, injury, and disability. CDC has various divisions including the National Center for Infectious Diseases (NCID) which specifically deals with EIDs and has divisions. [On-line]. Available: http://www.cdc.gov/. Under the NCID the Division of Vector-Borne Infectious Diseases serves as a national and international reference center for vector-borne viral and bacterial diseases. [On-line]. Available: http://www.cdc.gov/ncidod/dvbid/. The Division of Viral and Rickettsial Diseases includes the Special Pathogens Branch. [On-line]. Available: http://www.cdc.gov/ncidod/dvrd/spb. The Division of Bacterial and Mycotic Diseases has information on those pathogens. [On-line]. Available: http://www.cdc.gov/ncidod/dbmd. The Division of Parasitic Diseases has information on parasitic diseases. [On-line]. Available: http://www.cdc.gov/ncidod/dpd. The National Center for HIV, STD, and TB Prevention (NCHSTP) is responsible for public health surveillance, prevention research, and programs to prevent and control human immunodeficiency virus (HIV) infection and acquired immunodeficiency syndrome (AIDS), other sexually transmitted diseases (STDs), and tuberculosis (TB). [On-line]. Available: http://www.cdc.gov/nchstp.

Council of State and Territorial Epidemiologists. The surveillance and epidemiology of infectious diseases, chronic diseases and conditions, and environmental health concerns are priority areas for CSTE. Over 150 members serve as special topic consultants for a broad range of public health concerns such as HIV/AIDS and vaccine-preventable diseases. [On-line]. Available: http://www.cste.org.

EuroSurveillance. A European Union project dedicated to the surveillance, prevention and control of infectious and communicable disease.

Eurosurveillance produces two bulletins, Eurosurveillance Weekly and Eurosurveillance Monthly (in English, French, Spanish, Portuguese and Italian). [On-line]. Available: http://www.eurosurveillance.org.

The **Federation of American Scientists**' ProMED project is focused on surveillance of emerging human, animal and plant infectious diseases around the world. **ProMED**, the Program for Monitoring Emerging Diseases, is the premier discussion group for specialists in emerging infectious diseases. [On-line]. Available: http://www.fas.org/promed/

The **Global Health Network** (GHNet) is an alliance of experts in health and telecommunications who are actively developing the architecture for a health information structure for the prevention of infectious disease in the 21st century. [On-line]. Available: http://www.pitt.edu/~im/1/diabetes/ghnetcpa.txt

The **Hardin MetaDirectory of Internet Health Sources** web site offers extensive links to infectious disease and microbiology sites, access to electronic journals and Medline. Free access, no registration required. [On-line]. Available: http://www.lib.uiowa.edu/hardin/md/micro.html

Health Canada: Public health information site containing disease prevention and control guidelines, infectious disease fact sheets, upcoming events, and travel health. [On-line]. Available: http://www.hc-sc.gc.ca/hpb/lcdc/phi_e.html

Healthfinder: Infectious Diseases links to organizations, web resources and fact sheets. [On-line]. Available: http://www.healthfinder.org

Infection Control Nurses Association (ICNA) works in collaboration with medical, nursing, professions allied to medicine and commercial companies in the fight to control infection using a multi-national approach to ID control. [On-line]. Available: http://www.icna.co.uk/

Infections—MCW HealthLink—Information about infectious and communicable diseases from the physicians of the Medical College of Wisconsin. Numerous links to other infectious disease sites. [On-line]. Available: http://healthlink.mcw.edu/infections/

The **Infectious Disease Association of California** (IDAC), an affiliate of the Infectious Diseases Society of America, sponsors two symposia each year, distributes a quarterly newsletter, publishes a membership directory, and operates a surveillance e-mail network for sharing information on emerging infectious diseases. [On-line]. Available: http://home.idac.org/idac/idlinks.html

The **Infectious Diseases Society of America** strives to promote and recognize excellence in patient care, education, research, public health and the prevention of infectious diseases. Information on the Society, its meetings, and other related information. [On-line]. Available: http://www.idsociety.org

Infectious Diseases WebLink: Links to other Infectious Disease web sites, as well as clinical guidelines and treatment guidelines for infectious diseases. [On-line]. Available: http://pages.prodigy.net/pdeziel/

InfectNet, a Canadian bilingual website with facts about Infectious Disease, providing comprehensive, credible and readable information to the public and health care workers. Maintained by the Canadian Infectious Disease Society. [On-line]. Available: http://www.infectnet.com

International Association of AIDS Physicians. Covers international conferences and updates in HIV/AIDS therapy and policy. [On-line]. Available: http://www.iapac.org

International Society for Infectious Diseases brings together all individuals interested in ID. It aims to increase the knowledge base of infectious diseases through research and to enhance the professional development of the individual in this discipline; to extend and transfer technical expertise in microbiology and infectious diseases; and to develop, through partnerships, strategies for control and cost-effective management of infectious diseases. [On-line]. Available: http://www.isid.org/

International infectious disease societies link to more than 40 ID organizations. [On-line]. Available: http://www.idlinks.com/international_id/int_soc.html

The **Johns Hopkins Infectious Diseases** web site serves as a resource for physicians and other health care professionals in providing care and treatment to patients with any of a number of infectious diseases. [On-line]. Available: http://www.hopkins-id.edu

Karolinska Institute: An excellent, multi-award winning Swedish site with a very extensive list of infectious disease sites by categories and individual diseases. [On-line]. Available: http://www.mic.ki.se/Diseases/index.html

The **Ket-On-Line** Web site is an educational service designed to encourage peer-to-peer exchange of information in the specialty of infectious diseases and antimicrobial therapy. Includes a moderated group discussion, topical news summaries, resource links, and self-guided clinical cases. [On-line]. Available: http://www.ket-on-line.com

Medscape is an online service designed to provide clinicians with timely information that is directly applicable to their patients and practice. Information in Medscape is arranged by specialty, with extensive and timely coverage of infectious diseases, full text articles, and links to other infectious disease sites. Registration is free but required. [On-line]. Available: http://www.medscape.com/home/about.html

MedWebPlus is a comprehensive listing and linkage service of Biomedical Internet Resources. Membership is free. Provides links to many full text articles and infectious disease sites. [On-line]. Available: http://www.medwebplus.com

The **National Center for Infectious Disease** (NCID), CDC conducts surveillance, epidemic investigations, epidemiologic and laboratory research, training, and public education programs to develop, evaluate, and promote prevention and control strategies for infectious diseases. [On-line]. Available: http://www.cdc.gov/ncidod

The **National Foundation for Infectious Diseases** (NFID) supports basic and clinical research on infectious diseases; sponsors public and professional education programs; and aids in the prevention of infectious diseases. [On-line]. Available: http://www.nfid.org

The **National Institute of Allergy and Infectious Diseases** (NIAID, National Institutes of Health, provides the major support for scientists conducting research aimed at developing better ways to diagnose, treat and prevent infectious, immunologic and allergic diseases worldwide. [On-line]. Available: http://www.niaid.nih.gov

The **Open Directory Project** is a comprehensive directory of infectious disease sites available on-line. No registration required. [On-line]. Available: http://dmoz.org/Health/Conditions_and_Diseases/Infectious_Diseases/

The **Pan American Health Organization** (PAHO) is an international public health agency working to improve health and living standards of the countries of the Central and Latin America. [On-line]. Available: http://www.paho.org/

Partnership for Food Safety Education is a public-private partnership created to reduce the incidence of foodborne illness by educating Americans about safe food handling practices. [On-line]. Available: http://www.fightbac.org

The purpose of the **Pediatric Infectious Disease Society** is the advancement of knowledge of pediatric infectious diseases and its application to the care of children, including diagnosis, treatment and prevention of infectious diseases. [On-line]. Available: http://www.pids.org/

The Public Health and Infectious Disease Network: Public health, infectious diseases, and environmental health links directory. [On-line]. Available: http://imanurse.tripod.com

The **Public Health Laboratory Service** (PHLS) of England and Wales protects the population from infection by detecting, diagnosing, and monitoring communicable diseases. It provides evidence for action to prevent and control infectious disease threats to individuals and populations. [On-line]. Available: http://www.phls.co.uk/

The **United States Army Medical Research Institute for Infectious Diseases** (USAMRIID). As the Department of Defense's lead laboratory for medical aspects of biological warfare defense, USAMRIID conducts research to develop vaccines, drugs and diagnostics for laboratory and field use. In addition to developing medical countermeasures, USAMRIID formulates strategies, information, procedures, and training programs for medical defense against biological threats. [On-line]. Available: http://www.usamriid.army.mil/index.html

The **World Health Organization** (WHO) promotes technical cooperation for health among nations, carries out programs to control and eradicate disease and strives to improve the quality of human life. [On-line]. Available: http://www.who.int The mission of **WHO's Communicable Disease Surveillance and Response (CSR)** is to strengthen national and international capacity in the surveillance and control of infectious diseases that represent new, emerging, and re-emerging public health problems, and to mobilize a team of experts to outbreak locations. Access to the global infectious disease situation from the Disease Outbreak News is provided. [On-line]. Available: http://www.who.int/emc/

PUBLICATIONS: JOURNALS

Some are specific to infectious diseases, and others frequently have related materials. Other journals such as Annals of Internal Medicine are more general sources. Only a few of these are mentioned below. Some in this list are in print and some online. The online references are given to aid the reader in locating the journal.

American Journal of Epidemiology. [On-line]. Available: http://www.aje.oupjournals.org

American Journal of Infection Control. [On-line]. Available: http://www.apic.org/ajic/

American Journal of Public Health. [On-line]. Available: http://www.apha.org/journal/AJPH2.htm

American Journal of Tropical Medicine and Hygiene, and *Tropical Medicine and Hygiene News*. [On-line]. Available: http://www.astmh.org/journal.html

American Society for Microbiology Journals Online. [On-line]. Available: http://www.journals.asm.org

Annals of Epidemiology. [On-line]. Available: http://www.elsevier.com

Antimicrobial Agents and Chemotherapy. [On-line]. Available: http://aac.asm.org/

Applied and Environmental Microbiology. [On-line]. Available: http://aem.asm.org/misc/about.shtml

British Medical Journal. [On-line]. Available: http://www.bmj.com

Canadian Journal of Infectious Diseases. [On-line]. Available: http://www.pulsus.com/INFDIS/home.html

Clinical and Diagnostic Laboratory Immunology. [On-line]. Available: http://cdli.asm.org/misc/about.shtml

Clinical Infectious Diseases. [On-line]. Available: http://www.journal-s.uchicago.edu/CID/home.html

Clinical Microbiology Reviews. [On-line]. Available: http://cmr.asm.org/

Clinical Updates. [On-line]. Available: http://www.nfid.org/publica-tions/clinicalupdates/

Current Clinical Topics in Infectious Diseases. [On-line]. Available: http://www.medirect.com

Current Opinion in Infectious Diseases. [On-line]. Available: http://www.co-infectiousdiseases.com

Current Opinion Infectious Diseases. [On-line]. Available: http://www.currentopinion.com/

Diagnostic Microbiology and Infectious Disease. [On-line]. Available: http://www.elsevier.com/locate/diagmicrobio

Emerging Infectious Diseases. [On-line]. Available: http://www.cdc.gov/ncidod/eid/index.html

The *European Journal of Clinical Microbiology and Infectious Disease.* [On-line]. Available: http://link.springer.de/link/service/journals/10096/

Helicobacter. [On-line]. Available: http://www.blackwell-science.com

ID Linx. [On-line]. Available: http://www.idlinx.com

Infection. [On-line]. Available: http://link.springer.de/link/service/journals/15010/index.htm

Infection and Immunity. [On-line]. Available: http://iai.asm.org/

Infection Control and Hospital Epidemiology. [On-line]. Available: http://www.slackinc.com/general/iche/ichehome.htm

Infections in Medicine. [On-line]. Available: http://id.medscape.com/SCP/IIM/public/journal.IIM.html

Infectious Disease Alert. [On-line]. Available: http://www.ahcpub.com/ahc_root_html/products/newsletters/ida.html

Infectious Disease Clinics of North America. [On-line]. Available: http://www.harcourthealth.com

Infectious Disease in Children. [On-line]. Available: http://www.slackinc.com/child/idc/idchome.htm

Infectious Disease News. [On-line]. Available: http://www.slackinc.com/general/idn/idnhome.htm

Infectious Diseases in Clinical Practice. [On-line]. Available: http://www.infectdis.com

Infectious Diseases in Obstetrics and Gynecology. [On-line]. Available: http://www.interscience.wiley.com/jpages/1064-7449/info.html

Infecto.com. [On-line]. Available: http://www.infecto.com

International Journal for Parasitology. [On-line]. Available: http://www.elsevier.nl/homepage/sah/para/fp.sht

International Journal of Antimicrobial Agents. [On-line]. Available: http:/www.ischem.org

Journal of Antimicrobial Chemotherapy. [On-line]. Available: http://www.jac.oupjournals.org/

Journal of Applied Microbiology. [On-line]. Available: http://www.blackwell-science.com

Journal of Bacteriology. [On-line]. Available: http://jb.asm.org/

Journal of Clinical Microbiology. [On-line]. Available: http://jcm.asm.org/misc/about.shtml

Journal of General Virology. [On-line]. Available: http://vir.sgmjournals.org/

Journal of Hepatology. [On-line]. Available: http://www.jhep-elsevier.com

Journal of Hospital Infection. [On-line]. Available: http://www.harcourt-international.com/journals/jhin/

Journal of Infection. [On-line]. Available: http://www.harcourt-international.com/journals/jinf/

Journal of Infection and Chemotherapy. [On-line]. Available: http://www.harcourt-international.com/journals/jinf/default.cfm?/

Journal of Infectious Diseases. [On-line]. Available: http://www.journals.uchicago.edu/JID/

Journal of Medical Microbiology. [On-line]. Available: http://www.jmedmicrobiol.com

Journal of Medical Virology. [On-line]. Available: http://www.interscience.wiley.com/jpages/0146-6615/

Journal of Travel Medicine. [On-line]. Available: http://bcdecker.yy.net/cgi-bin/tangocgi.exe/tango/decker/journals/journal.qry?function=view&ID=15&_UserReference=166799826

Journal of Virology. [On-line]. Available: http://jvi.asm.org/misc/about.shtml

Journal Watch: Infectious Diseases. [On-line]. Available: http://www.jwatch.org/id/

Lancet. [On-line]. Available: [On-line]. Available: http://www.thelancet.com

Lancet Infectious Diseases. [On-line]. Available: http://www.infection.thelancet.com

Malaria and Infectious Diseases in Africa. [On-line]. Available: http://www.chez.com/malaria/indexan.htm

Medical Microbiology and Immunology. [On-line]. Available: http://www.link.springer.de/link/service/journals/00430/index.htm

Microbes and Infection. [On-line]. Available: http://www.pasteur.fr/infosci/publisci/mic-aims.html

Microbiology. [On-line]. Available: http://mic.sgmjournals.org/

Microbiology and Molecular Biology Reviews. [On-line]. Available: http://mmbr.asm.org/misc/about.shtml

Morbidity and Mortality Weekly Report. [On-line]. Available: http://www.cdc.gov/mmwr

Pediatric Infectious Disease Journal. [On-line]. Available: http://www.pidj.com

Public Health. [On-line]. Available: http://www.stockton-press.co.uk/ph/

Quarterly Journal of Medicine. [On-line]. Available: http://qjmed.oupjournals.org

Trends in Parasitology. [On-line]. Available: http://www.trends.com/pt/about.htm

Reviews in Tropical Medicine and International Health. [On-line]. Available: http://www.blackwell-science.com/

Weekly Epidemiological Record. [On-line]. Available: http://www.who.int/wer/

PUBLICATIONS: BULLETINS, NEWSLETTERS, REPORTS, AND FACTSHEETS

Australian Communicable Diseases Intelligence: a fortnightly joint publication of the National Centre for Disease Control, Commonwealth Department of Health and Aged Care and the Communicable Diseases Network Australia and New Zealand. It aims to provide timely information about the incidence of and risk factors for communicable diseases in Australia to inform and assist those with responsibility for communicable disease control in a wide variety of settings. [On-line]. Available: http://www.health.gov.au/pubhlth/cdi/cdihtml.htm

Canada Communicable Disease Report, is a publication of Health Canada, Population and Public Health Branch. [On-line]. Available: http://www.hc-sc.gc.ca/english/branches.htm

Communicable Disease Report Weekly is published by the Communicable Disease Surveillance Centre (CDSC) of England/Wales, and supplies news of communicable disease incidents, trends, guidelines, and policy, and current surveillance data. CDR Weekly is abstracted in Medline, and has a comprehensive annual index. [On-line]. Available: http://www.phls.co.uk/publications/cdr.htm

Current Infectious Disease Reports: Presents the views of experts on current advances in infectious diseases and provides selections of the most important papers from the great wealth of original publications, annotated by experts. All sections of this journal are available only to paid subscribers. [On-line]. Available: http://www.current-reports.com/cr_aims.cfm

Disease Outbreak News: Maintained by WHO, this on-line bulletin offers pertinent information about worldwide communicable disease outbreaks. [On-line]. Available: http://www.who.int/disease-outbreak-news/

Double Helix, the official newsletter of NFID, the National Foundation of Infectious Diseases. [On-line]. Available: http://www.nfid.org/

Emerging and Other Communicable Diseases Surveillance and Control (EMC): Fact sheets and references on worldwide emerging and re-emerging infectious diseases worldwide. [On-line]. Available: http://www.who.int/emc/index.html

EpiNorth. The online infectious disease bulletin of Northern Europe. [On-line]. Available: http://www.epinorth.org

European Communicable Disease Bulletin: Funded by DGV of the Commission of the European Communities, contains information and links regarding infectious diseases in Europe. [On-line]. Available: http://www.ceses.org/eurosurv_eng.htm

Eurosurveillance Monthly: A publication of the European Union, it is available free on the Internet in 5 languages. It publishes original articles on infectious diseases.[On-line]. Available: http://www.eurosurveillance.org

Eurosurveillance Weekly. Available free on the internet with searchable archives dating from 1997. Reports news of infectious disease outbreaks from the European Union and beyond. [On-line]. Available: http://www.eurosurveillance.org

Infectious Diseases News Brief: a weekly digest of national and international information about communicable disease incidents and issues published by the Population and Public Health branch of Health Canada. [On-line]. Available: http://www.hc-sc.gc.ca/pphb-dgspsp/bid-bmi/dsd-dsm/nb-ab/index.html

Infectious Facts: Fact sheets on infectious diseases from the Association of State and Territorial Directors of Health Promotion and Public Health Education. [On-line]. Available: http://www.astdhpphe.org/infect/

Kansas State University sponsors a site that provides links to information on *Cryptosporidium* and other parasitology related pages. [On-line]. Available: http://www.ksu.edu/parasitology/links

The *Ket-On-Line Newsletter* series provides highlights from key international scientific meetings relevant to infectious disease researchers and clinicians. [On-line]. Available: http://www.ket-on-line.com

National Foundation for Infectious Diseases' fact sheets about infectious diseases, appropriate for reproduction and distribution to patients. [On-line]. Available: http://www.nfid.org/library/

ProMED Digest: The International Society for Infectious Diseases' Program for Monitoring Emerging Diseases (ProMED) produces an online, daily-updated synopsis of current discussions on emerging infectious diseases. [On-line]. Available: http://www.promedmail.org

Science Central: Health Sciences: Infectious Disease and Epidemiology: Science news alerts, research news and infectious disease resources available in full text with a searchable index. [On-line]. Available: http://www.sciquest.com/

Weekly Epidemiological Record (WER): Serves as an essential instrument for the rapid and accurate dissemination of epidemiological information on cases and outbreaks of diseases under the International Health Regulations, other communicable diseases of public health importance, including the newly emerging or re-emerging infections, noncommunicable diseases and other health problems. [On-line]. Available: http://www.who.int/wer/

World Health Organization Communicable Disease Surveillance and Response. Has fact sheets and current information. [On-line]. Available: http://www.int/emc.index.html

Glossary

aerobic organisms—organisms that live and thrive in an oxygenated environment

aerosol—a fine mist containing minute particles

anaerobic organisms—ones that need little or no oxygen

arbovirus—a virus borne by arthropod vectors

arenavirus—a virus family whose members are usually transmitted to humans via rodents; members include the Lassa, Junin, Machupo, and Guanarito viruses, each causing a type of hemorrhagic fever

arthropod—a vector belonging to the phylum Arthropoda that transmits an organism from one host to another

authochthonous—locally acquired

biosafety level—specific combinations of work practices, safety equipment, and facilities to minimize exposure of workers to infectious agents; these range from level 1 for agents not usually causing human disease to level 4 for agents posing a high risk of life-threatening disease, such as the Ebola virus

biotype—organisms sharing a specific genotype

bunyavirus—a virus family among whose members are the hantaviruses and the Rift Valley fever virus

clade—a group or subtype of organisms of related isolates that are classified by genetic similarities

colonization—state of a microorganism living in or on a body without causing disease

endemic disease—one that is consistently present in a population or geographic location at a certain level

endotoxin—a toxin of internal origin that is separated from a microorganism on disintegration

enzootic—disease of animals that is consistently present in a certain animal population or locale

epidemic disease—one that occurs suddenly in numbers in excess of what is usually expected

epizootic—an epidemic in an animal population

exotoxin—one produced during microbial growth and released without disintegration

filovirus—a virus family infecting primates and humans that has only two members, Ebola and Marburg viruses

flavivirus—a virus family whose members include the dengue virus, West Nile virus, and the hepatitis C virus

fomite—an inanimate object on which pathogens live

host—organism on or within which microorganisms live

immunocompetent—a person with a functional immune system

immunocompromised—a person whose immune system does not function properly

incidence—measure of frequency with which a new case of a specific condition or disease occurs during a specified time period

incubation period—time from exposure to appearance of disease

index case—the earliest recognized case of a disease

isolate—a particular strain of a microorganism taken from an individual

microbes—microscopic living organisms such as bacteria, protozoa, and fungi

nosocomial infection—one that develops and is recognized in patients and employees in a health care institution

outbreak—occurrence of an unusually large number of cases of disease in a short period of time

pandemic—an epidemic disease of widespread prevalence usually in more than one continent

pathogen—a microorganism causing disease

pathogenicity—ability of an infectious agent to produce disease in a susceptible host

prevalence—number or proportion of persons in a given time period with a specific condition or disease

protozoa—a type of parasite

recurrence—the return of a disease or condition thought to be in remission

reservoir for infection—organism (such as humans, animal, plant, or inanimate material—often called fomite) in which a microbial agent normally lives and multiplies

retrovirus—a virus that has RNA as its genetic material and uses reverse transcriptase to copy its genome into host DNA; human immunodeficiency virus belongs to this group

serogroup—group of closely related microbes distinguished by a characteristic set of antigens

serotype—a particular strain of a microorganism

source of infection—organism or inanimate object or substance from which a microbial agent passes to a host

sporozoa—nonmotile protozoan parasites

vector—a living organism, usually an arthropod, that can transfer a microbe from one host to another

virulence—degree of pathogenicity

zoonoses—animal diseases transmitted from animals to humans; their ongoing reservoir is in nonhuman animals, and arthropods are usually involved in their transmission

Index